Dermatology Simplified

Jules Lipoff · Diego Ruiz Dasilva

Dermatology Simplified

Outlines and Mnemonics

Second Edition

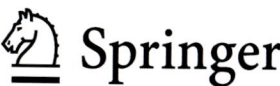

Jules Lipoff
Lewis Katz School of Medicine
Temple University
Philadelphia, PA, USA

Diego Ruiz Dasilva
Forefront Dermatology
Virginia Beach, VA, USA

Eastern Virginia Medical School
Virginia Beach, VA, USA

ISBN 978-3-031-66738-1   ISBN 978-3-031-66739-8   (eBook)
https://doi.org/10.1007/978-3-031-66739-8

1st edition: © Springer International Publishing Switzerland 2016
2nd edition: © The Editor(s) (if applicable) and The Author(s), under exclusive license to Springer
Nature Switzerland AG 2024

This Springer imprint is published by the registered company Springer Nature Switzerland AG
The registered company address is: Gewerbestrasse 11, 6330 Cham, Switzerland

If disposing of this product, please recycle the paper.

Preface

Dear Reader,

When I was little, I would follow my cardiologist father as he sat in doctors' lounges interpreting EKGs and dictating reports for hospitals. I was impressed by his ability to immediately rattle off a diagnosis after a brief glance, seemingly without thought. Later, as a medical student, when I was taught to approach EKGs in a methodical and algorithmic way, it occurred to me that my dad had begun this way first and then built upon his skills with experience and confidence. When I began my dermatology residency, I remembered these childhood memories and felt that same awe: my senior residents knew things instantly, yet I struggled without a method or algorithm to guide me.

Fortunately, I trained at a residency program with a master diagnostician and Socratic teacher, Dr. Michael Fisher, who emphasized the concept of reaction patterns. Though he rarely enumerated each category into lists or presented outlines, he provided a simple, effective, and efficient method to approach dermatology patients. Now as an attending dermatologist, this method guides my teaching and helps me develop a differential diagnosis when I get stumped by a particularly difficult case.

This guidebook is derived from notes first taken during my residency at the Albert Einstein College of Medicine and Montefiore Medical Center and expanded upon and refined in the 12 years I have practiced since as an attending dermatologist. I have compressed, simplified, and organized dermatologic diagnoses and treatment approaches, building upon the five reaction patterns taught by Dr. Fisher. This ever-growing collection of notes and snippets is comprised of outlines, buzzwords, factoids, mnemonics, and lists. While it is impossible to learn everything, my goal in formulating this collection was to capture everything that is most important to know in caring for patients.

The first step in my approach is to learn the big picture. There is plenty of time during a three-year dermatology residency to fill in the details as you gain experience. In this book's centerpiece medical dermatology outline section, dermatologic conditions are organized by clinical differential diagnosis or by pathophysiologic basis, prompting an immediate understanding of their place in the big picture. In the remaining sections, lists and mnemonics group diseases thematically to reinforce understanding in complementary ways. Finally, the last sections cover useful topics that are not disease-specific, with high-yield notes on medications, cosmetics, surgery, and basic science.

When studying dermatology, a great deal of knowledge must be memorized. While there is no escaping memorization, using an algorithmic, standardized approach will increase the amount of information that is retained much more effectively than a random "hit or miss" approach to learning factoids.

This second edition aims to update every section of the book to keep pace with the constant evolution and innovation in dermatology. It also seeks to integrate the principles of the modern Core and Applied board examinations, which have shifted focus from rote memorization of seemingly random factoids to clinically relevant management decisions in patient care. It combines notes and pearls from my experiences at the Albert Einstein College of Medicine and at the University of Pennsylvania and also capitalizes on my new co-editor, Dr. Ruiz Dasilva's, recent personal experience of going through the modern board certification pathway.

To that end, we hope this book can be used as a resource for medical students and dermatology residents diagnosing patients in clinic, senior dermatology residents studying for board exams, internal medicine and pediatrics residents learning dermatology, teachers creating educational presentations for students or residents, and practicing dermatologists seeking quick reference. Enjoy!

Jules Lipoff
Philadelphia, USA

Acknowledgments

There are innumerable people who I am incredibly lucky to have worked with and learn from, from residency to present. I continue to be indebted to a village of support for this new edition. First, as always, I must thank my amazing wife, Renee, who has always been a true partner. I also want to thank my young daughters, Zadie and Tess, who are a joy and inspiration for all that I do. My family has always been very supportive of my training and education, and I am in their debt.

In my residency training, I was inspired to enter dermatology by the great Dr. Michael Fisher, and his approach to dermatology led to this book. At Einstein, I was privileged to work with fantastic faculty and residents. I am especially thankful to Dr. Fisher, Dr. Ranon Mann, Dr. Steven Cohen, Dr. Karthik Krishnamurthy, Dr. Donald Rudikoff, Dr. Ryan Turner, and Dr. Adam Friedman for their teaching and support. At Penn, I was grateful for many brilliant colleagues, namely my mentors, Dr. William James and Dr. Carrie Kovarik.

Lastly, I wish to thank Dr. Diego Ruiz Dasilva, who generously accepted my invitation to collaborate and take on the task with me to update and co-edit this book to better suit a new generation of dermatologists in a new era of board studying and preparation—things change oh so quickly! I am honored by and grateful for your support.

Jules Lipoff

First, I have to thank my incredible wife, Tiffany, who has always been my role model and source of inspiration. I also want to thank my children, Wilder and River, who keep me grounded and help me appreciate what life is all about. These three have kept me going, even in the most difficult times of my life. I also want to thank my recently departed dogs, Prince and Nahla, who taught me the true meaning of unconditional love and compassion.

I am fortunate to have worked with so many influential figures in dermatology and am truly grateful for the pearls imparted on me by each of them, from powerhouses in our field to my own inspiring co-residents. At Penn Medicine, I was honored to work with cutting-edge faculty and residents. I am especially thankful to Drs. Nicholas Mollanazar, Roman Bronfenbrenner, William James, Misha Rosenbach, William Higgins, Cory Simpson, Cherie Ditre, Analisa Halpern, Victoria Werth, Robert Micheletti, Joseph Sobanko, Zelma Chiesa, Adam Rubin, and, of course, my co-author Dr. Jules Lipoff. Without them, I would not be the person or dermatologist that I am. I also want to thank my senior co-residents who supported me and paved the way—Drs. Jun Zhang, David Dunaway, Brittany Oliver, Courtney Rubin, Ashwin Agarwal, Lucas Cavallin, and Robert Smith.

Diego Ruiz Dasilva

Contents

I   Introduction

II   Medical Dermatology Outlines

III   Lists and Mnemonics

IV   High Yield Topics

List of Figures

List of Tables

Introduction

Introduction: The Starter Kit

Contents

© The Author(s), under exclusive license to Springer Nature Switzerland AG 2024
J. Lipoff and D. Ruiz Dasilva, *Dermatology Simplified*,
https://doi.org/10.1007/978-3-031-66739-8_1

1

Abstract

Mastering a complex field like dermatology can initially be quite intimidating. We recommend trusting your own past methods of studying while focusing on learning the essential building blocks of our field. You must be able to describe clinical dermatologic conditions, key features in dermatopathology. Then you are ready to construct a differential diagnosis.

Keywords

Approach to studying dermatology · Dermatology boards · Conceptual learning · Lumper-splitter dichotomy · Dermatologic disease definition · Dermatology teaching · Describing skin conditions · Differential diagnosis · Fitzpatrick skin phototype scale · Definitions of skin appearance · Common skin conditions · Skin classifications

1.1 General Advice on Studying

1.1.1 How to Study

Everyone has his own strategy for learning dermatology. Dermatology residents are often assigned to read textbooks, study unknown dermatopathology slides, and participate in teaching rounds, conferences, and grand rounds! These present a large amount of information, but of course, much of this knowledge is quickly forgotten.

If we have one piece of advice for studying dermatology, it's this: don't reinvent the wheel. Stick with whatever has worked for you in the past.

More and more, we are focusing our energy on "the new boards." Both the Core examinations and the American Board of Dermatology Applied exam were designed to test relevant clinical knowledge that all dermatologists should have by the end of training. Gone are the days of testing obscure facts and minutiae that are not vital to patient care or that are easily searchable and therefore not worth committing to memory. Still, you may be surrounded by residents whose impressive knowledge base about dermatologic disease is quite intimidating. Do not be afraid! It is great to learn trivia and excel at roundsmanship, but anybody can memorize facts if given the time. The important thing is to learn how to think like a master clinician and approach each patient in a logical, systematic manner. While certain facts must be memorized, try to organize and understand the concepts that support this knowledge. The best physicians know the facts (e.g. what the treatment for a disease is), but also have a broad understanding of the reasoning behind this choice (e.g. the targeted pathophysiology and the mechanism of action of the treatment). Conceptual learning provides the bedrock for memorizing and retaining facts. Fortunately, with the new examinations, this type of critical thinking that incorporates patient comorbidities, social determinants of health, goals of care and systematic frameworks of diagnosis and treatment is emphasized and therefore the American Board of Dermatology understands that producing a well rounded "master clinician" should be the goal of every training program as opposed to someone who can just recite every factoid in a textbook.

1.1.2 Logic of This Book

When confronted with the need to classify species in 1857, Charles Darwin wrote, "It is good to have hair-splitters and lumpers. Those who make many species are the 'splitters,' and those who make few are the 'lumpers.'" This line of thinking, the lumper-splitter dichotomy, is quite applicable to the categorization of dermatologic diseases.

A lumper believes there are many names for the same disease, perhaps because observers of that same disease are able to distinguish subtly different forms. It is simpler to learn a classification with fewer categories.

A splitter sees all the subtle differences and variations in disease processes and hopes to define optimal treatments by applying the scientific method to each separately categorized condition.

This book assigns merit to both the lumper and splitter worlds. There is value in lumping diseases into categories for the sake of easy learning and understanding, though admittedly sometimes this forces diseases into groups in which they may not cleanly fit.

On the other hand, splitting diseases by enumerating different names and distinctions permits more in depth learning about diseases in a broader category while defining distinctive features.

Despite being residents in different times and in different cities, we both found that textbook readings, lectures, and other didactics blended together unpredictably, and often specific topics were taught in very different ways by each professor. There was also a large amount of important information that was not clearly presented in textbooks or manuals. In order to gain focus, we compiled outlines and lists of everything we learned in an effort to unify various perspectives and points of view, and also to collect factoids and mnemonics that could be used to study important material the same way every time. Our notes reflect an organic mix of teachings during residency and as attending dermatologists including information from lectures, textbooks, clinical articles, and personal experience. Our goal is to combine and organize this information in a systematic and logical way so that it is easier to learn. To simplify the presentation, we have not listed references. In the main outlines, we have focused on the important high yield and key conceptual points, yet still the information is comprehensive. This second edition pro-

1

vides an updated trove of knowledge combining our pearls and experiences from the Albert Einstein College of Medicine in the Bronx and the Hospital of University of Pennsylvania in Philadelphia.

1.2 Describing Skin Conditions

Though it seems deceptively simple, learning to describe skin findings is a critically important skill. All physicians must learn to translate clinical observations into clear language to organize information and communicate effectively with colleagues.

A description should include the primary and secondary lesions, distribution, colors, configuration, nature of borders, and shape. If relevant, texture and patterns may provide diagnostic information.

- Remember: it is critically important to generate a complete differential diagnosis; this is far more important than getting the one right diagnosis. In theory, your description should allow a listener who has not seen the patient to develop a mental picture that would allow him or her to develop a comprehensive differential diagnosis.
- The description should lead to the differential, not the other way around. Often the first impression of diagnosis prompts the physician to describe features that match this initial impression (e.g. when we describe likely psoriatic lesions with "silvery scale"). This is a trap that limits the differential diagnosis.
- It is best to avoid descriptive terms that define themselves (e.g. verrucous, psoriasiform, acneiform, herpetiform). These terms also lead to closed-minded thinking. If you must use these terms (and we all do use them as a crutch), try to use them to supplement more descriptive terms.

1. Skin type: I to VI
   - The Fitzpatrick skin phototype scale runs from I to VI, describing a patient's complexion and sensitivity to sun exposure.

   Type I.   Very white, fair, red/blonde hair/blue eyes (Irish). Always burns, never tans.

   Type II.   White. Usually burns, rarely tans.

   Type III. White/olive skin. Sometimes burns, gradually tans.

   Type IV.   Brown skin, rarely burns, tans easily. (Mediterranean, Latino)

   Type V.   Dark brown skin, very rarely burns (Middle eastern, Indian)

   Type VI.   Black skin, never burns, always tans. (African).

   Note: this is a historical/stereotypical classification system but nonetheless does provide a framework from which to consider a patient's skin cancer risk or propensity for post-inflammatory pigmentary changes. In short, this system is flawed, but remains commonly used, so still important to know.

2. Distribution/Location
   - Where are the skin lesions located? Generalized, bilateral/unilateral, sun exposed, intertriginous, extensor/flexural surfaces, acral (distal body such as hands and feet)?

- Make sure you know the difference between distribution and configuration.
3. Configuration
    - How are lesions arranged? Confluent versus discrete, scattered, clustered/grouped, geometric/linear, dermatomal, serpiginous, Blaschkoid, nevoid
    - Certain shapes and configurations are almost always caused by external forces (e.g. geometric/linear) suggesting an "outside job," such as contact dermatitis or Koebner phenomenon
    - Blaschkoid = linear/whorled (like marble) along an embryologic line of Blaschko
    - Nevoid = A distinct configuration, well-demarcated, unilateral
4. Primary lesions
    - Primary lesions of skin disease are extremely valuable features that are unmodified by external forces (see ▶ Sect. 1.2.1).
5. Secondary lesions
    - Modification of primary lesion from evolution, trauma, or other external influence (see ▶ Sect. 1.2.2)
    - If an examination reveals only secondary lesions, the findings may be entirely secondary to external influences such as scratching, "an outside job." Tip: ask your patient, "Which came first, the itch or the rash?"
6. Color
    - This can be subjective, but describe each skin condition the best you can
    - Try to use specific colors with a description of normal skin color as a comparison rather than just "hyperpigmented" or "hypopigmented"
    - "Depigmented" (no color/white) should only be used to describe a finding if the Wood's lamp or biopsy have confirmed that pigment is completely lost. Wood's lamp enhances epidermal pigment change, but not dermal
    - Know the distinguishing features between these terms (especially erythema vs. purpura):
        Erythematous = red and blanches (on palpation or diascopy) since from vasodilatation
        Violaceous = purple (dermatologists may use "violaceous" rather than purple to avoid confusion with "purpuric")
        Purpuric = red/purple non-blanching caused by extravasation of blood
        Dusky = dark purple/grey (suggests necrosis)
    - It can be difficult to distinguish between purpura and early necrosis.
7. Borders
    - Regular versus irregular, blurred versus sharp/well-demarcated, scalloped, punched-out
8. Shape
    A. Annular (round with central clearing)
    B. Round/nummular/discoid (no central clearing)
    C. Ovoid (oval-like e.g. pityriasis rosea)
    D. Serpiginous (snake-like)
    E. Targetoid: refers specifically to erythema multiforme lesions with three zones: dusky or blistered center, surrounded by white ring, and then erythema (as opposed to urticaria, which displays central clearing)
    F. Polycyclic (multiple overlapping annular)

1

G. Arcuate (incomplete annular arc)
H. Polymorphous (many shapes).
9. Texture
   A. Soft (like fat)
   B. Firm
      – Calcium and gout are "rock hard" on palpation
   C. Indurated
      – Firm and bound-down on palpation
   D. Boggy
      – Edematous, suggests fluid between collagen bundles in the dermis
   E. Fleshy
      – Implies exophytic or pedunculated with soft texture
      Note: exophytic = growing outward, vegetative = growing
   F. Horny
      – Has thick pointy hyperkeratotic component (like a cutaneous horn)
   G. Vegetative
      – Growing upon itself, layered extension of a plaque/tumor
   H. Juicy
      – Suggests an edematous/fluid-filled appearance of fluid-filled, about to ooze
10. Patterns
   A. Follicular/folliculocentric
   B. Morbilliform ("measles"-like; macules and papules 2 mm to 1 cm)
      – The so-called "maculopapular" pattern is meant to specifically refer to toxic erythema of morbilliform drug eruptions and viral exanthems. Though many non-dermatologists may use this as a blanket term for any rash, it is meant to be highly specific.
   C. Reticular/reticulated (net-like throughout)
   D. Retiform (branching/angulated/stellate edged)
   E. Guttate (drop-like)
   F. Monomorphic/monomorphous (all lesions identical, in the same stage).

1.2.1 Primary Lesions (Defining Lay Terms)

Common lesions:

Note: For 1–7, most consider A < 1 cm, B > 1 cm, but definitions vary. Common primary lesions can be defined in lay terms and dermatologic terms (see ◘ Table 1.1).
1. Bump
   A. Papule
      – Dome-shaped, flat-topped, umbilicated/delled.
   B. Plaque

◻ Table 1.1 Primary lesions

Lay term	Derm term (<1 cm)	Derm term (>1 cm)
Bump (raised)	Papule	Plaque
Spot (flat)	Macule	Patch
Blister	Vesicle	Bulla
Blister with pus	Pustule	Lakes of pus
Lump (under the skin)	Nodule (nodule with fluid = cyst)	Tumor
Non-blanching red spot	Petechia	Purpura

2. Spot
   A. Macule
      – Technically, if you close your eyes, you should not be able to palpate a macule or observe it. Any component of elevation would preclude use of this term
   B. Patch
      – Note: technically, a patch is a large macule (flat), but many dermatologists use the term to indicate some thin substance. Also, some dermatologists use the term macule regardless of size of the lesion
3. Blister
   A. Vesicle—small blister
   B. Bulla—large blister
      – Flaccid (probably epidermal) versus tense (probably dermal)
      – On acral sites, epidermal blisters can appear tense given the thicker overlying stratum corneum
      – Tense blisters can evolve to flaccid, flaccid blisters cannot become tense.
4. Pustule (a pus-filled vesicle)
   A. Pustule
   B. Lakes of pus
      – An old school term for confluent pustules as can be seen in pustular psoriasis
5. Lump
   A. Nodule
      – Note: A cyst is a nodule filled with liquid or semi-liquid material (e.g. keratin)
   B. Tumor
      – This term does not imply that a lesion is neoplastic or malignant. Also, many dermatologists use the term nodule regardless of size.
6. Non-blanching red spot
   – Does not blanch because these represent extravasated red blood cells
   A. Petechia
   B. Purpura

1

Other specific lesions:

1. Hives
   A. Wheal (lesion)
      – Name of disease = urticaria
2. Single blanching superficial vessel/ gin blossom
   A. Telangiectasia/ectasia
3. Comedones
   A. Closed comedone (white-head)
      – Technically, singular form of comedones is "comedo"
   B. Open comedone (black-head)
      – Opens to expose keratin, which oxides and turns black
   C. Milia and epidermal inclusion cysts
      – In a sense, these are on a spectrum with comedones.
4. Burrow = think scabies
5. Boil = follicular abscess
   Mnemonic = (F)uruncle = (F)ollicle, (C)arbuncle = (C)ombo
   Note: these can begin as pustules in a cluster on a nodule (pointing), and progress to become soft and spewing pus (fluctuance)
   A. Furuncle = involving one hair follicle
   B. Carbuncle = involving multiple hair follicles

1.2.2 Secondary Lesions

Main lesions:

Mnemonic = ABCS
A: Atrophy and scarring
B: Breakage in skin: erosion, ulcer, fissure
C: Crap on skin: scale, crust (also, eschar)
S: Scratching: lichenification, excoriation.

Other secondary lesions:

Erosions are breaks in the skin limited to the epidermis; ulcers involve the dermis and fissures are linear erosions or ulcerations localized to skin folds or acral surfaces.
Ulcers may be "punched out" suggesting vaso-occlusive etiology, or may have "undermined borders" as in pyoderma gangrenosum
Crust = scab = dried exudates or plasma from vesicle, pustule, trauma
Scale = flakes/plates of compacted stratum corneum.
"Branny" scale = exfoliating scale that is bran flake-like
Eschars are thick black/necrotic crusts; commonly associated with rickettsialpox (endemic to the Bronx), anthrax, brown recluse spider bites, ecthyma gangrenosum (*Pseudomonas*), tularemia, bubonic plague
Atrophy: shiny = epidermal atrophy, wrinkled = dermal atrophy
Poikiloderma = triad of atrophy, hypo/hyperpigmentation, and telangiectasia

Collarette of scale: small circle of scaling, which you can deduce must be from ruptured/evolved vesicle or pustule

Trailing scale: occurs in pityriasis rosea and erythema annulare centrifugum (superficial type)

Exfoliation = peeling skin (stratum corneum)

Desquamation = scaling of skin (stratum corneum)

Denudation = loss of entire epidermis including basement membrane (as in TEN)

Epidermal change = scale, decreased/increased pigmentation, vesiculation, fissures, lichenification, epidermal atrophy (shiny, thin), verrucous/papillomatous change

Dermal change = dermal atrophy (wrinkling), anetoderma (loss of elastic tissue), erythema, papules, plaques, nodules, cysts, sclerosis/scar/keloid, peau d'orange

1.2.3 Other Non-specific Terms (Try to Limit Use, but Impossible to Avoid)

Eruption = breaking out of an exanthem or rash

Rash = an eruption of the skin

Dermatitis = inflammation of the skin

Dermatosis = disease of the skin

Lesion = an abnormal change in the structure of an organ due to aging, injury or disease

1.3 Describing Dermatopathology Findings

1.3.1 Dermatopathology Terminology

Layers of epidermis:

Cornified layer (stratum corneum) = top layer, basket weave in normal skin

Granular layer (stratum granulosum) = between corneum and spinous layer with visible keratohyaline granules

Spinous layer (stratum spinosum) = bulk of epidermis, with visible desmosomes = "spines"

Basal layer (stratum basale) = single layer of cells, includes keratinocytes and melanocytes

Other important terms:

Rete ridges = epidermal projections that extend downward between dermal papillae

Dermal papillae = dermal projections that extend upward between epidermal rete ridges

Parakeratosis = retention of nuclei in stratum corneum keratinocytes, suggests rapid turnover/movement to surface preventing normal maturation with loss of nuclei

Orthokeratosis=anuclear stratum corneum layer (the normal basket weave), compact orthokeratosis=flattened corneal layer

Hyperkeratosis = thickened stratum corneum

Spongiosis=intercellular edema (hallmark of all eczematous dermatitides)

Acantholysis=loss of keratinocyte cohesion (only in epidermis)

Acanthosis=thickening of the spinous layer of the epidermis

Psoriasiform hyperplasia = uniform/regular rete ridge elongation (versus irregular epidermal hyperplasia in lichen simplex chronicus)

Papillomatosis=outward growth of epidermis with associated elongation of dermal papillae

Pagetoid spread = individual upward cell spread of malignant cells in the epidermis (can be "buckshot" scatter)

Epidermotropism=presence of atypical lymphocytes in the epidermis, specifically refers to the migration of T lymphocytes in mycosis fungoides

Granuloma=collection of histiocytes, with or without giant cells

Suppurative=many neutrophils (pus), often infectious.

Pseudoepitheliomatous (or pseudocarcinomatous) hyperplasia=irregular downward proliferation of epidermis into dermis
  - This mimics the pattern seen in SCC
  - Can see in mycobacterial infections, deep fungal infections, pyoderma gangrenosum, pyoderma vegetans, borders of ulcers, prurigo, granular cell tumor, bromoderma

Interface=dermal–epidermal junction (DEJ) or basement membrane zone (BMZ); interface dermatitis includes lichenoid and vacuolar

Lichenoid inflammation=band-like inflammation at the interface which may obscure the dermal–epidermal junction

Vacuolar alteration=damage to basal keratinocytes with formation of vacuoles

Pigment incontinence=melanin deposits in dermal melanophages secondary to inflammation

Necrobiosis=altered/degenerated collagen

Civatte bodies/colloid bodies=apoptotic or dyskeratotic keratinocytes

Russell bodies=large eosinophilic homogeneous immunoglobulin-containing inclusions (think: pregnant plasma cells)

1.3.2 A Few Quick Tips

Bluish color=think mucin or elastosis

Purple color=think calcium

Frozen section=allows for slide preparation in 15 min. Poorer quality, but in acute situations (TEN) and Mohs surgery (for SCC, BCC), the quality is sufficient. Difficult to identify melanocytes on frozen sections (but can be done with Melan-A).

1.3.3 Approaching Histopathologic Description

1. Get oriented: Look at the slide so you don't miss a piece! Where are the epidermis and dermis? If it's broken into pieces, it might be fragments of tissue from curettage.
2. Type of biopsy = shave or punch?
3. Location—use site clues:
   - Thick stratum corneum/presence of stratum lucidum = likely acral (Thick stratum corneum can also just be from LSC)
   - Many hair follicles = likely scalp or face
   - Many sebaceous glands = face
   - No stratum corneum or granular layer (more specific), large and pale keratinocytes (filled with glycogen), many plasma cells could indicate mucosa
   - Thin skin with multiple vellus hairs could mean eyelid
   - Solar elastosis could mean older person in sun-exposed area
   - Otherwise guess "trunk or proximal extremities"—that's most of them!
4. Describe the epidermis: stratum corneum with normal basket weave?
5. Describe the dermis—look for common structures: hair follicles, sebaceous glands, eccrine glands, blood vessels
6. Describe the panniculus (subcutaneous fat)
7. Do you think this is inflammatory or neoplastic (Remember, neoplasms can be inflamed)? Do you think this is primarily an epidermal or dermal process, or both? What's the reaction pattern (e.g. superficial and deep perivascular)? What kind of cells are in the infiltrate: neutrophils (multi-lobed), histiocytes (large cells with grainy cytoplasm), eosinophils (pink granules), plasma cells (eccentric nucleus with "clock face" chromatin and perinuclear clearing), mast cells ("fried eggs"), or lymphocytes (the default small blue cell)?
8. Describe anything that looks unusual, with specifics as you know them.
9. Use the shape of the biopsy to give you clues about the clinical appearance: e.g. Was it a papule? Was it umbilicated? Secondary changes?

1.3.4 Immunofluorescence Findings

DIF = direct immunofluorescence; an antibody directly detects presence of a pathologic antibody in the skin

IIF = indirect immunofluorescence; serum is introduced to a substrate (e.g. monkey esophagus) in order to detect circulating pathologic antibodies

Salt-split skin = with NaCl, DIF is cleaved at lamina lucida (of dermal–epidermal junction)—Allows separation of roof/floor fluorescence—e.g. BP (roof) vs. EBA (floor)

- Precise type of basement membrane immunofluorescence pattern in a DIF may demonstrate a n-serrated pattern similar to salt-split roof fluorescence (bullous pemphigoid or linear IgA), or a u-serrated pattern similar to salt-split floor fluorescence (EBA or bullous lupus erythematosis)

1

Biopsy for DIF of blistering disease: Most advise sampling perilesional skin. In perilesional skin, the anatomy will still be intact for identifying what structures are bound by antibodies.

- This is placed in Michels solution, not formalin

1.4 Morphologic Reaction Patterns

- The point is to organize dermatologic entities into as few general categories as possible to make them easier to understand and memorize.
- Many dermatologic diseases will not fit into this classification, but this is helpful for inflammatory diseases.

The five basic inflammatory reaction patterns as taught by Dr. Michael Fisher:

1. PAPULOSQUAMOUS = red and scaly, papular
2. ECZEMATOUS =
   a. Acute (edematous, vesicular)
   b. Subacute (red, scaly)
   c. Chronic (lichenified)
3. VESICULOBULLOUS = vesicles/bullae/pustules
4. VASCULAR = deeper, red/purple color, minimal epidermal/surface change
5. DERMAL = deeper (can get fingers around, but not under), minimal epidermal/surface change; if can't get fingers around, suggests subcutaneous

Note:

1. Papulosquamous and subacute eczematous are both red and scaly, hard to distinguish (Some of your most common ddx will be this; for instance, tinea, psoriasis, and eczema can be hard to tell apart sometimes, which is why in this ddx, we usually perform a KOH at the bedside or a PAS stain for formalin fixed sections of tissue)
2. Acute eczematous and vesiculobullous both have vesicles, hard to distinguish.
3. Papulosquamous, eczematous, and vesiculobullous are the reaction patterns primarily confined to the epidermis
4. Vascular and dermal have overlap as vessels are in the dermis; ephemeral entities are more likely to be vascular
5. Subcutaneous entities can be grouped under dermal, but will feel "deeper," i.e. can't even get your fingers around it, let alone under it (like in panniculitis).

Medical Dermatology Outlines

Papulosquamous

Contents

© The Author(s), under exclusive license to Springer Nature Switzerland AG 2024
J. Lipoff and D. Ruiz Dasilva, *Dermatology Simplified*,
https://doi.org/10.1007/978-3-031-66739-8_2

2

Abstract

Papulosquamous diseases are mostly epidermal. They are distinguished as pink, raised, and scaly eruptions.

Keywords

Papulosquamous · Papulosquamous diseases

2.1 Psoriasiform

2.1.1 Psoriasis

- Clinically, mild defined as < 3% BSA, moderate 3–10%, severe > 10%
- Extent of psoriasis can be measured by different indices; one of the most commonly used is the PASI (Psoriasis Area and Severity Index), based on redness, thickness, and scaliness of lesions
- Nail findings include nail pitting, oil spots, onycholysis, thickened nails
- Associated with systemic inflammatory comorbidities (e.g. increased risk of cardiovascular disease)
- Pathogenesis = T-cell activation with cytokine mediated keratinocyte proliferation (Th1 and Th17), mostly CD8+ T-cells. IL17 and IL23 are the primary downstream elevated cytokines.
- Path: psoriasiform hyperplasia, parakeratosis, neutrophils in the epidermis (pathognomonic for psoriasis and AGEP) "Munro's microabscesses" in stratum corneum, "Spongiform pustule of Kogoj" in stratum spinosum
  Clinical signs:
- Koebner phenomenon = recurrence at site of trauma (also see in lichen planus, lichen nitidus)
- Auspitz sign = lesions bleed when scale is removed, from thinned suprapapillary plates and dilated papillary dermal vessels
- "Woronoff ring" = hypopigmented halo/ ring around plaques caused by inhibition of prostaglandin E2 (PGE-2)
- Can be triggered by meds (SIR BLAM): steroid rebound, interferon and ribavirin, beta blockers, lithium, anti-malarials
- Unlike atopic dermatitis, psoriasis plaques rarely impetiginized (perhaps because no decrease in antimicrobial peptides)
- Inflammatory linear verrucous epidermal nevus (ILVEN) may have clinical/ path overlap (*see also Keratotic Disease: Hyperkeratotic Eruptions*)
- Geographic tongue (benign migratory glossitis) can be associated; is psoriasiform on path

- Psoriasis will not directly cause hair loss from scalp involvement; however, "psoriatic alopecia" is a rare non-scarring or scarring alopecia that may be associated with TNF inhibitors
- Treatment: topical corticosteroids (TCS), topical calcineurin inhibitors (TCI), vitamin D analogs, PDE inhibitors, aryl hydrocarbon receptor agonists, phototherapy, acitretin, methotrexate, cyclosporine, TYK2 inhibitors, JAK inhibitors (JAKi), anti-TNF, anti-IL12/23, anti-IL-17, and anti-IL-23 biologics
- Treatment with prednisone discouraged given apparent risk of flare of pustular psoriasis upon withdrawal, although recent papers have disputed this dogma

Types of psoriasis:
a. Psoriasis vulgaris
 I. Chronic plaque psoriasis
b. Guttate psoriasis
 – Associated with *Strep* pharyngitis
 – May respond to treatment with antibiotics
c. Inverse psoriasis
 = Distributed in inframammary and inguinal folds, axillae
d. Pustular psoriasis
 – Ddx candidiasis, AGEP, also Sneddon-Wilkinson
 – *See also Vesiculobullous: Subcorneal Blisters.*
  I. Palmoplantar pustular psoriasis (Barber-Königsbeck)
  II. Acrodermatitis continua suppurativa (Hallopeau)
   = Aka dermatitis repens
   – Chronic, localized to fingers, toes, nail beds, usually limited to one digit
  III. Generalized pustular psoriasis (von Zumbusch)
   – Lakes of pus, fever, erythroderma; can be provoked by prednisone withdrawal
   – Check for hypocalcemia
   – First choice treatment = biologics (anti-IL-17 or anti-IL-36 now preferred over acitretin or methotrexate)
  IV. Impetigo herpetiformis (pustular psoriasis in pregnancy)
   – Can use cyclosporine or prednisone for tx
e. Scalp psoriasis
f. Nail psoriasis
 – Onycholysis, thickening of nail plate, oil drop spots (nail bed involvement), irregular pitting (from proximal nail matrix involvement)
g. Palmoplantar psoriasis
h. Erythrodermic psoriasis
i. Psoriatic arthritis
 – 5–30% of patients with psoriasis affected

2

- – Risk of arthritis with psoriatic nail findings, intertriginous disease, or scalp disease
- – Skin findings usually precede arthritis
- – With IP joint erosion, can see "pencil-in-cup" deformity 5 types:
    - I.   Mono and asymmetric oligoarthritis
        - – Most common type
        - – DIPs and PIPs, usually not MCPs
        - – Can make "sausage digits" when DIP plus PIP involved
    - II.   Arthritis of distal interphalangeal joints (DIPs)
        - – Exclusively DIP involvement
    - III. Rheumatoid arthritis-like presentation (symmetric)
        - – Especially PIP, MCP, wrists, ankles, elbows
        - – Usually seronegative
    - IV.   Arthritis mutilans
        - – Most severe form and rarest
        - – Can see "telescoping of digits"
    - V.   Spondylitis and sacroilitis
        - – Like ankylosing spondylitis
- j. Sebopsoriasis
    - – A hedge diagnosis of limited psoriasis to some areas of the scalp that is clinically consistent also with exuberant seborrheic dermatitis. Psoriasis typically makes discrete plaques and may not be limited to the scalp, whereas seborrheic dermatitis typically involves more diffuse scaling without discrete plaques and is limited to the scalp and seborrheic areas.
- k. Acute generalized exanthematous pustulosis (AGEP)
    - – A pustular drug eruption, perhaps a drug-induced pustular psoriasis (not an exacerbation of underlying psoriasis)
    - – *See also Vesiculobullous:Subcorneal Blisters and Vascular:Drug Eruptions.*

2.1.2 Seborrheic Dermatitis

- ▪ Classically affects the "seborrheic areas": scalp, nasolabial folds, eyebrows, ears; also, may affect axilla, infra-scapular back, inguinal folds, chest
- ▪ Associated with yeast *Malassezia;* evidence has shown removal of yeasts with antifungals does lead to remission, and relapse associated with reappearance of yeasts
- ▪ In infants, can begin at 1 week after birth (as opposed to atopic dermatitis at 2–3 months), on scalp called "cradle cap"
- ▪ Infantile form ddx: atopic dermatitis, irritant diaper dermatitis, infantile psoriasis, Wiskott-Aldrich syndrome, Langerhans cell histiocytosis, tinea capitis, crusted scabies
- ▪ Can be exuberant in HIV/AIDS, Parkinson's, patients on antipsychotics
- ▪ In the ear = seborrheic otitis

- "Petaloid" seborrheic dermatitis = presents with arcuate/polycyclic pink/hypopigmented plaques with minimal scale
- Has features of both papulosquamous and eczematous
- Path: mounds of scale/crust at lips of follicular infundibula, "shoulder parakeratosis," psoriasiform
- Treatment: TCS, antifungals, anti-dandruff shampoos, and oral fluconazole in recalcitrant cases

Note: Pityriasis/Tinea amiantacea [ami ann tay sha] = massive white scaling pattern (not a disease) that can be seen in psoriasis, seb derm, tinea capitis; means "asbestos-like"

2.1.3 Parapsoriasis

- Both forms characterized by lymphoid infiltrates (predominantly CD4+); a controversial entity, debate continues about the relationship between MF and parapsoriasis
  a. Small plaque parapsoriasis
     - Clinically may see a "digitate" (finger-like) pattern.
     - Will not progress to MF
  b. Large plaque parapsoriasis
     - May represent a clonal dermatitis not yet progressed to MF
     - May see more in bathing suit distribution, poikiloderma
     - Clinically can have wrinkled "cigarette paper" quality
     - On a spectrum with MF
     - Treatment: TCS, TCI, phototherapy, and oral bexarotene in recalcitrant cases

2.1.4 Mycosis Fungoides (MF)

- Papulosquamous/erythrodermic/eczematous eruption; perhaps "smudgy" (not well demarcated) patches/plaques
- MF is the most common form of CTCL, but CTCL is a more general term
- *See also Neoplastic:Lymphomas*
- Treatment: TCS, imiquimod, topical carmustine, topical nitrogen mustard, topical retinoids, phototherapy, radiation, isotretinoin, bexarotene, methotrexate, brentuximab, mogalizumab, interferon and ECP

2.1.5 Reactive Arthritis (Formerly Reiter's Syndrome)

- Try not to call Reiter's (Nazi doctor who killed hundreds)
- Triad: arthritis, urethritis, conjunctivitis/uveitis/keratitis

2

- Associated with HLA-B27, GI/GU infection, check HIV
- Psoriasiform/pustular lesions in 5%; called keratoderma blennorrhagica
- See mostly on soles, extensor legs, penis
- On glans penis, called balanitis circinata

2.1.6 Pityriasis Rubra Pilaris (PRP)

- Erythroderma with "islands of sparing," red-orange palmoplantar keratoderma, "cornuba wax"-dipped hands, follicular papules with "nutmeg grater" appearance
- Path: psoriasiform hyperplasia, "checkerboard" of orthokeratosis and parakeratosis
- Tx = retinoids, methotrexate, anti-TNF, anti-IL-12/23, anti-IL-17, anti-IL-23, phototherapy. Prednisone and cyclosporine out of favor.
- Types: Type I (classic adult) > 55% of cases, Type II (atypical adult), Type III (classic juvenile), Type IV (circumscribed juvenile) ~25%, Type V (atypical juvenile)
- Type VI in HIV patients

2.1.7 Palmoplantar Keratoderma

See also Keratotic Diseases

2.2 Pityriasiform

Note: "Pityriasis" means scaling

2.2.1 Pityriasis Rosea (PR)

- Associated with HHV-6 and 7; may be a viral exanthem? Has been reported during pandemic from both COVID-19 and the vaccines
- Herald patch (precedes eruption)
- Clears within 6–8 weeks
- Tends to be in body folds, e.g. "Christmas tree" distribution
- Usually spares lower extremities
- Follow pregnant patients closely (may be at increased risk of miscarriage)
- Variant: inverse PR (involves face, axillae, inguinal areas)—may be more common in darker skin types
- Always check an RPR in PR (Ddx secondary syphilis)

- Path: cannot differentiate from spongiotic derm, but is not psoriasiform; may have focal mounds of parakeratosis, RBCs
- PR-like drug eruption: from ACEIs, gold, terbinafine
- Treatment: TCS, antihistamines, ?acyclovir, erythromycin

2.2.2 Secondary Syphilis

See also Infectious Diseases: Bacterial : Treponemes

2.2.3 Tinea/Dermatophytosis

- Most common: Trichophyton, Microsporum, Epidermophyton
- *T. rubrum* most common; in tinea capitis, think *T. tonsurans*
See also Infectious Diseases: Fungal

2.2.4 Pityriasis (Tinea) Versicolor

- Caused by *Malassezia furfur* (and *globosa*)
- Hyphal and yeast forms seen on KOH, "spaghetti and meatballs"
- Treatment: topical antifungals, oral fluconazole

2.2.5 Pityriasis Rotunda

- Type I has been associated with malnutrition, mycobacterial disease (TB and leprosy), malignancy (most common: hepatocellular carcinoma or gastric cancer), hepatic cirrhosis
- Type II has a strong hereditary association with no underlying systemic illness or malignancy

2.3 Lichenoid

2.3.1 Lichen Planus (LP)

- Classic Ps: pruritic, purple, polygonal, planar, papular
- Many types: actinic, annular, atrophic, bullous, hypertrophic (shins), linear (Blaschkoid), ulcerative/erosive (mucous membranes), nail, oral, lichen plano-pilaris (LPP)
- Strong association with HCV, especially with oral LP
- Wickham's striae = white/grey streaks over LP lesions

- Nail findings: longitudinal ridging/splitting, dorsal pterygium (adhesion of proximal nail fold to nail plate/nail bed)
- Always examine nails and mouth if LP in ddx
- On genitals, ddx lichen sclerosus, psoriasis
- Path: lichenoid infiltrate, sawtooth rete ridges, hypergranulosis, rarely has eos or parakeratosis (see more in lichenoid drug); also, apoptotic keratinocytes that may stain on DIF
- Max-Joseph spaces = artifactual subepidermal clefts
- "Cytoid bodies" or "colloid bodies" = IgM + fibrinogen in papillary dermis; "Civatte" bodies = apoptotic keratinocytes in epidermis (Mnemonic: Ci = inside epidermis, Co = outside)
- Koebnerizes
- Graham-Little-Piccardi-Lasseur Syndrome = LPP, KP, axillary/genital non-scarring alopecia
  Other types of lichen planus:
  - LP may include erythema dyschromicum perstans (EDP) (controversial), which some consider post-inflammatory LP
  - LP pigmentosus = a postinflammatory hyperpigmented form of LP that may be similar to EDP
  - LP actinicus = a photosensitive variant presenting with annular, dyschromic, or violaceous plaques in sun-exposed areas
  - LP pemphigoides (LP/BP overlap)
    - From anti-BPAG2 antibodies
    - Bullae on previously uninvolved skin (unlike bullous LP, in which bullae occur in longstanding LP lesions)
  - Treatment: TCS, TCI, ILK, topical JAKi, phototherapy, systemic steroids, retinoids, dapsone, hydroxychloroquine, apremilast, cyclosporine, MMF, metronidazole, MTX, anti-TNF, systemic JAKi, and more

2.3.2 Lichenoid Drug Reaction

- Most commonly from beta-blockers, ACE-inhibitors, penicillamine, also TNF-α inhibitors
- Path: lichenoid, with parakeratosis, often with eosinophils
- *See also Vascular: Toxic erythema*

2.3.3 Lichen Nitidus

- Unlike LP, lichen nitidus is NOT pruritic
- Esp. on flexor wrists/forearms, penis. Can be diffuse
- Path: "ball and claw" (extended rete ridges around localized lymphohistiocytic granulomatous infiltrate)

2.3.4 Lichen Striatus

- Overlap with linear lichen planus, Blaschkitis (in adults)
- Typically in children (median age 2–3)
- Usually on extremity, presenting over days/weeks, resolves after 1 year or more
- Path: lichenoid with periadnexal inflammation common

2.3.5 Graft Versus Host Disease (GVHD)

- Chronic GVHD can resemble lichen planus and lichenoid drug eruptions
- *See also Vascular: Other Reactive Toxic Erythema*

2.3.6 Keratosis Lichenoides Chronica

- Violaceous keratotic lichenoid papules, linear/reticulated on limbs/trunk; may have associated facial seb derm-like rash

2.4 Erythroderma/Exfoliative Dermatitis

- Defined as erythema and scale > 90% of skin surface
  Mnemonic = pretty please don't make beets, dear (psoriasis, PRP, dermatitis, MF, blistering disease, drug eruptions)
  Note: with erythroderma,
  1. Risk of inability to maintain temperature
  2. Risk of high output heart failure given vasodilatation
  1. Psoriasis
  2. Pityriasis rubra pilaris (PRP)
  3. Dermatitis (Atopic, Contact, Seborrheic, Stasis)
  4. Mycosis fungoides
  5. Blistering (Pemphigus foliaceus, urticarial BP)
  6. Drugs
     - Consider drug eruptions first!
  7. Other- paraneoplastic, lichen planus, Norwegian scabies, GVHD, rarely sarcoidosis
  8. Infantile erythroderma
     - Do not forget immunodeficiencies, SSSS, ichthyoses

2

2.5 Other (Not Traditionally Thought of as Papulosquamous, but May Be Pink, Raised, and Scaly)

1. Subacute eczematous dermatitis
   See also Eczematous
2. Lupus
   – SLE, DLE, subacute lupus
   See also Connective Tissue Disease
3. Sarcoidosis
   – Macular or papular sarcoid, including psoriasiform
   See also Dermal:Granulomatous
4. Malignant epidermal neoplasms
   – Squamous cell carcinoma (SCC), actinic keratosis (AK), basal cell carcinoma (BCC)
   See also Neoplastic:Keratinocytic Neoplasms
5. Porokeratosis
   See also Keratotic Disease
6. Lichen planus-like keratosis (LPLK)
   – Aka benign lichenoid keratosis (BLK)
   – Solitary lichenoid papule on sun-damaged skin, hard to diagnose clinically
   – Usually appears as BCC, SCC, SK, or melanocytic clinically
   – Path: lichenoid papule on sun-damaged skin
7. Dermatomyositis
   – Can strongly resemble psoriasis with extensor involvement
   – Gottron's papules = lichenoid papules over MCPs, DIPs, PIPs
   – Gottron's sign = pink/red/purple atrophic or scaling eruption over knuckles, knees, elbows
   – Shawl sign = erythema and scale ± poikiloderma over shoulders
   See also Connective Tissue Diseases
8. Pityriasis lichenoides spectrum
   – Characterized by recurrent crops of spontaneously regressing erythematous papules; PLEVA and PLC considered on a spectrum, whereas LyP has clinical overlap but is distinct
   – More in children
   – Preponderance of CD8+ cells (unique to PLEVA), CD8+ or CD4+ in PLC
     a. Pityriasis lichenoides et varioliformis acuta (PLEVA)
        – Mucha-Habermann disease is severe ulcerative variant known as febrile ulceronecrotic Mucha-Habermann disease
        – Ddx varicella (varioliformis means like smallpox), papular eruptions
        – Path: mnemonic PLEVA = parakeratosis, lichenoid, extravasated RBCs, wedge(v)-shaped hypergranulosis, apoptotic keratinocytes
        – Tx = topical steroids, azithromycin/erythromycin and tetracycline (as anti-inflammatory rather than as antibiotic), phototherapy, systemic steroids, MTX

    b. Pityriasis lichenoides chronica (PLC)
      – More mild and chronic, scaly rather than crusted compared to PLEVA
    c. Lymphomatoid papulosis (LyP)
      – Formerly classified as a CTCL, now a benign lymphoproliferative disorder
      – Clinical overlap, but distinct disease from PLEVA and PLC, which are considered on a spectrum
      – CD30 positive (excludes PLEVA/PLC), like anaplastic large cell lymphoma (ALCL), Hodgkin's
      – May be assoc. with MF, ALCL, Hodgkin's
      – Treatment: TCS, TCI, ILK, phototherapy, MTX andsurgery, brentuximab, radiation or HSCT in recalcitrant cases

9. Erythema annulare centrifugum—superficial type
   See also Vascular: Gyrate Erythemas
10. Norwegian (crusted) scabies
    See also Infectious Disease

Eczematous

Contents

J. Lipoff and D. Ruiz Dasilva, *Dermatology Simplified*,
https://doi.org/10.1007/978-3-031-66739-8_3

3

Abstract

Eczematous diseases are mostly epidermal. They are defined by "spongiotic dermatitis" on pathology, and clinically they may present in one of three stages (acute, subacute, or chronic) and in different contexts (types). The word "eczema" is derived from ancient Greek, meaning "to boil," a reflection of the acute vesicular stage. Though many physicians and lay people use the word "eczema" synonymously with "atopic dermatitis," the word "eczema" in this book is used differently. "Eczema" (or "dermatitis") here is defined as a spongiotic reaction pattern that may present in different locations and contexts, with different names applied. For instance, in the context of atopy, a spongiotic dermatitis could be called atopic dermatitis. Other diseases including pityriasis rosea and dermatophytosis can also cause a spongiotic dermatitis.

Keywords
Eczematous diseases · Eczema

3.1 The Three Stages of Eczema

3.1.1 Acute

- Clinical = edematous, red, vesicular, weeping eruption
- Ddx vesiculobullous disease
- Path: stratum corneum = basket weave, epidermis = intraepidermal vesicles/spongiosis, dermis = mild infiltrate

3.1.2 Subacute

- Clinical = red and scaly eruption, may have crusting
- Ddx papulosquamous disease
- Path: stratum corneum = scale/crust, epidermis = acanthosis, exocytosis, dermis = denser infiltrate

3.1.3 Chronic

- Clinical = dry, lichenified eruption
- Path: stratum corneum = hyper/parakeratosis, epidermis = less spongiosis/more psoriasiform, dermis = fibrosis

3.2 Types of Eczema

CANDID SCALES mnemonic[1]
= Contact, Atopic, Nummular, Dyshidrotic, Id reaction and Infectious eczematoid, Drug, Stasis, CTCL, Asteatotic, LSC, Erythroderma, Seborrheic

Classic clues to distinguishing different eczematous disorders
> Location:
>> Legs—asteatotic eczema, stasis dermatitis
>> Hands/feet—dyshidrotic eczema, contact dermatitis
>> Ankles/neck—lichen simplex chronicus
>> Antecubital/popliteal fossae/face—atopic dermatitis
> Pattern:
>> Round weepy plaques—nummular eczema
>> Lichenified plaques—lichen simplex chronicus, atopic dermatitis
>> Linear or patterned mostly on hands/feet—contact dermatitis
>> Generalized—atopic dermatitis, cutaneous T-cell lymphoma, drug reaction
> Associated disease:
>> Asthma/allergic rhinitis—atopic dermatitis
>> Venous stasis—stasis dermatitis
>> Wound—contact dermatitis (neomycin), infectious eczematoid
>> Lower extremity infection or dermatitis—id reaction
>> Psychiatric disorder or "neurodermatitis"—lichen simplex chronicus

3.2.1 Contact Dermatitis

a. Allergic contact dermatitis (ACD)
b. Irritant contact dermatitis (ICD)
c. Photoallergic contact dermatitis
d. Phototoxic contact dermatitis
   - Contact dermatitis can be divided by the type and specificity of the eruption
     Irritant dermatitis causes 80% of reactions, allergic only 20%

---

[1] This mnemonic is used with permission by Dr. Steven Cohen.

3

a. Allergic contact dermatitis
   - An immunologic response in some individuals, type IV hypersensitivity reaction, 24–48 h after contact (on re-exposure)
   - Clinical suspicion with patterned, linear, or geometric shapes; anatomical restriction to hands or feet, for instance. Eyelids are easily affected
   - Patch testing may be indicated to detect allergen; most common test is TRUE test = Thin-layer Rapid Use Epicutaneous test

Common contact allergens:
  Plants
  Metals
  Fragrances
  Preservatives
  Textiles
  Personal care products
  Topical medications

Plants:
  Four main genera of plants responsible for allergic contact dermatitis, all start with the letter A (Mnemonic AAAA):
  Anacardiaceae
  Alstroemeriaceae
  Asteraceae
  Alliaceae

  Anacardiaceae (Cashew and Sumac Family)
   - *Toxicodendron* is the poison ivy genera, formerly *Rhus* (reaction was called *Rhus* dermatitis)
   - #1 plant cause of allergic contact dermatitis = poison ivy
   - Allergen = sap containing urushiol (a mixture of catechols)
   - Common cross reactants (all in *Anacardiaceae* family): cashew (*Anacardium occidentale*), mango rind (not fruit), gingko tree (leaf pulp, not supplement), lacquer tree of Japan, Brazilian pepper tree, Indian marking tree
   - Mnemonic: sounds like Ana Kardashian, the lesser known Kardashian that stings and burns

  Alstroemeriaceae (Peruvian lily)
   - #1 cause of contact dermatitis in florists
   - Sensitizer = tuliposidase A

  Asteraceae
   - Star-shaped plants ("aster" = star in Latin) = chrysanthemum (#2 cause of contact in florists), ragweed, feverfew, artichoke
   - Sensitizer = sesquiterpene lactones (SQLs)
   - Permethrin is made from chrysanthemums

Alliaceae
  = Onions, garlic, chive
  – Mnemonic: "Allia" like aioli
  – Allergen = diallyl disulfide (a thiocyanate)
  – May also cause irritant dermatitis

Others
  Latex
    – Increased in atopic, spina bifida pts
    – Cross-reactants: mnemonic "Passion on your BACK" = passion fruit, banana, avocado, chestnuts, kiwi
    – Derived from *Hevea brasiliensis* tree extract

Metals:
  Nickel
    – Most common contact allergy
    – Dimethylglyoxime test for detection of nickel
    – Co-sensitization with cobalt
  Potassium dichromate (chromates)
    – In leather tanning, wet cement, green pigment (Mnemonic: beat down on the cement curb with leather shoes because you hustled at pool (green felt))

Fragrances:
  Balsam of Peru
  Fragrance mix #1 and #2

Preservatives:
  Formaldehyde
    – May see in wrinkle–free shirts
  Formaldehyde releasers (formaldehyde releasing preservatives) = Quaternium-15, DMDM hydantoin, imidazolidinyl urea, diazolidnyl urea
    – If allergic to formaldehyde, probably allergic to releasers
  Isothiazolinones
  Methylisothiazolinone (known for causing contact dermatitis in baby wipes)
  Parabens
    – Often in cosmetics, topical medications
  Iodopropynyl butylcarbamate
    – In many cosmetics and personal products
  Thimerosal
    – In vaccines
  Glutaraldehyde
    – Used in cold sterilization, may cause contact dermatitis in dentists

3

Textiles:
>Rubber
>>Thiuram mix (gloves), disulfiram cross-reactant
>>Mercaptobenzothiazole (shoes, latex)
>>Black rubber mix
>>>– Includes para-phenylenediamine (PPD), in tires
>>Carba mix
>>Mixed dialkyl thioureas
>>>– In neoprene gloves
>Nail products
>>Nail polish (resin) = toluene-sulfonamide-formaldehyde
>>Artificial nails = cyanoacrylate, methyl methacrylate (acrylics/glues)
>Dimethyl fumarate
>>– In preservative packets, Chinese sofas
>Colophony
>>– A resin found in gum, paper

Personal care products:
>Hair products:
>>Hair dye (and black henna)
>>Para-phenylenediamine (PPD)
>>>– Cross-reacts with HCTZ, PABA, sulfas, esters
>>Shampoos
>>>– Cocamidopropyl betaine (thickening agent/surfactant)
>>Permanent wave formula—glycerol thioglycerate
>>Bleaching agent—ammonium persulfate
>Cosmetics
>>– #1 fragrance mix, #2 preservatives
>Lanolin
>>– In Aquaphor (wood alcohol)
>Toothpaste
>>– Allergen = cinnamic aldehyde
>Deodorant
>>– Clinically more likely to affect axillary vault versus contact from clothing/other allergens

Topical medications
>Neomycin/bacitracin
>Corticosteroids:
>>Note: usually testing with tixocortol pivolate and budesonide will confirm most topical steroid allergies
>Ethylenediamine
>>– In topical antihistamine creams; cross-reacts with hydroxyzine, theophylline
>Propylene glycol
>>– Frequently a component of topical medications

Sunscreen
- Para-aminobenzoic acid (PABA), most sunscreens have now eliminated this

b. Irritant contact dermatitis
- From direct corrosive effect (not immune mediated); e.g. acids, alkalis
- Often occupational: hairdressers, bakers/chefs, florists
- Symptoms typically more burning/stinging than itching

c. Photoallergic contact dermatitis
= Only select few are allergic and react with sun exposure
  I. Chronic actinic dermatitis
  - Aka actinic reticuloid (severe) versus photosensitive eczema/dermatitis (mild)
  - Can be in leonine facies ddx
  - Patch and photo-patch testing may be helpful, should also consider checking HIV
  - Note: actinic prurigo is a PMLE variant, but may appear eczematous, *see also Dermal:Inflammatory:Lymphocytic*
  - Treatment: TCS, TCI, photoprotection, naltrexone, MMF, MTX, dupilumab, JAKi

d. Phototoxic contact dermatitis
Note: non-immunologic, everyone reacts
  I. Sunburn (solar erythema)
  = Erythema, possible blistering, desquamation
  - Caused more by UVB than UVA (the lower the wavelength, the more superficially the light penetrates, leading to more potent erythema)
  - Path: may see "sunburn cells" = apoptotic keratinocytes
  - UVA not blocked by windows, UVB is; UVC blocked by ozone
  - UVB required for vitamin D synthesis, causes mutations linked to skin cancers (BCC and SCC, not MM); UVA's role in skin cancer less understood but plays role in photoaging
  Sun tanning:
  - Immediate darkening due to alteration/oxidation of existing melanin (from UVA)
  - Delayed tanning (peak 3 days later) from increased melanocytes and melanin synthesis (from UVB)
  - Sunless tanning most commonly from dihydroxyacetone
  Sunscreen ingredients:
  Benzophenones— good UVA absorbers, most common ingredients of chemical blockers
    - Oxybenzone blocks UVB and UVA2
    - Avobenzone blocks UVA1 and UVA2, not UVB
  Inorganic/physical blockers (both UVA/UVB):
    Titanium dioxide
    Zinc oxide
  II. Phytophotodermatits (Berloque dermatitis)
  - Require allergen exposure, then light exposure

- Most common agents = furocoumarins (e.g. psoralens)
- Notable for bizarre-shaped hyperpigmentation
  1. *Apiaceae* (*Umbilliferae*)—most common
     - Dill, celery, parsley, fennel, parsnip (Mnemonic—all dainty yuppie vegetables)
     - "Strimmer"/"weed wacker"/"weed eater" dermatitis from lawn trimming
  2. *Rutaceae* (citrus)
     - Lemon, lime, grapefruit, bergamot in perfume
III. Phototoxic drug reactions
  - Most associated with tetracyclines, NSAIDs
    1. Exaggerated sunburn
    2. Radiation recall
       - Can see with methotrexate, other chemotherapy, eruption in previously irradiated area
    3. Radiation enhancement
    4. Ultraviolet recall
    5. Photo-onycholysis
       - Classically from tetracyclines
IV. Photo-associated eruptions
  1. Photodistributed drug eruptions
     - Commonly photolichenoid, drug-induced SCLE,pseudoporphyria (classically from naproxen)
     - See also Vascular:Toxic Erythema:Drug Eruptions
  2. Autoimmune connective tissue disease-associated photosensitivity (*see also Connective Tissue Disease*)
  3. Pellagra (niacin deficiency)
     - *See also Nutritional Disease*
e. Systemic contact dermatitis
  I. Baboon syndrome
     - Aka symmetrical drug related intertriginous and flexural exanthema (SDRIFE) or recurrent flexural erythema = Symmetric well-demarcated erythema of gluteal or inguinal areas related to ingestion of a contact allergen

3.2.2 **Atopic Dermatitis**

- Familial, chronic inflammatory skin disease that commonly presents during early infancy and childhood but can persist or start in adulthood
- Characterized by:
  1. Skin barrier defects
  2. Immune dysregulation, classically thought of as Th2 mediated disease (IL-4,5,13), with some Th1 predominance in chronic lesions
- Associated with atopy (allergic rhinitis, food allergies and asthma)

- Hanifin-Rajika criteria require at least three or more features for diagnosis: pruritus, typical morphology, chronic or chronically relapsing dermatitis, personal or family history of atopy
- Per history, classically "the itch that rashes"—the itch precedes the eruption
- Classically affects flexural antecubital/popliteal fossae
- Clinical associations: Dennie-Morgan lines (double infraorbital folds), atopic shiners, pityriasis alba, ichthyosis vulgaris, xerosis, headlight sign (perinasal pallor), atopic salute
- In kids, onset usually after two months, ddx seborrheic dermatitis, which can start 1 week after birth
- Associated with decreased antimicrobial peptides (β-defensins, cathelicidins (LL-37)); could explain high rate of impetiginization (fascinating contrast with psoriasis, which has increased antimicrobial peptides and low rate of impetiginization)

3.2.3 Nummular Dermatitis

= Coin-shaped lesions, typically crusted
- May respond to antibiotics if crusted/weepy

3.2.4 Dyshidrotic Dermatitis/Pompholyx

- "Tapioca pudding-like vesicles" on palms/soles, lateral aspects of fingers
- May be exacerbated by excessive hand washing
- "Hand dermatitis" is a general category that may include dyshidrotic eczema, irritant and allergic contact dermatitis, and atopic dermatitis of the hands

3.2.5 Id Reaction (Autosensitization or Autoeczematization Dermatitis)

- A secondary dissemination of eczema, associated with stasis or craquele dermatitis, and with fungal infection; classically on arms/hands from initial dermatitis on legs/feet

3.2.6 Infectious Eczematoid

- Eczematous eruption secondary to contact with purulent drainage

3

3.2.7 Drug Dermatitis

— Local reaction from contact with a topical medication or a generalized eruption from a systemic medication

3.2.8 Stasis Dermatitis

— Classically, on the legs from edema; may be consulted for "bilateral cellulitis"
— Clinically, may see varicose veins
    a. Acroangiodermatitis (aka pseudo-Kaposi's sarcoma)
— A variant of stasis dermatitis, hyperplasia of existing vessels that may mimic Kaposi's

3.2.9 Cutaneous T-Cell Lymphoma (CTCL)/Mycosis Fungoides (MF)

— May appear eczematous both clinically and on pathology
— See also *Papulosquamous:Psoriasiform* and *Neoplastic:Lymphomas*

3.2.10 Asteatotic Dermatitis (Eczema Craquele)

— Aka "winter eczema"
— On a spectrum with xerosis
— Classically on shins, "cracked river bed"

3.2.11 Lichen Simplex Chronicus (LSC)/Prurigo Nodularis

— *See also Keratotic Disease:Lichen Simplex*

3.2.12 Exfoliative Dermatitis (Erythroderma)

— *See also Papulosquamous:Erythroderma*

3.2.13 Seborrheic Dermatitis

— A psoriasiform disease (*see also Papulosquamous:Psoriasisiform*)

3.2.14 **Other Eczemas**

a. Juvenile plantar dermatosis
   - Shiny/scaly balls of feet in kids > age 3, usually spares middle foot; path shows chronic eczema
   - From repeated maceration of feet
b. Meyerson phenomenon
   - Eczematous inflammation surrounding a melanocytic nevus

- Experts are discussing a simplification of classification of all these related conditions into "atopic spectrum disease" given their shared pathophysiology and response to treatment. In clinical practice, there is a challenge to get medications approved depending on the way disease is coded (medication may be approved for atopic dermatitis but denied for nummular dermatitis). Many would argue (lumpers) that these are the same disease.
- Treatment: TCS, TCI, topical JAKi (ruxolitinib), phototherapy, systemic steroids, traditional immunosuppressants (cyclosporine, MMF, AZA), IL-4/13 blocker (dupilumab), IL-13 blocker (tralokinumab), systemic JAKi (upadacitinib, abrocitinib)

Vesiculobullous

Contents

4

Abstract

Vesiculobullous diseases are characterized by the presence of blisters and erosions on mucous membranes and/or skin. Blisters are caused by splits in either the epidermis or dermis. They can be classified by the level of this split and type of associated inflammation.

Keywords

Vesiculobullous diseases · Vesicobullous disease · Blistering diseases

Clinically it can be difficult to distinguish the level of a blister. However, one can infer the level of the split based on certain findings:

- If mostly flaccid bullae are seen, it is more likely to be intraepidermal
- If most blisters are tense and intact, and if there are associated milia and scarring, it is more likely to be subepidermal.
- Yet for blisters on hands and feet, keep in mind that all blisters tend to remain tense given the thickened stratum corneum.
- With time, tense blisters can become flaccid, but flaccid blisters cannot become tense.
- Hemorrhagic blisters presumably are subepidermal, since vessels are in the dermis.
- Blisters caused by infection or inflammation should start on an erythematous base.

When performing biopsies to diagnose blistering diseases: for H&E, perform a biopsy of lesional skin; for direct immunofluorescence (DIF), most recommend biopsy of perilesional skin; the rationale for perilesional in this case is that normal structures will be intact without blister, and for a DIF, intact anatomy is important for identifying the targeted antigen.

Three primary causes of blisters in the epidermis:

Acantholysis (loss of keratinocyte cohesion)

Spongiosis (intercellular edema)

Ballooning degeneration (viral).

Clinical signs suggestive of suprabasilar split or full epidermal necrosis:

Nikolsky's sign = slight tangential pressure of skin causes denudation; seen in TEN and pemphigus; implies epidermal separation

Asboe-Hansen sign = aka pseudo-Nikolsky's sign, an extension of blister with pressure applied on top.

4.1 Subcorneal Blisters/Superficial

1. Pustular psoriasis and palmoplantar pustulosis
   - These are two separate entities; psoriasis should have physical findings beyond palmoplantar pustules
   - With palmoplantar pustulosis, consider SAPHO syndrome
   - Path = subcorneal neutrophilic pustules, ddx AGEP, candidiasis
   - *See also Papulosquamous: Psoriasiform*
   - Treatment: TCS, TCI, topical PUVA, doxycycline, and other typical psoriasis therapies
2. Acute Generalized Exanthematous Pustulosis (AGEP)
   - Non-follicular, sterile pustules on erythematous background, may start on face/axilla/inguinal folds, then generalize; ddx pustular psoriasis, candidiasis
   - Caused most commonly by beta-lactams, macrolides, terbinafine
   - <4 days after exposure, non-antibiotics have longer latency period
   - Can be associated with neutrophilia/elevated WBC (18–25), fever
   - Patch testing positive in 80%
   - *See also Vascular: Toxic Erythema: Drug Eruptions*
3. Infections (not Viral)
   a. Bacterial infections
      I. Bullous impetigo (*S. aureus*)
         - Can be considered a localized form of SSSS
         - Increased incidence in atopic dermatitis
         - See also Infectious Disease: Bacterial
      II. Staphylococcal scalded skin syndrome (SSSS)
         - See primarily in children <5
         - Can see in adults in context of renal failure (unable to clear toxin) or immunosuppression
         - Can present with erythroderma, scarlatiniform eruption
         - Caused by *Staph* exfoliative toxin A, from *Staph* (group 2, phage 71) against Dsg1
         - Path: granular layer split (unlike apoptotic keratinocytes in TEN, in entire epidermis)
         - *See also Infectious Disease: Bacterial and Vascular: Toxic Erythema: Drug Eruptions: Scarlatiniform*
   b. Superficial fungal infections
      I. Bullous tinea
         - *See also Infectious Disease: Fungal*
      II. Bullous candida/ candidiasis.
         - *See also Infectious Disease: Fungal*
   c. Bullous syphilis
      - *See also Infectious Disease: Treponemes and Spirochetes*
4. Pemphigus Foliaceus
   - Can be subcorneal or intraepidermal
   - Antigen = desmoglein-1 = 160kD

4

- Clinically scale/crust can resemble "cornflakes"
- Path: may see cling-on keratinocytes attached to the roof of the blister (aka "the dingleberry")
- DIF = intercellular IgG and complement
- IIF done on guinea pig esophagus
- Antibodies can cross placenta in pregnancy, but do not cause neonatal skin disease since Dsg3 more present in neonate skin (mucosa-like skin)
   a. Pemphigus erythematosus (Senear-Usher syndrome)
      - A controversial entity that was formulated to describe an overlap syndrome of pemphigus foliaceus and SLE; however, more accepted now as just a localized variant of pemphigus foliaceus
      - Scaly, crusted lesions in malar, scalp, chest, back (seborrheic distribution)
      - Only rare patient has features of both pemphigus and SLE and considered to have both conditions simultaneously; but classical description includes positive ANA, DIF with DEJ and intraepidermal involvement
   b. Fogo selvagem (endemic pemphigus foliaceus in Brazil)
      - Associated with the black fly (*Simulium*)
      - Fogo selvagem means "wild fire" in Portuguese
      - May be autoimmune? No clear infectious etiology yet identified
5. Subcorneal Pustular Dermatosis (Sneddon-Wilkinson Disease)
   - Annular or polycyclic plaques and subcorneal pustules in flexures (especially axillae)
   - May have associated IgA paraproteinemia
   - Responds to dapsone (unlike pustular psoriasis) vs. acitretin
   - Immunofluorescence should be negative
6. IgA Pemphigus
   a. Subcorneal pustular dermatosis type
      - Might include Sneddon-Wilkinson, which is clinically and histologically indistinguishable, with only difference being a positive DIF
      - Antigen target = desmocollin-1 (110 kD)
      - DIF shows intercellular IgA deposition
   b. Intraepidermal neutrophilic type.
      - Sunflower-like configuration
      - May have IgA Ab against Dsg1 or 3
      - Treatment: TCS, dapsone, sulfasalazine, or MMF in recalcitrant cases
7. Infantile Blisters/Pustules
   a. Erythema toxicum neonatorum (ETN)
      - Extremely common (50% of full term neonates)
      - Presents with papules, vesicles, macules
      - Clinically can do a Wright stain to check for eosinophils to confirm diagnosis
   b. Infantile acropustulosis
      - Typically more acral distribution
      - Ddx scabies, Gianotti-Crosti
      - May be induced post-scabetic

    c. Transient neonatal pustular melanosis (TNPM)
       – Presents at birth, ddx ETN (may be a variant?)
       – Vs. ETN, has neutrophils, leaves hyperpigmentation behind for months
    d. Miliaria crystallina
       – *See also Vesiculobullous: Other: Miliaria*

4.2 Intraepidermal Blisters

1. Herpes
   – Infects keratinocyte nuclei causing "ballooning degeneration": keratinocyte necrosis leads to formation of multi-nucleated giant cells with chromatin margination, molding of nuclei (3Ms)
   – Clinically, herpes may show umbilicated vesicles (like poxviruses)
     a. Herpes simplex virus (HSV).
     b. Varicella zoster virus (VZV).
   – *See also Infectious Disease: Viral*
2. Acute Eczematous Dermatitis
   – Classic example = allergic contact dermatitis to poison ivy
   – Blisters caused by spongiosis
   – On path, ddx arthropod assault, drug ("drug or bug")
   – *See also Eczematous*
3. Friction/trauma Blisters
   – Path: intraepidermal blister on acral skin, minimal inflammation
4. Epidermolysis bullosa simplex (Weber-Cockayne type).
5. Incontinentia pigmenti
   – Four stages: 1. Vesicular, 2. Verrucous, 3. Hyperpigmentation, 4. Hypopigmentation
   – Aka Bloch-Sulzberger syndrome
   – First three stages usually in infancy, in lines of Blaschko; fourth stage (hypopigmented, atrophic streaks) may persist indefinitely
   – X-linked dominant disease, lethal in males
   – Can have dental (conical or peg teeth), eye (coloboma, strabismus), neurologic, musculoskeletal abnormalities
   – Defect in NEMO, NF-κB essential modulator; thus lose regulation of apoptosis
   – Path (vesicular stage) = eosinophilic spongiosis, necrotic keratinocytes, dyskeratosis, dermal eosinophilic infiltrate

4.3 Suprabasilar Blisters

1. Pemphigus vulgaris (PV)
   – Antigen = desmoglein-3 (Dsg3) = 130kD
   – DIF = "chicken wire fence" (intercellular IgG in epidermis)
   – IIF on monkey esophagus

4

– Can see acantholysis down hair follicles

2. Pemphigus Vegetans
   – Pemphigus with vegetating eruptions in flexural areas (classically in axillae)
3. Paraneoplastic Pemphigus
   – Most associated with non-Hodgkin's lymphoma (40%), CLL (30%), Castleman's disease (10%), thymomas
   – May have antibodies to multiple antigens: Dsg3, Dsg1, envoplakin, periplakin, desmoplakin I and II, BPAG1
   – Pathogenesis may be from tumoral inhibition of keratinocyte junctional antigen tolerance
   – Prominent mouth involvement (classically, intractable stomatitis); not in eyes (in ddx is SJS, but likely to see both eyes and mouth involved)
   – Path may show PV-like, EM-like, and LP-like features, overlapping
   – IIF on rat bladder epithelium (transitional epithelium differentiates from classic pemphigus, whose antibodies only bind to stratified squamous epithelium)
   – Can have systemic effects in kidneys, upper GI, respiratory tract (bronchiolitis obliterans is feared complication)
   – Typically poor response to pemphigus therapies and requires treatment of underlying trigger/neoplasm
4. Hailey-Hailey Disease
   – Aka benign familial chronic pemphigus
   – Autosomal dominant, erosions/vesicles in intertriginous areas (e.g. axillary/inguinal folds)
   – Defect in ATP2C1 (mnemonic "to see one Halley's comet in a lifetime"), calcium pump
   – Path: "dilapidated brick wall"—acantholysis, rare dyskeratosis
   – Low-dose naltrexone may be helpful
5. Acantholytic Dyskeratotic Dermatoses
   Note: Darier's and Grover's can look identical on path
   Types of dyskeratotic keratinocytes:
   Corp grains = in corneum, abundant keratohyalin granules, hard pink cytoplasm, like "seeds"
   Corp ronds = in spinous, granular layers: round bodies, dark nuclei, perinuclear halo
   Note: do not forget SCC can present with atypia and acantholysis, and herpes can also cause acantholysis
   a. Darier's disease (aka keratosis follicularis, a misnomer)
      – Pruritic keratotic/crusted papules/plaques in seborrheic areas, whitish papules in oral mucosa
      – Usually first presents in adolescence/childhood
      – Nail changes: red and white parallel bands, V-nicking
      – Defect in ATP2A2 (AD), ER calcium ATPase (SERCA2)
      – Can be linear; may include palmoplantar keratoderma
      – 3Ds: Darier's has Dis-hesion, Dyskeratosis
      – Lithium can induce Darier's (avoid in patients with Darier's)

- May have acrokeratosis verruciformis of Hopf (autosomal dominant flat wart-like lesions on dorsal hands and feet)
- Tx = topicals (TCS, retinoids), systemic retinoids (acitretin, isotretinoin) first line, prednisone, apremilast, naltrexone, dupilumab in recalcitrant cases

  b. Grover's disease (transient acantholytic dermatosis)
- Pruritic non-follicular crusted papules/papulovesicles on trunk (usually upper), may be acute/transient or persistent (despite name), typically in older white men
- Worsened by heat, sweat, friction, sunlight
- Path: acantholysis, different patterns (pemphigus vulgaris-like, Hailey-Hailey-like, Darier's-like)
- Treatment: TCS, TCI, phototherapy (can flare initially so should combine acute therapy such as cyclosporine or prednisone), naltrexone, systemic retinoids, dupilumab

  c. Warty dyskeratoma
- Papule with focal acantholytic dyskeratosis (FAD)
- Usually head/neck, cup-shaped invagination, arises from hair follicle

4.4 Subepidermal Blisters

4.4.1 Neutrophilic

a. Dermatitis herpetiformis
- Aka Duhring's disease
- Cutaneous manifestation of celiac disease/gluten sensitivity
- Papulovesicles on elbows/knees/extensor forearms/back/ buttocks/scalp (rarely see intact vesicles since so pruritic)
- Over 90% have evidence of gluten-sensitive enteropathy, whereas only 20% are symptomatic for celiac disease
- Increased risk of autoimmune thyroid disease, diabetes, pernicious anemia and enteropathy-associated T-cell lymphoma
- Intense "climbing up the wall" pruritus, cases of suicide reported
- Exacerbated by iodides (like SSKI)
- DIF = granular IgA in dermal papillae
  Tx − dapsone + gluten-free diet (avoid wheat/flour, may eat corn, rice, and oats); TCS occasionally helpful

b. Linear IgA disease/ chronic bullous dermatosis of childhood (CBDC)
- Most commonly caused by drugs, especially vancomycin
- Ab to BPAG2 (97 kD segment); also a sub-lamina densa form with Ab against collagen VII
- May show rosette-like configuration (vesicles at periphery), start in flexures, face; described as "crown of jewels" of vesicles, especially in flexures, groin

4

- DIF = linear IgA (hence the name, which is unrelated to clinical presentation)
- *See also Vascular: Toxic Erythema: Drug Eruption and Mnemonics: Drug Eruptions*
- Treatment: Discontinue culprit med, TCS, TCI, dapsone (1st line), colchicine, doxycyline, prednisone, traditional immunosuppressives in recalcitrant disease (MTX, MMF, AZA) vs IVIG or rituxumab

c. Bullous lupus erythematosus
  - Some consider this EBA occurring in a patient with SLE
  - DIF = granular IgG, C3
  - *See also Connective Tissue Disease: Lupus*
  - Treatment: Dapsone is first line (in addition to traditional SLE meds)

d. Epidermolysis bullosa acquisita (EBA)
  - Ab to collagen VII (NC1 non-collagenous domain), similar to bullous lupus
  - Association with IBD, esp Crohn's disease
  - *See also Vesiculobullous: Other*
  - Treatment: same as BP or LABD but with lower rate of success.

4.4.2 Lymphocytic

a. Bullous erythema multiforme
  - Path = vacuolar interface dermatitis, acute (normal) stratum corneum, necrotic keratinocytes
  - *See also Vascular: Erythema multiforme*

b. Fixed drug eruption
  - Path = vacuolar interface dermatitis, acute changes of normal stratum corneum, but also chronic changes (papillary dermal fibrosis, perivascular melanin incontinence); first occurrence could be in ddx with EM
  - *See also Vascular: Toxic Erythema: Drug Eruptions*

c. Polymorphous light eruption (PMLE).
  - *See also Dermal: Lymphocytic*

d. Bullous lichen sclerosis
  - *See also Connective Tissue Disease: Sclerotic Disease*

e. Stevens-Johnson syndrome/ Toxic epidermal necrolysis (SJS/TEN)
  - Can see subepidermal blister with spare perivascular lymphocytic infiltrate
  - See also Vascular: Erythema Multiforme.

4.4.3 Eosinophilic and Mixed

a. Bullous pemphigoid
  - Infiltrate of eosinophils > neutrophils, may be cell-poor
  - Clinically, may first appear in flexural areas
  - May have early urticarial pre-bullous phase or rarely is non-bullous

- On path, can see eosinophils lining up along DEJ, even before blister formation
- Ab against BPAG2 = 180kD = collagen XVII (NC16A domain) > BPAG1 = 230kD
- DIF = IgG, C3 at DEJ, salt-split skin on roof (epidermal)
- Ddx = linear IgA, cicatricial pemphigoid (DIF, IIF and clinicopathologic correlation is needed to differentiate)

Rarer variants:

I. Anti-p200 pemphigoid
   - Clinically similar to bullous pemphigoid, but DIF shows antibodies against a different 200 kD protein of the DEJ
II. Pemphigoid vegetans
   - Rare intertriginous variant of bullous pemphigoid with vegetative plaques and nodules
III. Pemphigoid nodularis.
   - Presentation of BP with prurigo nodularis-like clinical appearance

b. Herpes gestationis (pemphigoid gestationis)
   = A pemphigoid variant in pregnancy
   - Pruritic annular, urticarial bullae/vesicles in pregnancy
   - Ab to BPAG2, late 2nd/3rd trimester
   - DIF = linear C3 at DEJ
   - Maternal antibodies can transfer and cause neonatal HG
   - Late in pregnancy (or immediately post-partum)
   - Increased risk of prematurity (not so in PEP)
   - May flare subsequently with OCPs or worsen with future pregnancies
   - Patients have an increased risk for Graves disease
   - Ddx: PEP, which is on striae

c. Cicatricial pemphigoid
   - A pattern of clinical subepidermal blistering disease that affects
   - Ab often BPAG2 (180 kD), laminin-5, α6β4-integrin
   - DIF = IgG, IgA and/or C3 in basement membrane, salt-split skin on roof or floor (differentiates from BP which is roof only)

I. Brunsting-Perry (limited to head and neck skin)
   - Ab to BPAG2, laminin-5, collagen VII
   - Minimal mucosal involvement, may have scarring alopecia
   - May overlap EBA as localized variant
   - Treatment: Dapsone considered first line
II. Mucosal membrane
   - Ab to anti-laminin-5/332 aka epiligrin
   - Anti-epiligrin pemphigoid may have increased risk of malignancies (check age appropriate screening)
III. Ocular-specific (ocular cicatricial pemphigoid)
   - Ab to α6β4-integrin (β4 in particular)
   - Symblepharon = fibrous tract between bulbar and palpebral conjunctival surfaces
   - First-line tx = cyclophosphamide, IVIG or rituximab

   d. Arthropod reaction
- Tics/fleas (neutrophilic)
- Other bites (lymphocytic with eosinophils)
- On path, infiltrate often very deep and diffuse

   e. Polymorphic eruption of pregnancy (PEP)
- Formerly known as pruritic urticarial papules and plaques of pregnancy (PUPPP)
- Most common of the pregnancy-specific dermatoses (up to 1:160), usually in late term, ddx herpes gestationis
- Usually begins on abdominal striae, with periumbilical sparing (unlike herpes gestationis); may have microvesiculation
- No maternal or fetal risks, rarely recurs; may have higher risk with twins
- Path: usually fewer eosinophils than herpes gestationis, DIF negative

   f. Epidermolysis bullosa acquisita (EBA).
- *See also Vesiculobullous:Other*

4.4.4 Non-inflammatory/Cell-Poor

   a. Dystrophic epidermolysis bullosa (EB)
- *See also Vesiculobullous:Other*

   b. Porphyria cutanea tarda (PCT)
- Cell poor subepidermal blisters on sun-exposed areas
- Can see erosions, milia, hypertrichosis on cheeks, PIPA, sclerodermoid changes
- Path: "festooning of dermal papillae," "caterpillar bodies"=Type IV collagen (basement membrane), colloid bodies
- DIF=IgG, C3 around DEJ and papillary dermal vessels
- Deficiency of uroporphyrinogen decarboxylase
- Confirm diagnosis with blood and urine porphyrin testing
- Can be triggered by alcohol, HCV, HIV
- Strong association with HCV
- Can remember as a fisherman's disease: imagine a fisherman drinking in the sun, getting a hook in his hand (alcohol, UV, trauma)
- Tx=phlebotomy, antimalarials (remarkably important to note this is dosed twice weekly in this population to prevent a risk of fulminant liver failure)

   c. Pseudoporphyria (pseudoporphyria cutanea tarda)
- Clinically and histologically indistinguishable from PCT, but cannot detect abnormalities in porphyrin metabolism
- Commonly see in chronic renal failure, and with medications (NSAIDs esp. naproxen, furosemide, antibiotics—tetracyclines, dapsone)

   d. Bullous pemphigoid
- Can be eosinophilic (see above), neutrophilic, or cell poor

4.5 **Other**

1. Epidermolysis bullosa (EB) (mechanobullous disease)
   - EB includes different inherited (not autoimmune) blistering disease differentiated by the specific defect
   - Can potentially affect any epithelial-lined tissue (skin, mucous membranes, GI tract excluding the stomach, GU tract)
   a. EB acquisita (EBA) (immune mediated)
      - Not a type of inherited EB; but included here to differentiate
      - Ab to collagen VII (NC1 non-collagenous domain), similar to bullous lupus
      - Rarely may have association with Crohn's disease
      - *See also Vesiculobullous:Subepidermal blisters*
   b. Inherited EB (inherited deficiency)
      I. EB simplex (K5 and 14 deficiency) (EBS)
          - Can present later in life
          1. Generalized (Koebner).
          2. Localized (Weber-Cockayne).
             - On hands/feet
          3. Herpetiform (Dowling-Meara)
             - The most severe form of EBS
          4. EB Simplex with Mottled Pigmentation
             - Ab to just K5
      II. EB junctional type (hemidesmosome proteins)
          1. Herlitz type (severe type)
             - Compound heterogeneous mutations in laminin-5/332/epiligrin
          2. Non-Herlitz Type (Mild Type)
             - Aka GABEB (generalized atrophic benign EB)
             - Mutation in laminin-5 or BPAG-2
      III. EB dystrophic type (collagen VII—anchoring fibrils).
          - Can see absence of nails, contractures
          - Hard to distinguish de novo or germline dominant mutations versus recessive inherited
          - Mortality initially primarily from superinfection/sepsis, but once survive to adolescence, SCCs cause most mortality
          1. Recessive Dystrophic EB
             - Can see multiple cutaneous SCCs in scars (especially in Hallopeau-Siemens)
             - "Mitten hands"
          2. Hallopeau-Siemens Subtype
             - Rarely, renal failure
          3. Dominant dystrophic EB
          4. Transient bullous dermolysis of the newborn (TBDN)
             - Blistering confined to first 1–2 years of life, then rapid resolution

4

      5. EB Pruriginosa
        – Rare subtype with extreme pruritus and resultant scarring
  IV Other EB types/variants
      1. EB with muscular dystrophy
        – Ab to plectin (Think: weak pecs)
        – Hemidesmosomal/ simplex
      2. EB with pyloric atresia
        – Ab to $\alpha6\beta4$-integrin
        – Hemidesmosomal/junctional
        – Usually lethal with extreme skin fragility; may have urologic abnormalities and rudimentary ears
      3. Kindler syndrome
        – Poikiloderma with EB-like features
      4. Bart's syndrome
        – EB with aplasia cutis congenita

* Important to note that these syndrome names and accompanying mutations are no longer emphasized on board examinations due to the ever-evolving and variable nature of clinical manifestations of these disorders. Broad genetic testing is performed at centers who care for these children in the neonatal period before labeling with a particular diagnosis. Treatment is mostly comprised of supportive care however several drugs are in development or have been reported in the recent literature such as kinase inhibitors (erlotinib), baricitinib, IV gentamicin, gene replacement therapy and a few others.

2. Miliaria

    Miliaria are caused by occlusion of eccrine sweat ducts (a, b, c) or apocrine sweat ducts (d).

    Note: Milia = benign, keratin-filled cysts (small epidermoid cysts), *see also Acneiform Disease:Follicular Cysts*

    a. Miliaria crystallina
      – In neonates, superficial (stratum corneum) ductal occlusion; also common in ICU patients
      – Clear vesicles
    b. Miliaria rubra
      – Aka "Prickly heat"
      – In heat, intermediate (lower epidermis) ductal occlusion
      – Erythematous papules or pustules (pustulosa)
    c. Miliaria profunda
      – Deeper (D-E junction) ductal occlusion
      – White papules
    d. Fox-Fordyce disease (apocrine miliaria)
      – Usually pruritic, in the axillae of females

3. Erosive Pustular Dermatosis of the Scalp
   - Extensive crusting and pustules on the scalp, in areas of chronic sun exposure, may be triggered by injury or surgery
   - Has also been reported on the legs
   - Treatment: Clobetasol first line, TCI, TCS/calcipotriene, isotretinoin, dapsone, PDT has also been reported
4. Coma Blisters
   - Characterized by necrosis of eccrine glands, subepidermal > intraepidermal
5. Bullosis Diabeticorum
   - Usually tense subepidermal blisters in context of diabetes, classically on feet
6. Necrolytic Erythemas
   Note: the necrolytic erythemas may present as erosive/crusted eruptions by the mouth, genital/perineal, and intertriginous areas.
   a. Necrolytic migratory erythema (glucagonoma syndrome).
      - In absence of glucagonoma, called pseudo-glucagonoma syndrome
      - *See also Neoplastic: Paraneoplastic syndromes*
   b. Necrolytic acral erythema
      - Hyperpigmented acral plaques seen in some patients with hepatitis C
   c. Acrodermatitis enteropathica/ zinc deficiency
   d. Other nutritional deficiency dermatosis.
      - *See also Nutritional Disease*
7. Acne (Pustular)
   - *See also Acneiform Diseases: Acne*
8. Sucking Blisters
   - Can see on upper lip/hands/forearms of neonates and infants in first weeks of life
9. Bullous Amyloidosis
   - *See also Dermal: Depositional: Amyloid*
10. Bullous Mastocytosis
    - *See also Dermal: Inflammatory: Mastocytic*

Vascular

Contents

© The Author(s), under exclusive license to Springer Nature Switzerland AG 2024
J. Lipoff and D. Ruiz Dasilva, *Dermatology Simplified*,
https://doi.org/10.1007/978-3-031-66739-8_5

5

Abstract

Vascular diseases are mostly dermal because the skin's blood vessels are in the dermis. They are distinguished from other dermal diseases (other inflammatory, depositional, neoplastic), by their red and purple colors caused by vasodilatation, extravasated red blood cells, and vascular inflammation.

Keywords

Viral exanthems · Drug eruptions · Erythema multiforme · Vasculitis

5.1 Toxic Erythema

5.1.1 Viral Exanthems (Children ≫ Adults)

- Path = vasodilatation ± sparse perivascular infiltrate (same as morbilliform drug eruption).
  a. Classic childhood exanthems
    I. First Disease – rubeola/measles – paramyxovirus
    II. Second Disease – scarlet fever – *Streptococcus* pyogenes (not viral)
    III. Third Disease – rubella – togavirus
    IV. Fourth Disease – "Duke's disease" – not specific
    V. Fifth Disease – erythema infectiosum – parvovirus B19
    VI. Sixth Disease – roseola/exanthem subitum – HHV-6/7
    VII. Others
        1. Gianotti-Crosti syndrome
            – Aka papular acrodermatitis of childhood
            – Typically symmetric papular eruption of extremities, face, and buttocks
            – Usually spares trunk (does not exclude)
            – Associated with EBV, HBV > numerous viruses
        2. Unilateral laterothoracic exanthem
            – Ddx Gianotti-Crosti, often starts in axilla
            – Aka asymmetric periflexural exanthem of childhood (APEC)
            – Unclear etiology, thought to be viral
        3. Varicella (chickenpox)
            See also Infectious Disease: Viral
  b. Other viral exanthems
      – Classically associated with enteroviruses

- Acute HIV seroconversion (classic morbilliform) (*see also Infectious Disease: Viral*)
- Pityriasis rosea thought perhaps to be a viral exanthem from HHV-6 or 7 (*see also Papulosquamous: Pityriasiform*)

5.1.2 Drug Eruptions (Adults ≫ Children)

Note: the typical toxic erythema eruption presents a ddx of viral exanthem versus morbilliform drug eruption. Drug eruptions of any type, beyond that of simple morbilliform eruptions, are also listed here.

a. Morbilliform drug eruption
   - Aka exanthematous drug eruption, maculopapular eruption
   - Classically occurs 5–14 days after exposure; commonly from
   - PCN/sulfa/anti-convulsant/allopurinol/cephalosporin
   - Occurs faster upon reexposure
   - Will occur when PCN given for mononucleosis (not an allergy)
   - Thought to be caused by a delayed type IV hypersensitivity reaction
   - Path = vasodilatation ± sparse perivascular infiltrate (same as viral exanthem)
b. DRESS (Drug reaction with eosinophilia and systemic symptoms)
   - Aka drug-induced hypersensitivity syndrome
   - Eruption is typically morbilliform, but may have myriad presentations
   - Typically 2–8 weeks after exposure
   - Most commonly from aromatic antiepileptic agents (phenytoin, carbamazepine, and phenobarbital – these three cross-react), the sulfonamides, allopurinol, dapsone (dapsone hypersensitivity syndrome), minocycline
   - Clinically, facial edema may be hallmark
   - Usually see elevation in transaminases (liver most commonly involved)
   - May see eosinophilia (despite name DRESS, only in ~60%)
   - May also cause myocarditis, pericarditis, nephritis, pharyngitis, pneumonitis
   - Possible role of HHV-6 and 7 has been proposed – some will check HHV-6 viral load when diagnosis in question
   - Monitor TFTs for 12 wks; hypothyroidism possible
   - 10% mortality, mostly from hepatic necrosis or myocarditis
   - Treatment: TCS, long taper of high dose systemic steroids (2–4 mg/kg daily tapered over 2–3 months), MMF, MTX, IVIG, JAKi in recalcitrant cases
c. Serum-sickness-like eruption
   - Fever, arthralgias, urticarial or morbilliform rash
   - Can occur 1–3 wks after cefaclor > other abx most commonly
d. Drug-induced urticaria/angioedema
   - Most common cause of anaphylaxis: ASA
   - *See also Vascular: Urticaria*

e. Drug-induced vasculitis
   - *See also Vascular: Purpura: Vasculitis*
   - ANCA-associated vasculitis can be induced by PTU (propylthiouracil), methimazole, hydralazine, minocycline, levamisole
f. Erythroderma
   - *See also Papulosquamous: Erythroderma/exfoliative dermatitis*
g. Stevens-Johnson syndrome/toxic epidermal necrolysis (SJS/TEN)
   - *See also Vascular: Erythema Multiforme*
   - 5–21 days after exposure
h. Fixed drug eruption
   - One or a few, round, sharply demarcated erythematous and edematous plaques sometimes with grey, dusky, violaceous hue, central blister
   - Common sites: mouth (lips and tongue), genitalia, face, and acral areas
   - Occurs < 48 h after re-exposure, but 1–2 weeks after first exposure
   - Can have non-pigmenting variant with pseudoephedrine
   - Can see disseminated fixed drug eruption that could resemble SJS
   - *See also Lists: Other Lists: Drug Eruption Mnemonics*
i. Acute generalized exanthematous pustulosis (AGEP)
   - A pustular drug eruption
   - Non-follicular, sterile pustules on erythematous background, may start on face/axilla/inguinal folds, then generalize; ddx pustular psoriasis, candidiasis
   - Often caused by beta-lactams, macrolides, terbinafine
   - <4 days after exposure, non-antibiotics have longer latency period
   - Can be associated with neutrophilia/elevated WBC (18–25), fever
   - Patch testing positive in 80%
   - Can see upregulated IL-8 (neutrophil chemoattractant)
   - Treatment: TCS and drug cessation often adequate but sometimes systemic corticosteroids are necessary
j. Linear IgA disease
   - Most commonly from vancomycin
   - *See also Vesiculobullous: Subepidermal blisters, Lists: Other Lists: Drug Eruption Mnemonics*
k. Drug-induced bullous pemphigoid
   - *See also Vesiculobullous: Subepidermal blisters, Lists: Other Lists: Drug Eruption Mnemonics*
l. Lichenoid drug eruption
   - Most commonly from beta-blockers, ACE-inhibitors, penicillamine, also TNF-α inhibitors
   - *See also Papulosquamous: Lichenoid and Lists: Other Lists: Drug Eruption Mnemonics*
m. Drug-induced interstitial granulomatous dermatitis
   - May be drug-induced, e.g. from ACE inhibitors, calcium channel blockers, other

- Typically occurs after many years on a drug, and may take months-years after drug cessation before resolution (making establishment of a drug association often difficult)
- *See also Dermal:Granulomatous*
n. Pemphigus-like drug eruption
- Thiol groups in drugs (ACEIs, penicillamine) can mimic desmogleins
- *See also Vesiculobullous:Suprabasilar blisters, Lists:Other Lists:Drug Eruption Mnemonics*
o. Drug-induced lupus
- *See also Connective Tissue Disease:Lupus, Lists:Other Lists:Drug Eruption Mnemonics*
p. Drug-induced acne
- *See also Acneiform Disease:Acne*
q. Halogenoderma (includes iododerma)
- From bromides, fluorides, iodides; acneiform or bullous eruption
- Ddx folliculitis, dimorphic fungal infections, pyoderma gangrenosum, Sweet's syndrome, pemphigus vegetans
r. Cutaneous lymphoid hyperplasia (formerly pseudolymphoma)
- *See also Dermal:Lymphocytic and Neoplastic:Lymphomas*
- Reported from anticonvulsants, antipsychotics
s. Chemotherapy and radiation-induced drug reactions
    I. Acral erythema of chemotherapy
    - Lumped category of many different chemo reactions on hands and feet
    - Includes erythrodysesthesia
    - Aka hand-foot syndrome
    - Often from cytarabine, bleomycin
    II. Sweet's syndrome (acute febrile neutrophilic dermatosis)
    - Can be caused all-*trans*-retinoic acid (ATRA), G-CSF, or GM-CSF, but drugs only represent < 5% of Sweet's cases
    - *See also Dermal:Inflammatory:Neutrophilic*
    III. Neutrophilic eccrine hidradenitis
    - Necrosis of eccrine coils with neutrophilic infiltrate
    - Associated especially with cytarabine in AML, but also other chemotherapy agents
    IV. Serpentine supravenous hyperpigmentation
    - Local reaction from IV 5-fluorouracil
    V. Radiation recall
    - An eruption in previously irradiated area that occurs with a new systemic medication (e.g. classically methotrexate)
    VI. Radiation enhancement
    - An eruption from a medication exacerbated synergistically with radiation
    VII. Acneiform eruption and paronychia
    - EGFR inhibitors most common culprit

VIII. Lichenoid eruptions associated with PD-1 inhibitors
– Reports of lichen planus and LP-like eruptions common
IX. Inflammatory dermatoses
– E.g. eczema, granulomatous, lichenoid, psoriasis, urticaria, pemphigoid
– Immunotherapy can cause any of these

5.1.3 Scarlatiniform Eruptions

a. Scarlet fever
– Caused by Group A *Strep*, erythrogenic toxins A, B and C
– Clinically, see rough sandpaper erythema, strawberry tongue, Pastia's lines in body folds, axilla, circumoral pallor
– *See also Infectious Diseases: Bacterial*
b. Staphylococcal Scalded Skin Syndrome (SSSS)
– See primarily in children < 5
– Dsg1 affected by *Staph* toxin
– Path: granular layer split (unlike apoptotic keratinocytes in TEN)
– *See also Vesiculobullous: Intraepidermal Blisters and Infectious Diseases: Bacterial*
c. Toxic shock syndrome (*Staph aureus* or *Strep pyogenes*)
   I. Staph
– TSST-1, was originally associated with superabsorbent tampons, now more commonly nasal packing
   II. Strep
– From Group A *Strep*
– *See also Infectious Diseases: Bacterial*
d. Kawasaki disease (mucocutaneous lymph node syndrome)
– Dx criteria = high fever (>102°F) × 5 days plus 4/5 of:
   1. Conjunctivitis
   2. Lip/oral changes
   3. Hand/foot swelling/erythema
   4. Cervical LAD
   5. Polymorphous rash (scarlatiniform, urticarial, or EM-like)
– Unknown etiology, likely infectious
– Early finding: perineal eruption common with early desquamation two days later
– Must check echocardiogram to r/o coronary aneurysm
– May clinically mimic SJS in children
– Tx = ASA and IVIg

5.1.4 Other Reactive Toxic Erythema

a. Graft versus host disease (GVHD)

Acute = (< 3 months) often like morbilliform drug eruption

Chronic = (> 100 days) can have lesions resembling lichen planus, sclerotic lesions like lichen sclerosus, morphea, scleroderma, eosinophilic fasciitis, and poikilodermatous changes

– Acute GVHD typically begins on head/acral sites first
– Chronic GVHD usually lichenoid (early), sclerodermoid (late)
– Induced by donor immunocompetent T cells (predominantly CD8 +) against host that cannot reject them
– Affects primarily the liver (cholestatic hepatitis), GI tract (diarrhea), and skin
– Most often from allogeneic stem cell or bone marrow transplant for leukemia/lymphoma
– GVHD actually associated with clinical benefit despite morbidity (anti-tumor effects)
– Severe form can resemble TEN with positive Nikolsky's
– Tx = systemic corticosteroids in addition to tacrolimus/cyclosporine/MMF/MTX; oral ruxolitinib is now approved; also extracorporeal photopheresis (ECP)
– *See also Papulosquamous: Lichenoid and Connective Tissue Disease: Sclerotic Disease*

b. Eruption of lymphocyte recovery

– Transient, can have associated fever, but no GI/liver effects
– Thought to be from the return of immunocompetent lymphocytes to circulation after chemotherapy-induced lymphopenia
– May be misdiagnosed as acute GVHD

5.2 Figurate Erythemas (Annular or Gyrate Erythemas)

Note: Path usually cannot reliably differentiate the figurate erythemas; may see parakeratosis, spongiosis, "tight cuffing" of perivascular lymphs

1. Erythema migrans (Lyme disease)
   – Ddx Southern tick-associated rash illness (STARI)
   – *See also Infectious Diseases: Treponemes and Spirochetes*
2. Erythema annulare centrifugum
   – Superficial (trailing scale) and deep types (infiltrated edge)
   – A hypersensitivity reaction
   – May have many different associations (systemic diseases, medications, paraneoplastic, pregnancy, blue cheese ingestion)
   – *See also Papulosquamous: Other*

5

3. Erythema marginatum (rheumatic fever)
   – Rapidly expanding, evanescent rash, in < 10% of patients with rheumatic fever (reactive from *Strep*)
   – Path: may see interstitial and perivascular neutrophils (unlike other gyrate erythemas)
   – Reticulate erythema ddx: erythema marginatum, Still's disease, erythema infectiosum (Parvovirus)
   – *See also Infectious Diseases: Bacterial*
4. Erythema gyratum repens
   – Extremely rare, associated with malignancy
   – "Wood grain" appearance
   – Paraneoplastic most common with lung cancer
   – Rapid migration, up to 1 cm/day
   – *See also Neoplasms: Paraneoplastic syndromes*
5. Eosinophilic annular erythema
   – A rare disease of unknown etiology, typically in adults but also seen in children, may present as a figurate erythema
   – May be a form of Well's syndrome, *see also Dermal: Eosinophilic*

5.3 Urticaria

- Individual raised lesion caused by edema and vasodilatation, called "wheal"; may have pale center and surrounding erythema ("flare"); may appear target-like
- Although of similar etiology, depth of swelling distinguishes urticaria (more superficial), angioedema (deeper in dermis/subq), and anaphylaxis
- Type I hypersensitivity reaction
- Path = vasodilatation and edema ± sparse perivascular infiltrate
- Acute urticaria defined as < 6 weeks, chronic urticaria ≥ 6 wks
- Often caused by: idiopathic, drug, food, infection (GAS, viral, parasites)
- Primary effector cell = mast cell; Ag binds to IgE bound to mast cells leading to degranulation of mediators that cause inflammation
- IgE bound to high affinity IgE receptors ($F_c\varepsilon$ receptor I)
- Pre-formed mediators = histamine, heparin, tryptase, chymase
- Newly formed mediators = prostaglandins, leukotrienes, PAF (platelet activating factor)
- Stem cell factor, complement C5a anaphylatoxin, and substance P can cause degranulation by binding to receptors independent of $F_c\varepsilon RI$
  1. Physical Urticaria
     a. Dermatographism
     b. Pressure urticaria
     c. Cold urticaria
     d. Cholinergic urticaria
        – Caused by sweat-inducing stimuli (including heat)

 e. Solar urticaria
  – Acute (lasts only hours) compared to PMLE (lasts for days), exact photoallergen not identified
 f. Contact urticaria
  – Most common plant cause = stinging nettles (*Urtica* family), contain histamine/serotonin/acetylcholine within sharp hairs
  – Includes aquagenic urticaria (from water contact), not histamine mediated
  – Allergic contact urticaria can be caused by celery, latex
  – *See also Eczematous:Contact Dermatitis*

2. Angioedema
 – Look for stridor, GI/respiratory symptoms
 – Notably can be caused by ACE inhibitors
 a. C1 esterase inhibitor deficiency (inherited)
  – Never causes urticaria
  – Screen for with C4 level (will be low; in absence of inhibitor of esterase, cannot prevent C4 from being degraded)
  – Treated with danazol in the past, now with several modern recombinant factors, enzyme replacement and receptor blockers
 b. Acquired angioedema (acquired C1EI deficiency)
  – Acquired from association with lymphoproliferative disorders (lymphomas, monoclonal gammopathy) (type I), or from antibodies against C1EI or immune complex consumption (type II)
  – See decreased C4 and C1q (from antibodies or immune complex-medicated consumption)

3. Anaphylaxis

4. Non-immunologic urticaria (anaphylactoid drug reaction)
 – Caused by direct mast cell granulation
 – Mnemonic PROMS = polymyxin B, radiocontrast, opioids, muscle relaxants, salicylates/NSAIDS
 – *See also Lists:Other Lists:Drug Eruption Mnemonics*

5. Urticarial vasculitis
 – Clinically indistinguishable from urticaria, but lasts > 24 h
 – Consider vasculitis work-up as well as CH50, C3, C4, C1q, antibodies to C1q
 – *See also Vascular:Purpura:Palpable Purpura/Vasculitis*
 a. Hypocomplementemic urticarial vasculitis syndrome
  – Defined by low serum complement levels plus presence of anti-C1q precipitin (in 100%), decrease in C1 activity; highly associated with SLE
 b. Schnitzler's syndrome
  – *See also Vascular:Urticaria:Urticarial syndromes*

6. Urticaria multiforme (giant annular urticaria)
 = an entity that describes presentation of large plaque urticaria with ecchymotic centers often confused for EM (can also have arthralgia and edema).
 – Most commonly seen in infants/young children, associated with viruses, immunizations, antibiotics

5

7. Urticarial syndromes
   a. Schnitzler's syndrome
      – Chronic non-pruritic urticaria, FUO, disabling bone pain, hyperostosis, monoclonal IgM gammopathy (most commonly = IgM-κ), which can progress to neoplasia (Waldenström's)
      – Can cause urticarial vasculitis
   b. Muckle-Wells syndrome
      – Acute febrile inflammatory episodes with arthritis, urticaria, abdominal pain, multiorgan amyloid; autosomal dominant, also causes sensorineural deafness
      – Defect in pyrin/NOD
      – Tx = anakinra, canakinumab, rilonacept
   c. Familial Mediterranean fever
      – Some clinical similarity to Muckle-Wells syndrome
      – Defect in pyrin/NOD
   d. Neonatal-onset multisystem inflammatory disease (NOMID)
      – Defect in cryopyrin
      – Tx = anakinra, canakinumab, rilonacept
   e. TNF receptor-associated periodic syndrome (TRAPS)
      – Defect in TNF receptor-1

5.4 Erythema Multiforme (EM)

Note: EM, SJS, and TEN are terms that have evolved in meaning given a greater understanding of their etiologies over time. In the past, these terms have been used differently and interchangeably. Here is the current paradigm:

- EM is an acute but self-limited skin disease affecting mucous membranes and mostly acral surfaces
- EM is associated with infections, especially HSV and *Mycoplasma*, and only very rarely drugs (even then many consider this more of an EM-like morbilliform eruption)
- SJS and TEN are acute skin diseases almost always associated with new drug exposure (exception – a markedly similar process named reactive infectious mucocutaneous eruption, or RIME, has been associated with *Mycoplasma* and several viruses)
- SJS and TEN are considered diseases on a spectrum; EM will never progress to SJS/TEN
- EM and SJS/TEN are different diseases, but may have clinical and histologic overlap
- SJS and TEN have significant mortality, so the culprit drug must be identified quickly
- Treatment of SJS and TEN targets the causes of mortality, with special attention on preventing sepsis and fluid/electrolyte imbalances
- 1 in every 1000 pts with HIV will have SJS/TEN, an 1000 fold increased risk

- Target lesion = Typically < 3 cm in diameter, has a regular round shape and a well-defined border, three distinct zones: (1) central dusky or bullous zone, surrounded by (2) white halo, and (3) surrounding erythema; tend to occur on face, mucosal, acral sites, genitalia; most commonly seen in EM, may see atypical targets in SJS/TEN (although a distinguishing factor is that they are not palpable in SJS/TEN)
- Nikolsky sign = A clinical test to demonstrate epidermal detachment by placing tangential mechanical pressure on erythematous areas. If induces cleavage between epidermis and dermis, it is positive. Suggests SJS/TEN, but not specific.
- Asboe-Hanson sign ("pseudo-Nikolsky") = extension of a blister to unaffected skin on direct pressure
- BSA = body surface area of epidermal detachment, not just areas of involvement
  1. Erythema multiforme minor
     - #1 cause = HSV; outbreak precedes EM by 3–14 days
     - No systemic or mucosal involvement, may not need treatment
     - Path = vacuolar degeneration, necrotic keratinocytes, with vasodilatation, sparse perivascular infiltrate
  2. Erythema multiforme major
     - Caused by infection in 90% (HSV, *Mycoplasma*), very rarely drugs
     - Has systemic and/or mucosal involvement, may require systemic steroids in acute flare, and antivirals if recurrent and associated with HSV
     - Full development of all lesions in 24–72 h, last at least a week
     - Does not progress to TEN
     - Recalcitrant cases may require dapsone, azathioprine, mycophenolate, IVIG, TNFi or JAKi
  3. Stevens-Johnson syndrome (SJS)
     - BSA < 10%, 10–30% = considered SJS-TEN overlap
     - Almost always has mucosal involvement and systemic symptoms
     - 1–5% mortality
     - Almost always caused by new medication exposure, on a spectrum with TEN
  4. Toxic epidermal necrolysis (TEN)
     - BSA > 30%
     - Pathophysiology: thought to be from Fas or granulysin-mediated apoptotic mechanism, oxidative stress may also be involved. Cytokines may amplify apoptotic pathways. IVIG is thought to inhibit the Fas–Fas ligand interaction (death receptor).
     - Almost always has mucosal involvement (usually on at least two mucosal sites) and systemic symptoms
     - 25–35% mortality
     - Path: apoptotic keratinocytes to full epidermal necrosis
     - Frozen section (or rushed path) may be necessary, empiric therapy often started before path confirmation

5

- Treatments: wound care and IVIG, steroids (controversial, with experts feeling strongly for one or the other but no definitive evidence), etanercept
- Check IgA to consider IVIG (IgA deficient individuals can have anaphylactic reaction); somewhat historical as most IVIG is now IgA depleted, however worth consideration
- Severe renal insufficiency (unless on dialysis) and decompensated CHF can becontraindications to IVIG (IVIG can cause fluid overload, and sucrose preparations can cause osmotic nephrosis). Must also be cautious in a hypercoagulable state given risk of VTE
- SCORTEN (severity scale) = points for age > 40, HR > 120, hx cancer, BSA > 10% on day 1, serum urea > 10 mmol/L, bicarb < 20 mmol/L, glucose > 14 mmol/L
- Mortality mainly due to infections (*Staph, Pseudomonas*), but fluid loss, altered insulin metabolism leading to hemodynamic instability are factors

5.5 Purpura

- Purpura, caused by extravasation of blood, may occur in many scenarios: a clotting defect such as low platelets, vessel walls weakened by inflammation (PPD or LCV), poor dermal support of vessels (solar purpura, scurvy, amyloid, chronic steroids, trauma), etc.

5.5.1 Palpable Purpura/Vasculitis

- Clinically, palpable purpura is essentially pathognomonic for leukocytoclastic vasculitis
- Important to distinguish:
  Vasculitis = inflammation of vessels
  Vasculopathy = occlusion of vessels with minimal inflammation
- Path of leukocytoclastic vasculitis (LCV) triad =
  (1) Fibrinoid necrosis (fibrin in vessel walls)
  (2) Neutrophilic perivascular inflammation/karyorrhexis (nuclear dust, aka leukocytoclasis)
  (3) Extravasated RBCs
- When working up for possible vasculitis, use these four steps:
  1. Confirm clinical diagnosis with pathology (biopsy for H&E + DIF)
  2. Assess extent of disease (check U/A with micro—the most important lab test; also stool guaiac, CBC, CMP to r/o systemic involvement)
  3. Attempt to establish etiology (work-up with labs for possibilities: consider hepatitis panel, HIV, ASO, ANA, RF, C3/C4, ANA, cryoglobulins, SPEP)
  4. Start therapeutic ladder/treatment (likely first with prednisone)

Traditionally, types of vasculitis can be classified by size of vessel. This book will conform to that standard, but will present two other ways first (by clinical reaction pattern and by etiology).

Reaction Pattern Approach to Vasculitis
1. "Hypersensitivity" vasculitis
    – This clinical pattern of vasculitis classically presents with many lesions of palpable purpura bilaterally symmetric on the legs.
    – This reflects immune complex disease reactive to a drug, infection, connective tissue disease, etc.
    – Path shows classic leukocytoclastic vasculitis/small vessel involvement
2. "Septic" vasculitis
    – This clinical pattern of vasculitis classically presents with very few lesions of palpable purpura or purpuric ulcers on distal sites (toes, fingers)
    – May be associated with "punched-out" ulcers, nodules, livedo reticularis
    – This reflects embolic disease leading to vasculopathy/vasculitis, or vasculitis affecting medium vessels
3. Retiform purpura
    – This clinical pattern demonstrates branching or stellate purpuric plaques
    – This reflects an underlying thrombotic vasculopathy or medium vessel involvement of several possible etiologies

Etiology-Based Approach to Vasculitis
1. Connective tissue disease
    – SLE, RA ≫ other CTD
    – *See also Connective Tissue Disease*
2. Medications
    – Many drugs, can be serum sickness-like (hydralazine, minocycline, PTU, cocaine, antibiotics, diuretics, phenytoin, allopurinol)
3. Infections
    – Hepatitis C (and cryoglobulinemia types II and III), *Strep*, HIV, HBV
4. Neoplasms/malignancy
    – Multiple myeloma, leukemia/lymphoma, Hodgkin's disease
5. Granulomatous
    – Includes ANCA positive vasculitis: Polyangiitis with granulomatosis (Wegener's), eosinophilic granulomatosis with polyangiitis (Churg-Strauss), microscopic polyangiitis
    – Others include: erythema induratum, Kawasaki's disease
6. Thrombotic disorders
    – TTP, DIC, septic emboli, HSP (related to Strep) and Finklestein's, antiphospholipid antibody syndrome, cryoglobulinemia (I)
7. Other syndromes
    – Schnitzler's (urticarial vasculitis), Muckle-Wells

Mnemonic for etiologies of vasculitis:

CTD SING =
CTD (SLE, RA)
Thrombotic (TTP, DIC, septic emboli, HSP, cryo)
Drugs (including serum sickness)
Syndromes (Schnitzler's, Muckle-Wells)
Infection (HCV, HBV, Strep, GC, HIV)
Neoplasms (Hodgkin's, multiple myeloma, leukemia)
Granulomatous (EGPA/Churg-Strauss, GPA/Wegener's, also MPA)

Traditional Size of Vessel-Based Approach to Vasculitis
1. Large vessel vasculitis
    – In general, extremely rare in dermatology to consider large vessel vasculitis in the differential.
    a. Temporal arteritis (giant cell arteritis)
        – Can be associated with polymyalgia rheumatica (PMR), jaw claudication, vision loss, scalp tenderness/necrosis
    b. Takayasu arteritis (pulseless disease)
        – Skin manifestations rare but include EM, EN, EI, PG, or non-specific ulcerated papules/nodules
    c. Buerger's (thromboangiitis obliterans)
        – Associated with smoking (tobacco primarily but also other substances)
        – Ulceration, gangrene of distal digits is the classic presentation
2. Medium vessel vasculitis
    – Clinically, typically see "punched out" ulcers, nodules, livedo reticularis, retiform purpura, digital gangrene

ANCA review:
    – ANCA = anti-neutrophil cytoplasmic antibody
    – c-ANCA = Cytoplasmic-ANCA against proteinase-3 (PR3), has strongest association with granulomatosis with polyangiitis (GPA), sensitive not specific
    – p-ANCA = Perinuclear-ANCA against myeloperoxidase (MPO), can see in many rheumatologic diseases, nonspecific inflammation
    – If both p-ANCA and c-ANCA positive, suggests an exogenous or medication-induced process (like levamisole in cocaine-associated vasculopathy)
    – Note: ANCA-assoc. vasculitis can be induced by PTU (propylthiouracil), methimazole, hydralazine, minocycline, levamisole
    a. Polyarteritis nodosa (PAN)
        – Systemically, may also see abdominal pain, arthropathy, mononeuritis multiplex (e.g. foot drop); can have some overlap with MPA; typically spares lungs
        – Rarely ANCA positive
        – Classically 5-10 mm subcutaneous nodules along blood vessels in context of livedo reticularis
        – Can develop hypertension from renal artery aneurysms (classic to have narrowing and aneurysms of vessels)

– Tx = corticosteroids ± cyclophosphamide (added with major internal organ involvement), maintenance with AZA > MTX. For limited cutaneous disease, colchicine is first line

1. Classic PAN
   – Association with HBV
2. Cutaneous PAN (benign cutaneous PAN)
   – 10% of PAN, common in children, usually benign, chronic course
   – limited to the skin without internal organ involvement, but may be recalcitrant
   – Cases reported with minocycline

b. Microscopic polyangiitis (MPA)
   – Up to 60% p-ANCA(+), 30% c-ANCA(+)
   – Characterized by renal involvement (90%) with necrotizing glomerulonephritis; also pulmonary capillaritis that may lead to alveolar hemorrhage
   – Lacks upper respiratory involvement or granulomas (compared to GPA)

c. Medium vessel granulomatous vasculitis
   1. Granulomatosis with polyangiitis (GPA, formerly Wegener's)
      – Wegener's name discouraged given his association with Nazis
      = Necrotizing granulomatous inflammation of upper and lower respiratory tract, glomerulonephritis, and systemic vasculitis.
      – Most often presents with nasal/sinus symptoms ("pulmonary renal syndrome")
      – "Strawberry gingiva" = red, friable, granular classic appearance in Wegener's
      – Up to 80% c-ANCA(+)
      – Tx = corticosteroids + cyclophosphamide/MMF (or rituximab), maintenance with MTX, MMF or AZA
   2. Eosinophilic granulomatosis with polyangiitis (EGPA, formerly Churg-Strauss)
      – Associated w/asthma, eosinophilia, can be p-ANCA(+)
      – ACR criteria: 4/6 of asthma, eosinophilia, mononeuritis multiplex, pulmonary infiltrates, sinusitis, eosinophil-associated vasculitis
      – Presents initially as adult-onset asthma/allergic rhinitis, then develop fever and peripheraleosinophilia, then ultimately develop granulomas
      – Tx = corticosteroids ± cyclophosphamide, AZA, MTX or MMF. Mepolizumab (anti-IL-5) with significant promise.

d. Kawasaki disease

e. Erythema induratum/nodular vasculitis
   – *See also Dermal:Inflammatory:Granulomatous and Dermal:Subcutaneous/Panniculitis and Infectious Disease:Mycobacteria:Typical Mycobacteria*

f. Septic vasculitis
   – *See also Vascular:Purpura:Vasculopathy and Infectious Disease:Bacterial*

3. Small vessel vasculitis
   – Clinically, see mostly palpable purpura
   a. Leukocytoclastic vasculitis (LCV)
      – Aka cutaneous small vessel vasculitis (CSVV)

5

  - General histopathologic reaction pattern of small vessel vasculitis: caused by infections, inflammatory diseases, drugs, neoplasms
b. IgA vasculitis/Henoch-Schönlein purpura (HSP)
  - Clinical tetrad: abdominal pain, hematuria, palpable purpura, arthritis
  - May be associated with preceding *Strep* infection (check ASO)
  - DIF shows perivascular IgA, C3
  - Steroids help with all manifestations but controversial whether it prevents renal disease; dapsone/colchicine with evidence as an alternative treatment
    1. Acute hemorrhagic edema of infancy (Finklestein's disease)
       - Some consider this a variant of HSP in < 2 y.o. children without systemic symptoms
       - Clinically, classically has "cockade" (band of ribbons) appearance, annular, or targetoid purpuric lesions
c. Cryoglobulinemia
   Type I: monoclonal immunoglobulin (IgM or IgG).
     - Causes vasculopathy > vasculitis
     - Protein aggregates, clogs vessels
   Type II: mixed with monoclonal component.
     - Monoclonal IgM against polyclonal IgG
   Type III: mixed; without monoclonal component.
     - Polyclonal IgM against IgG
     - I = clinically more livedo, retiform purpura
     - II/III = clinically more palpable purpura
     - II/III = Ab against other Igs (immune complex disease), causing vasculitis, and thus glomerulonephritis, palpable purpura
     - II/III associated with HCV
     - II and III antibodies are rheumatoid factors (antibodies that bind to Fc fragment of IgG); thus rheumatoid factor is a simple test to screen for II/III cryoglobulinemia – Rf should be positive in II/III
     - May be associated with lymphoproliferative disorders or CTD (more II)
d. Urticarial vasculitis
   - Clinical appearance overlaps with urticaria, but lesions last > 24 h, leave a bruised appearance and pathology shows vasculitis
   - Consider vasculitis work-up as well as CH50, C3, C4, C1q, antibodies to C1q
   - Can be associated with syndromes:
     1. Schnitzler's syndrome
     2. Muckle-Wells syndrome
     3. Hypocomplementemic urticarial vasculitis syndrome (HUVS)
        - Defined by low serum complement levels plus presence of anti-C1q precipitin (in 100%), decrease in C1 activity
        - SLE always present in HUVS patients

e. "Unexpected" vasculitis
   – LCV can be found in these entities, though not necessarily a character-istic feature
   – *See also Dermal:Inflammatory:Neutrophilic*
      1. Granuloma faciale
      2. Erythema elevatum diutinum (EED)
      3. Sweet syndrome

5.5.2 Macular Purpura

a. Pigmented purpuric dermatosis (PPD)
   – Aka benign pigmented purpura (BPP)
   – Caused by inflammation of the capillaries (capillaritis) with mild hemor-rhage
   – Various types described, distinguished by clinical presentation; pathology is all similar
   – Path: superficial perivascular infiltrate, extravasated RBCs
   – Classically in children/adolescents = lichen aureus and Majocchi's
   – Classically in adults = Schamberg's, Gougerot Blum (lichenoid form), and Doucas-Kapetenakis (eczematous form)
   – Classically abrupt onset = Majocchi's, Doucas-Kapetenakis, lichen aureus
   – Some cases of persistent PPD have eventually been diagnosed with MF (?precursor or overlap?); raised suspicion in disseminated PPD > classic lower extremity
      I. Schamberg's disease
         – Most common type of PPD and archetype
         – Pigmentation from hemosiderin
         – "Cayenne pepper" clinical appearance
      II. Lichen aureus
         – Sudden appearance of lichenoid golden macules on legs, usually solitary
      III. Eczematoid pigmented purpura (Doucas-Kapetenakis)
      IV. Lichenoid pigmented purpura (Gougerot-Blum)
         – May resemble Kaposi's or pseudo-Kaposi's
      V. Majocchi's disease (purpura annularis telangectoides)
         – Usually in young adults
      VI. Rare benign pigmented purpura types
         1. Itching purpura of Lowenthal (aka disseminated pruriginous angio-dermatitis)
         2. Granulomatous pigmented purpura
            – Classically in Asians on dorsal feet
b. Thrombocytopenic purpura
   – Can occur with either platelets < 50 K (usually not until < 20 K) or abnor-mal platelet function

5

c. Solar (senile) purpura
d. Ecchymosis (trauma)
  – Consider procoagulant effect, vitamin C deficiency, and poor dermal support of vessels (corticosteroids, systemic amyloidosis, Ehlers-Danlos)
e. Perifollicular petechiae (vitamin C deficiency/scurvy)
  – *See also Nutritional Disease*
f. Gardner-Diamond syndrome (psychogenic purpura)
  – Factiticial disorder with painful, swollen ecchymoses at sites of trauma; usually underlying psychiatric illness
g. Early leukocytoclastic vasculitis
  – Upon early acute presentation, LCV may present with macular purpura prior to evolving into palpable purpura

5.5.3 Vasculopathy

- Most types of vasculopathy may present with clinical signs associated with medium vessel vasculitis (livedo reticularis, ulcers, nodules, digital gangrene) or retiform purpura (branching or stellate purpuric plaques)
  a. Livedo reticularis
    – Term often interchangeably used with livedo racemosa, though reticularis initially meant to refer to physiologic type, racemosa to pathologic type
    – Can be associated with amantadine, quinidine, catecholamines
    – Ddx, remember reticulate erythema triad: erythema marginatum, Still's, Parvovirus; even erythema ab igne
    – *See also Connective Tissue Disease*
      I. Polyarteritis nodosa (PAN)
        – *See also Vascular: Vasculitis: Medium Vessel Vasculitis*
      II. Sneddon syndrome
        – Livedo reticularis, labile hypertension, and CNS disease (usually TIAs, CVAs, or dementia)
      III. Cutis marmorata (physiologic transient livedo reticularis)
        – Particularly see in neonates, infants, children
        – Should improve with warming
      IV. Cutis marmorata telangiectatica congenita (CMTC)
        – Aka congenital phlebectasia
        – Persistent cutis marmorata with atrophic lesions, may be associated with hypoplasia of affected limb
        1. Adams-Oliver syndrome
          = CMTC with aplasia cutis congenita
  b. Livedoid vasculopathy (aka atrophie blanche)
    – From venous insufficiency; often see with lipodermatosclerosis
    – Favors lower extremities (especially ankles), painful punched-out ulcers; white/round/stellate scars with peripheral telangiectasias, reticulate purpuric erythema

- Treatment is CHAP: calcium channel blocker (nifedipine, amlodipine), hydroxychloroquine, aspirin, pentoxifylline
c. Purpura fulminans/disseminated intravascular coagulopathy (DIC)
  - Widespread purpura of any type in septic patients or DIC (a reaction pattern, not a disease), especially meningococcemia, *Strep*, pneumococcemia, gonococcemia
  - In obstetrics, think abruptio placenta
  - In elderly, think any malignancy
  - In pediatrics, think Kasabach-Merritt syndrome
d. Warfarin (Coumadin) necrosis
  - Usually occurs on 2nd to 5th day on warfarin (by 10th day)
  - Typically overlies areas with abundant subcutaneous fat, such as the breast, hip, buttock, or thigh
  - Synthesis of Vitamin K dependent factors (II, VII, IX, X, proteins C and S) is inhibited by warfarin, but since anti-coagulant proteins C and S have shortest half-life, in first few days on warfarin, remember that patients are prothrombotic
  - Predisposed to by protein C deficiency
e. Heparin-induced thrombocytopenia (HIT)
  - Thrombosis is a classic sign of HITT
f. Cryoglobulinemia (types I > II/III)
  - Distinguish from cryofibrinogen or cold agglutinin, which are also causes of cryoagglutination
  - *See also Vascular: Vasculitis: Small Vessel Vasculitis*
g. ANCA-associated vasculitides
  - Granulomatous vasculitides, MPA, PAN
  - *See also Vascular: Vasculitis: Medium Vessel Vasculitis*
h. Antiphospholipid syndrome
  - Divided into two main groups: lupus anticoagulants (LAs) and anticardiolipin antibodies (ACAs)
  - Classically with arterial/venous thrombosis, thrombocytopenia, and recurrent fetal loss
  - Screening test = PTT; also, dilute Russell viper venom time (dRVVT), not affected by factor deficiencies or pregnancy
  - Assoc. with livedo reticularis, ulcers (may simulate PG), gangrene/necrosis, Raynaud's (skin first sign in 40%)
  - Tx = warfarin, DOACs (anticoagulation)
  - *See also Connective Tissue Disease*
i. Calciphylaxis
  - *See also Dermal: Deposition: Calcium*
j. Septic vasculitis
  - Do not forget about the possibility of septic emboli from endocarditis or other when presented with a patient with a clinical presentation of vasculopathy
  - *See also Vascular: Vasculitis: Small Vessel Vasculitis and Infectious Disease: Bacterial*

k. Cocaine-associated retiform purpura (levamisole induced)
  – Given levamisole (an antihelminthic medication used in veterinary medicine and previously in pediatrics) is apparently in 70% of cocaine in US, thought to cause classic purpura of ears, cheeks, retiform purpura on extremities; cocaine may also play a role in pathogenesis
  – Can be associated with neutropenia, classically both p and c-ANCA positive, may be anti-phospholipid Ab positive
  – Path: thrombotic vasculopathy ± vasculitis
l. Cholesterol emboli
  – Abrupt onset, livedo reticularis > retiform purpura
  – Commonly see after arterial/coronary catheterization (hours to weeks after); or in prolonged anticoagulation or acute thrombolytic therapy
  – Peripheral eosinophilia is common (80%); can see toe cyanosis, renal failure
  – Path: cholesterol clefts in vessel
m. Degos disease (malignant atrophic papulosis)
  – Vaso-occlusive/endovasculitic disorder that affects the skin, gastrointestinal tract, and central nervous system
  – Skin lesions consist of small erythematous papules that heal with atrophic white scars with peripheral ectatic rims
n. SLE pernio (Chilblain lupus)
  – *See also Connective Tissue Disease*
o. Pernio (Chilblains)
  – Abnormal vascular reaction to cold in acral skin, especially feet
  – Path: dermal edema, perivascular lymphs on acral skin (think of with dermal edema on acral skin)
  – Treatment: TCS, topical nitroglycerin, pentoxifylline > CCBs
p. Oxalosis
  – Presents with urolithiasis; in skin may present like live do reticularis, retiform purpura
  – In patient with renal failure, could confuse with cholesterol embolus,calciphylaxis
  – Biopsy, history of urolithiasis should distinguish from calciphylaxis
q. Thumbprint purpura
  – Seen in disseminated *Strongyloides* infection

5.6 Regional Erythema

1. Cellulitis
  a. Cellulitis
    – Classically caused by *Staphylococcus* and *Streptococcus*, but can be caused by many infectious agents including *Cryptococcus*
    – *See also Infectious Diseases:Bacterial:Gram Positive Bacteria:Staphylococcus and Streptococcus*

b. Erysipelas
- Aka "St. Anthony's fire"
- Superficial, well demarcated (usually *S. pyogenes*)
- Painful, often on face, though more on lower extremities

c. Erythrasma
- *Corynebacterium minutissimum* infection in intertriginous areas
- Coral red fluorescence with Wood's lamp from coproporphyrin III
- *See also Infectious Diseases:Bacterial*

2. Nevus flammeus (port wine stain)
- From dilated, tortuous capillaries; a capillary malformation
- early laser treatment (PDL, Nd:YAG) is key as these darken over time and become hypertrophic and recalcitrant to treatment during puberty
- Differs from a nevus simplex AKA "stork bite" on neck or "angel kiss/salmon patch" on forehead which is just a dilation of capillaries that fades over time

a. Sturge-Weber syndrome
- PWS in a CN V distribution, V1 or V2 usually, associated with calcification of brain vessels; seizures, developmental delay, glaucoma
- "Tram-track calcifications" in brain on X-ray

b. Klippel-Trenaunay syndrome (angio-osteohypertrophy syndrome)
- Manifests as a triad of capillary malformation, congenital varicose veins, and hypertrophy of underlying tissues, particularly skeletal overgrowth
- Now considered part of the PIK3CA-related overgrowth spectrum (PROS) with newly approved treatment PI3K inhibitor alpelisib

c. Phakomatosis pigmentovascularis
- Syndrome characterized by vascular (nevus anemicus) and melanocytic nevi (nevus spilus)
  CM = capillary malformation (port wine stain or cutis marmorata)
  Type 1: CM + epidermal nevus
  Type 2: CM + dermal melanocytosis ± nevus anemicus
  Type 3: CM + nevus spilus ± nevus anemicus
  Type 4: CM + dermal melanocytosis + nevus spilus ± nevus anemicus
  Type 5: Cutis marmorata telangiectatica congenita + dermal melanocytosis

3. Telangiectasia
  One lay term for telangiectasia = "gin blossom"
  a. Diseases characterized by telangiectasias
  I. Generalized essential telangiectasias
  II. Cutaneous collagenous vasculopathy
  - Clinically, cannot distinguish from generalized essential telangiectasias, but pathology may show fine hyaline pink material in small vessel walls
  III. Connective tissue disease
  - *See also Connective Tissue Disease*

5

1. Limited cutaneous systemic sclerosis (formerly CREST syndrome)

IV. Hereditary hemorrhagic telangiectasia (HHT)
   – Aka Osler-Weber-Rendu disease
   – Multiple mucocutaneous and GI telangiectasias (actually AVMs); notably on lips, tongue; epistaxis
   – Defect in HHT1 (endoglin), HHT2 (ALK-1 = activin-like kinase receptor 1) = TGF-β receptors

V. Ataxia-telangiectasia
   – *See also Vascular: Regional Erythema: Telangiectasia: Genodermatoses with Early Aging, Often Telangiectasia*

VI. Telangiectasia macularis eruptiva perstans (TMEP)
   – Actually, few to no telangiectasias
   – *See also Dermal: Inflammatory: Mastocytic*

VII. Angioma serpiginosum
   Serpiginous/unilateral/not purpuric vs. PPD

VIII. Nevus araneus (spider angioma)
   More common in liver cirrhosis, high estrogen states (pregnancy)
   Pulsations can occasionally be felt

IX. Unilateral nevoid telangiectasia
   – Congenital and acquired forms; associated with high estrogen states (pregnancy, liver disease)

X. Rosacea – erythematotelangiectatic type
   – *See also Acneiform Disease: Rosacea*

XI. TEMPI syndrome
   = Telangiectasias, Elevated erythropoietin level and erythropoiesis, Monoclonal gammopathy, Perinephric-fluid collections, and Intrapulmonary shunting
   – Associated with IgG-κ gammopathy
   – *See also Neoplastic: Skin diseases associated with monoclonal gammopathy*

XII. Other
   = Alcoholism, high estrogen states (pregnancy, OCPs)

b. Poikiloderma
   = Triad of telangiectasia, atrophy, hypo/hyperpigmentation (reticulate or mottled pigmentation)
   – Classic path: epidermal thinning (atrophy), telangiectasia, and pigment incontinence/alteration ± band-like lymphoid infiltrate, basal layer vacuolar alteration/hydropic degeneration depending on etiology
   Three major categories:
   I. MF/CTCL (poikiloderma atrophicans vasculare)
      – *See also Neoplasms: Lymphoma*
   II. Connective tissue disease
      1. Dermatomyositis
      2. Lupus
         – *See also Connective Tissue Disease*

III. Genodermatoses
1. Rothmund-Thomson syndrome (poikiloderma congenitale)
2. Bloom syndrome
3. Dyskeratosis congenita
IV. Other
1. Poikiloderma of Civatte
  – Benign poikiloderma on V of neck, probably from chronic UV exposure
2. Kindler's syndrome
  – Inherited syndrome with poikiloderma and EB-like changes
3. Radiation dermatitis
  – Path: telangiectasias, bizarre "stellate" fibroblasts, loss of adnexal structures
4. Other
c. Genodermatoses with early aging, telangiectasia, sun sensitivity
DNA helicase mutations:
  Bloom, Rothmund-Thompson, Werner/Adult progeria
Diffuse hyperpigmentation:
  Dyskeratosis congenita, Fanconi anemia
Nucleotide excision repair defects:
  Cockayne, xeroderma pigmentosum
Early aging: progeria, adult progeria, ataxia-telangiectasia
I. Ataxia-telangiectasia
  – Aka Louis-Barr syndrome
  – ATM gene, encodes kinase that senses DNA damage
  – Clinically, ataxia first sign, telangiectasias by age 3–6 (first on bulbar conjunctiva), progeric changes
  – Primary immunodeficiency leading to chronic/recurrent sinopulmonary infections in 80%; most common cause of death = bronchiectasis with respiratory failure
  – Those who live to adolescence have 40% chance of malignancy, especially lymphoid
II. Bloom syndrome
  – Photosensitive telangiectatic erythema (may resemble lupus) in first 2 years of life
  – Immune deficient, increased risk for all cancers, short stature, but normal intelligence
  – BLM gene, recQ3 DNA helicase (similar to Rothmund-Thomson), caused by sister chromatid exchange
III. Cockayne syndrome
  – Dwarfism, beaked nose, deafness, loss of subcutaneous tissues ("cachectic dwarf"), basal ganglia calcification, retinopathy
  – Defect in nucleotide excision repair (NER), but not global (compared to xeroderma pigmentosum)
  – No increase in cutaneous or internal malignancies, but usually die by 30 from neurologic degeneration

5

- Shares some features with trichothiodystrophy (PIBIDS), but no ichthyosis or tiger-tail hairs
- Retinitis pigmentosa (salt and pepper), like Refsum syndrome

IV.   Dyskeratosis congenita
- First presents with thin dystrophic nails in childhood (5–15), then leukoplakia (premalignant)
- Lacy, reticulate pigmentation on neck/chest, poikiloderma
- Triad = nail dystrophy, reticulated hyperpigmentation, leukoplakia (premalignant)
- Predisposed to mucosal SCC, leukemia, Hodgkin's; bone marrow failure
- DKC1 dyskerin; interacts with telomerase (in X-linked recessive, the most common form, usually male)
- hTERT and hTR mutations in AD form; these two form the enzyme telomerase

V.   Fanconi anemia
- Diffuse pigmentation of skin, absence of thumbs, severe hypoplastic anemia
- Associated with aplastic anemia, myelomonocytic leukemia (AML), SCC, hepatic tumors
- No hypersensitivity to UVR, XR, chemicals
- Usually autosomal recessive, caused by defects in various DNA repair proteins

VI.   Progeria (Hutchinson-Gilford syndrome)
- Accelerated aging, dwarfism, alopecia, generalized atrophy; usually fatal by 2nd decade
- Lamin A gene (LMNA) – encodes lamin A and C, components of nuclear membrane structure
- Usually de novo

VII. Rothmund-Thomson syndrome (poikiloderma congenitale)
- Early poikiloderma (at 3–6 months) on cheeks/hands/feet/buttocks
- Sun sensitivity (with bullae or erythema), spares antecubital/popliteal fossae
- Increased risk for osteosarcoma (in 10–30%)
- RECQL4 gene, DNA helicase (similar to Bloom)

VIII. Werner syndrome (adult progeria)
- Premature aging and growth at puberty, senile cataracts in 20 s and 30 s, premature balding/graying, scleroderma-like lesions of skin
- The movie *Jack* starring Robin Williams as a rapidly aging child was supposed to be based on this (clearly not medically accurate)
- RECQL2 aka WRN gene, encodes DNA helicase
- Autosomal recessive

   IX. Xeroderma pigmentosum
        – Extreme sun sensitivity, freckling, and skin cancers (often before
          10 years old)
        – Global defect in nucleotide excision repair (NER), cannot re-
          move DNA damage
    X. Acrogeria (Gottron syndrome)
        – A poikilodermatous syndrome with prominent veins, delayed
          growth, but no increased malignancy/photosensitivity, normal
          life span
        – Mostly females, can be associated with elastosis perforans ser-
          piginosa
   XI. Trichothiodystrophy
        – Autosomal recessive, sulfur-deficient brittle hair
        – "Tiger-tail banding" on hairs
        – DNA-repair gene mutations (XP-B, XP-D in nucleotide excision
          repair)
        – Severe neurologic and developmental abnormalities
        – PIBIDS = photosensitivity, ichthyosis, brittle hair, infertility, de-
          velopmental delay, short stature
        – May have same genes mutated as in xeroderma pigmentosum
          and Cockayne syndrome
4. Flushing
   = An exaggerated physiologic response
     a. Rosacea
        – *See also Acneiform Diseases: Rosacea*
     b. Carcinoid syndrome
        – R/o with 5-HIAA urine test
     c. Pheochromocytoma
        – R/o with urine and plasma metanephrines
     d. Scombroid fish poisoning

5.7 Vascular Tumors

— *See also Neoplastic: Vascular tumors*

5.8 Other

1. Still's disease/juvenile rheumatoid arthritis (JRA)
   – Evanescent salmon-colored eruption that could resemble a viral exanthem
2. Nevus anemicus
   – Hypopigmented macule or patch that cannot become erythematous due to
     localized hypersensitivity to catecholamines (alpha-adrenergic always activated,
     so blood vessels do not dilate)

– *See also Pigmentary Disorders:Hypopigmented entities*
– Borders usually not well demarcated
   a. Phakomatosis pigmentovascularis
3. Erythema ab igne
   – Reticular pattern from heat injury (e.g. heating pads, laptop)
4. Blueberry muffin baby
   a. Extramedullary hematopoiesis
      = Dermal infiltrate of red and white cell precursors, megakaryocytes; usually around superficial vessels.
      – Note: extramedullary hematopoiesis in adults most commonly caused by myelofibrosis
         I. Prenatal infections (TORCHeS)
            – Toxo, Other (HIV, Listeria), Rubella, CMV, HSV, Syphilis
         II. Congenital anemias
            – Hemolytic disease of newborn
            – Hereditary spherocytosis
   b. Malignancy (these are not extramedullary hematopoiesis)
      I. Neonatal neuroblastoma
      II. Congenital leukemia
      III. Congenital rhabdomyosarcoma
      IV. Congenital Langerhans cell histiocytosis
   c. Benign
      I. Hemangiomas
         – Hope it's just this!
         – Rule out liver involvement with US if 5 or more
5. Erythromelalgia
   = Erythema/painful burning usually in acral sites precipitated by heat, relieved by cooling
   – Causes include myeloproliferative disorders with high platelets, drug-induced, neurological small fiber neuropathy, hereditary, or autoimmune
   – Type I effectively treated with ASA, otherwise therapeutic ladder includes compounded ketamine, amitriptyline, lidocaine (KAL) cream, compounded midodrine cream, gabapentinoids, SSRI/SNRI, beta blockers, calcium channel blockers, or mexiletine
6. Superior vena cava syndrome
   – Facial erythema/edema without sun exposure
   – Expect breathing problems, weight loss, cough
   – Usually from bronchogenic carcinoma (in 90%)/Pancoast tumor
   – Vertically oriented dilated veins on chest wall
7. Hematoma
   a. Subungual hematoma
      – From acute trauma; can r/o fracture with X-ray and if painful, can drain blood by burring a hole through the nail with needle or punch tool (trephination); if no pain, no treatment needed
      – Electrocautery contraindicated with acrylic nails (flammable)

b. Talon noir/black heel and palm
  – From trauma, blood within thickened stratum corneum
  – Note: RBCs intact, so iron stains (e.g. Prussian blue for hemosiderin) will be negative
8. Lichtenberg figures
  = Fern-like branching erythema pattern as a result of lightning strike
9. Lymphocytic dermatoses
  – These may have clinical overlap with vascular entities
  – *See also Dermal:Inflammatory:Lymphocytic*
10. Neutrophilic dermatoses
  – These may have clinical overlap with vascular entities
  – *See also Dermal:Inflammatory:Neutrophilic*

Dermal

Contents

© The Author(s), under exclusive license to Springer Nature Switzerland AG 2024
J. Lipoff and D. Ruiz Dasilva, *Dermatology Simplified*,
https://doi.org/10.1007/978-3-031-66739-8_6

6

Abstract

Dermal diseases are centered in the dermis, whether the condition is related to inflammation, neoplasia, deposition, or other processes. When epidermal change is noted, it is not a dominant feature. Given that the depth tends to obscure specific features, the various dermal processes often cannot be differentiated on clinical grounds without a biopsy.

Keywords

Dermal inflammatory diseases · Depositional · Panniculitis

6.1 Inflammatory

Dermal inflammatory diseases are best categorized by their predominant cell type. Clinically, these infiltrative processes display morphologic clues that distinguish them. For instance, it may be possible to confidently diagnose a dermal granulomatous eruption, but it may be difficult to distinguish granuloma annulare from cutaneous sarcoidosis without a biopsy. When examining dermal inflammatory eruptions, use all historical and physical diagnostic clues before asking yourself: what cell line might this represent?

6.1.1 Lymphocytic

- Mnemonic: dermal lymphocytic processes can be remembered as the "Ls": Lupus, Leukemia/Lymphoma, polymorphous Light eruption, benign Lymphocytic infiltrate, pseudoLymphoma, Lyme, Lues (syphilis)
- Lymphocytic dermatoses tend to be erythematous dermal plaques (however relatively skin colored or hyperpigmented in skin of color)
  a. Lupus
     – *See also Connective Tissue Disease: Lupus*
  b. Leukemia/lymphoma
     – *See also Neoplastic: Lymphomas*
  c. Polymorphous light eruption (PMLE)
     – Papules/plaques > vesicles > EM-like (each patient only has one morphology) within hours of sun exposure (UVA or UVB), lasts a few days
     – Ddx LE (but no positive serology), EPP (but not painful), EM (but no interface), solar urticaria (but not ephemeral)

- Path: papillary dermal pallor, superficial and deep perivascular lymphocytes
- One form = "juvenile spring eruption" basically PMLE on the ears of kids
- Usually most severe in spring or early summer, frequently responds to HCQ
- A delayed-type hypersensitivity to unclear antigen
- ANA, Ro, La positive in 10–40% (Ro correlates best of all Ab with photosensitivity)
   I. Hydroa vacciniforme
      - Rare, childhood onset, sunlight-provoked disorder
      - Intermittent, scarring
      - May be a scarring form of PMLE
      - Associations with chronic and latent EBV
   II. Actinic prurigo
      - May be a variant of PMLE, but distinct
      - Most commonly seen in Native Americans; also cheilitis, conjunctivitis
      - HCQ not effective, thalidomide is treatment of choice traditionally but recent success with dupilumab
   III. Actinic folliculitis (formerly Acne aestivalis/Mallorca acne)
      - Monomorphous eruption of red papules/pustules on the face from UVA light, no comedones
      - Path with neutrophilic follicular destruction rather than lymphocytes of typical PMLE
      - Treated with sun avoidance, topical and oral retinoids, polypodium leucotomas, HCQ
d. Benign lymphocytic infiltrate of Jessner's
   - On head, neck, upper back; papules/plaques, often annular with no secondary changes
   - Overlaps tumid lupus
   - Sometimes grouped with pseudolymphomas
   - Topical steroids and HCQ are mainstay of tx
e. Pseudolymphoma (lymphocytoma cutis, benign cutaneous lymphoid hyperplasia
   - Benign mimicker clinically/histologically of lymphoma
   - Idiopathic, caused by drugs, insect bites, infections (Lyme, HSV), rosacea
   - Includes lymphomatoid drug eruption, lymphomatoid contactdermatitis, arthropod-induced pseudolymphoma, actinic reticuloid, lymphocytoma cutis, acral pseudolymphomatous angiokeratoma of children (APACHE), Kikuchi syndrome (flu-like illness with polymorphous eruption, LAD, from a virus?)
   - Path: follows normal anatomical structures, mixed cell types, polyclonal (unlike lymphoma -> no regard for anatomy, often destroys structures; monotypic, often atypical morphology, monoclonal); is "top heavy" rather than more monomorphic, "bottom heavy" infiltrate of lymphoma
   - Treat with doxycycline, ivermectin, cryotherapy, ILK, HCQ and TCS, excision in recalcitrant cases

6

   f. Other superficial and deep perivascular lymphocytic
-     I. Figurate/gyrate erythemas (including Lyme, another L)
-    II. Syphilis (aka Lues, another L)

6.1.2 Granulomatous/Histiocytic

Granulomatous dermatoses tend to be red-brown/orange dermal plaques, even "apple jelly"-colored, which may be appreciated on diascopy

a. Sarcoidosis
- Most common in lungs; 1/3 have skin findings
- Most frequently in African-Americans, highest incidence in Sweden
- Can involve any organ system, especially pulmonary, skin, ocular, renal, cardiac
- Consider CXR/CT/PFTs, eye exam, CBC, CMP, U/A, cardiac evaluation (in 20%, may cause complete heart block); note, ACE level, vitamin D not diagnostic
- Path: non-caseating "naked" granulomas
- Kveim test = skin test for sarcoid (not used anymore)
  - I. Macular/papular type
  - II. Subcutaneous nodular sarcoidosis (Darier-Roussy type)
  - III. Löfgren's syndrome
    - Triad: hilar LAD, erythema nodosum, arthritis; also uveitis, fever
    - Mnemonic to distinguish Löfgren from Loffler = Grrr...sarcoid... Löfgrrrrren's
    - Note: Loffler syndrome = respiratory illness associated with eosinophilia, *Ascaris* and *Strongyloides*
  - IV. Lupus pernio
    - Affects coldest areas (nose, ears, cheeks)
    - Associated with chronic sarcoid of the lungs (~75%) and upper respiratory tract, cystic lesions on distal phalanges
    - May be recalcitrant to treatment
  - V. Heerfordt's syndrome (uveoparotid fever)
    - = Parotid gland involvement, uveitis, fever, cranial nerve palsies (usually the facial nerve)
  - VI. Mikulicz syndrome
    - Bilateral enlargement of lacrimal, parotid, sublingual and submandibular glands (sarcoidosis is thought to be one cause, though Mikulicz now being lumped into IgG4-related disease as a larger category)
  - VII. Angiolupoid sarcoid
    - Can resemble rosacea
  - VIII. Infiltration of scars, injection sites, tattoos (TAGU = tatoo granuloma and uveitis)

IX. Other
- Annular, hypopigmented, ulcerative, erythrodermic, ichthyosiform (classically on shins), alopecia, morpheaform, mucosal
- Treatment: TCS, TCI, ILK, phototherapy, systemic steroids, HCQ, tetracyclines, pentoxifylline, dapsone, isotretinoin, MTX, MMF, TNFi, JAKi
- Worth noting that most non-infectious granulomatous disorders will respond to at least one of the above treatments however TNFi and JAKi seem most efficacious

b. Granuloma annulare (GA)
- 2/3 of patients under age 30, most on hands/feet/legs
- Path: palisading granuloma around mucin/degenerated collagen
  I. Localized GA
  - May include interstitial GA subtype, which on path shows less clearly formed granulomas (interstitial)
  II. Disseminated/Generalized GA
  - Associated with thyroid dysfunction, hyperlipidemia, diabetes (controversial)
  III. Interstitial GA
  IV. Subcutaneous GA
  V. Perforating GA
  VI. Arcuate dermal erythema/ Patch GA
  VII. Annular elastolytic giant cell granuloma (actinicgranuloma/GA)
  - There is controversy whether this is a form of GA
  - Path: granuloma without collagen alteration or mucin

c. Interstitial granulomatous inflammation
- Distinguishing these three entities may be difficult as clinical and pathologic presentations have considerable overlap.
  I. Interstitial granulomatous dermatitis (IGD)
  - May be drug-induced, e.g. from ACE inhibitors, calcium channel blockers, other
  - May be associated with connective tissue disease (RA, SLE, others)
  - Typically occurs after many years on a drug, and may take months-years after drug cessation before resolution (making establishment of a drug association often difficult)
  - Path: interstitial infiltrate of histiocytes, perhaps with eosinophils or interface
  - *See also Vascular; Toxic Erythema; Drug Eruptions*
  II. Interstitial granuloma annulare
  - Path: may show interstitial infiltrate of histiocytes with some mucin, with or without degenerated collagen
  III. Palisaded neutrophilic and granulomatous dermatitis (PNGD)
  - Path: neutrophilic infiltrate, abnormal collagen,granulomas, and leukocytoclastic debris
  - Seen in context of connective tissue disease (usually SLE or RA)

6

d. Necrobiosis lipoidica
  – Aka necrobiosis lipoidica diabeticorum (NLD)
  – Most common on shins; violaceous to red-brown atrophic, yellow–brown centered plaques with telangiectasias, may ulcerate
  – Path: "layer cake" of horizontal palisading granulomas around degenerated collagen, "square biopsy"
  – Seen in 0.3% of all diabetics
  – ~60% patients diabetic, ~15% hyperglycemic at presentation

e. Leprosy (Hansen's disease)
  I. Lepromatous
     – Low cell-mediated immunity, many symmetric lesions, late nerve damage, Th2 predominant response
  II. Borderline (BL, BB, BT)
  III. Tuberculoid
     – High cell-mediated immunity, few lesions < 5, anesthetic lesions, Th1 predominant response
     – *See also Infectious Disease: Mycobacterial: Typical Mycobacterial*

f. Tuberculosis
  Types of cutaneous TB:
  I. Exogenous source
     1. Primary inoculation
     2. Tuberculosis verrucosa cutis
     3. Tuberculosis cutis orificialis (orificial TB)
  II. Direct extension
     1. Scrofuloderma
  III. Hematogenous source
     1. Lupus vulgaris
        – Primarily from hematogenous spread > lymphatic, other
     2. Miliary tuberculosis
  IV. Tuberculid eruptions (reactive)
     1. Papulonecrotic tuberculid
     2. Lichen scrofulosorum
     3. Erythema induratum
        – *See also Infectious Disease: Mycobacterial: Typical Mycobacterial*

g. Xanthomas
  – Xanthomas develop from deposition of lipid; this is seen histologically as lipid-laden macrophages (foam cells) in the dermis
  – *See also Dermal: Depositional: Lipid*

h. Other granulomatous
  I. Granulomatous rosacea
     – *See also Acneiform Disease: Rosacea*
  II. Lupus miliaris disseminatus faciei
     – *See also Acneiform Disease: Rosacea*
  III. Rheumatoid nodule
     – Path: palisading granuloma around fibrin
     – *See also Connective Tissue Disease*

IV. Foreign body granuloma
- From ruptured cyst (#1), suture, silicon, silica, tattoo
- Polarize to see birefringent material; note that presence of polarized material does not exclude sarcoidosis

V. Infectious granuloma (suppurative)
- Includes deep fungal, mycobacterial, leishmaniasis

VI. Cheilitis granulomatosis (Melkersson-Rosenthal syndrome)
- Triad of: fissured tongue/scrotal tongue, lip swelling (lower > upper), Bell's palsy
- Path: non-caseating granulomas
- Note: cheilitis glandularis is a lower labial salivary gland hyperplasia (increased risk of SCC)

VII. Cutaneous Crohn's disease/metastatic Crohn's disease
- Clinical: erythematous plaques, often on genitals/buttock (labial/scrotal edema/erythema theclassic presentation in kids, could mimic childabuse)
- May see "knife-cut" ulcers

VIII. Blau syndrome
- Rare autosomal dominant inherited disease withgranulomatous arthritis, uveitis; may mimic sarcoidosis and granuloma annulare

i. Histiocytoses
- Note: Histiocytoses are diseases caused by infiltration of histiocytes.They appear more inflammatory than neoplastic (no evidence of clonality), but can be very infiltrative and life-threatening
- Note: there are indeterminate forms of histiocytosis with mixed immunohistochemistry between LCH and non-LCH

I. Langerhans cell histiocytoses (LCH)
   Note: spectrum from HPD to EG to HSCD to LSD
   - Eponyms are now historical as experts have moved to degree of organ system involvement as primary classifications
   - Aka Histiocytosis X
   - Rash can appear in the skin as hemorrhagic seborrheic dermatitis or like multiple JXGs
   - Path: proliferation of histiocytes in papillary dermis, identified by kidney bean (reniform) shaped nuclei, Birbeck granules (tennis rackets) on electron microscopy
   - Immunohistochemistry = S100(+) (sensitive, non-specific), CD1a(+), langerin(+) (CD207),
   - Langerin — transmembrane protein needed to form Birbeck granules; receptor-mediated endocytosis
   - Malignancies: increased incidence of ALL and retinoblastoma
   1. Hashimoto-Pritzker disease (limited to skin)
      - Aka congenital self-healing reticulohistiocytosis
      - Can relapse, so monitor long-term

2. Eosinophilic granuloma (unifocal)
   – Expanding proliferation on bone, skin, lungs, orstomach
   – Age 7–12 years
3. Hand-Schüller-Christian disease (multifocal, unisystem)
   – Classic triad of exophthalmos, diabetes insipidus (DI), and osteolytic bone lesions (most common at mastoid)
   – DI from infiltration of posterior pituitary by LCH cells
   – Mnemonic: "Popeye the pisser with a hole in his head"
   – Age 2–6 years
4. Letterer-Siwe disease ("See wee") (multifocal, multisystem)
   – LAD, hepatosplenomegaly, seborrheic dermatitis- like eruption
   – Age < 2 years
   – Treatments: excision, TCS, imiquimod, topical nitrogen mustard, phototherapy, MTX, AZA, cytotoxic chemotherapy

II. Non-Langerhans cell histiocytoses (NLCH)
   – Macrophage disorders
   – No Birbeck granules on EM (ddx LCH)
   – Immunohistochemistry: typically see HAM56(+),CD68(+) [a macrophage marker], factor13a(+), CD1a (-), usually S100(-) (exception = Rosai-Dorfman)
   1. NLCH, cutaneous self-healing
      a. Juvenile xanthogranuloma (JXG)
         – Most common histocytosis
         – Usually on head/neck > extremities
         – Associated with NF-1 and JMML (juvenile myelomonocytic leukemia)
         – Path: Touton giant cells (not specific) -> may not be in early JXG
         – When multiple, need eye exam to r/o hyphema, glaucoma (can cause blindness) – only 0.5%, but 40% of those had multiple JXGs
         – Internal: most common eye > lung
      b. Benign cephalic histiocytosis
         – Brown papules on face, age 1–3, self-limited
   2. NLCH, cutaneous persistent/progressive
      a. Papular xanthoma
   3. NLCH, systemic
      a. Multicentric reticulohistiocytosis (MRH)
         – Periungual "coral bead" papules/nodules, arthritis mutilans (can be like RA),malignancy association (in 28%, bronchial, breast, stomach and cervical carcinomas)
         – Path: large histiocytes with "ground glass"or "dusty rose" cytoplasm
         – Immunohistochemistry: CD68(+), S-100(−), CD1a (−)

    b. Xanthoma disseminatum
- Normolipemic
- Eruption of hundreds of xanthomas over the body
- Can develop diabetes insipidus

    c. Rosai-Dorfman disease (sinus histiocytosis with massive LAD)
- Massive painless cervical LAD; usually benign, resolves spontaneously
- Path: emperipolesis: histiocytes with engulfed lymphocytes; also S100 (+), CD1a (-)

    d. Necrobiotic xanthogranuloma (NXG)
- Ddx: xanthelasma, amyloidosis
- Usually periorbital, yellow papules/plaques
- Associated with paraproteinemia (>80% ofcases, most often IgGwith κ light chains), multiple myeloma in a minority
- Path: degenerated collagen surrounded bygiant cells (could look like NLD, but notpalisaded histiocytes), cholesterol clefts in collagen
- May be similar to plane xanthoma (which has a stronger association with multiple myeloma)
- *See also Neoplastic:Skin diseasesassociated with monoclonal gammopathy*

    e. Erdheim-Chester disease
- Rare systemic infiltrative disease of histiocytes with significantmorbidity/mortality
- Rarely may have xanthoma or xanthelasma-like skin lesions
- Consider same treatments as for LCH but also HCQ or dapsone

6.1.3 Neutrophilic

Neutrophilic dermatoses tend to be erythematous/edematous/ pseudovesicular dermal plaques and ulcers, may demonstrate pathergy

    a. Sweet's syndrome – acute febrile neutrophilic dermatosis
- Favors head/neck/upper extremities
- Edematous/erythematous papules/plaques that may appear as vesicles/ bullae, "juicy," but are firm (pseudovesiculation)
- Major criteria.
  1. Abrupt onset of cutaneous lesions
  2. Path consistent with Sweet's
- Minor criteria:
  1. Associated with infection/malignancy
  2. Fever/constitutional symptoms

3. Leukocytosis
4. Responsive to prednisone
- Path: diffuse neutrophilic dermal infiltrate, papillary dermal pallor, can have LCV
- Most associated with malignancies (AML), IBD
- Can be caused all-*trans*-retinoic acid or G-CSF or GM-CSF, but drugs only represent < 5% of cases
- Other associations include post-*Strep*, minocycline, Bactrim, furosemide
- Can have pathergy
- Variant: neutrophilic dermatosis of the dorsal hands

b. Erythema elevatum diutinum
- Note: diutinum is pronounced [Die Oo Tin Um]
- Violaceous, red-brown, or yellowish papules/plaques/nodules on extensor elbows, hands, and knees
- Can be associated with *Strep*, HIV, IgA monoclonal gammopathy, many diseases
- Path: neutrophilic with eosinophils, onion-skin fibrosis, acral skin, ddx granuloma faciale, may have LCV

c. Pyoderma gangrenosum
- Classic clinical presentation = non-healing ulcer with gun-metal grey to violaceous undermined, rolled border; may heal with characteristic cribiform pattern
- Types: ulcerative (most common), bullous (2nd most common), pustular, superficial granulomatous/vegetative
- Triad of common associations: 1. IBD, 2. Connective Tissue Disease (mostly RA), and 3. Hematologic malignancy
- Ulcerative often associated with disease in majority (IBD, RA, monoclonal gammopathy, malignancy – usually hematologic)
- Pustular often in active IBD, bullous in myelodysplastic disease, vegetative does not have strong associations
- Can have pathergy
- May present peristomal in IBD patients s/p ileostomy
- Can be associated with IgA monoclonal gammopathy
    I. Pyostomatitis vegetans
        - May be PG variant orally in UC > Crohn's
        - "Snail-track" ulcers in mouth
    II. PAPA syndrome
        - Sterile *p*yogenic *a*rthritis, *p*yoderma gangrenosum, and *a*cne
        - *See also Acneiform Disease*
    III. PAPASH syndrome
        - *P*yogenic *a*rthritis, *p*yoderma gangrenosum, *a*cne, and *h*idradenitis *s*uppurativa
        - *See also Acneiform Disease*

d. Behçet syndrome
- Major criteria: recurrent aphthous ulcers

- Minor criteria: recurrent genital aphthous ulcers, eye lesions (classically posterior uveitis, also hypopyon), skin lesions (erythema nodosum-like or follicular), pathergy
- Associated with HLA-B51
  I. Aphthous ulcers
     - Aka aphthous stomatitis/recurrent aphthous ulcers ("canker sores")
     - Associated with Behçet's disease, inflammatory bowel disease, cyclic neutropenia, B12 deficiency, HIV
     - May be trauma-induced
     - Ddx herpes
  II. Lipshütz ulcers
     - Ddx aphthous ulcers, pathologically similar
     - Large vaginal/labial ulcers associated with viral infection (e.g. EBV)
     - *See also Infectious Disease: Viral*
 e. Bowel-bypass syndrome
    - Aka BADAS = bowel-associated dermatitis-arthritis syndrome
    - Seems to be caused by bacterial overgrowth and immune response; responds to antibiotics or surgery
 f. Granuloma faciale (more mixed infiltrate)
    - Path: Mixed infiltrate of neutrophils, eosinophils, lymphocytes, histiocytes, often LCV, with Grenz zone; can be confused with EED
    - No granulomas! Not just on face
    - Tx = ILK, TCS, TCI, dapsone
 g. Neutrophilic dermatosis of the dorsal hands
    - Limited to hands, may represent a localized form of Sweet's.
 h. Rheumatoid arthritis neutrophilic dermatosis
    - *See also Connective Tissue Disease*
 i. Palisaded neutrophilic and granulomatous dermatitis (PNGD)
    - *See also Dermal: Inflammatory: Granulomatous/Histiocytic*
 j. Neutrophilic eccrine hidradenitis
    - Necrosis of eccrine coils with neutrophilic infiltrate
    - Associated with chemotherapy (especially cytarabine in AML)
 k. Idiopathic palmoplantar hidradenitis
    - A variant of neutrophilic eccrine hidradenitis
    - Primarily a disease of children, not associated with underlying disease; classically in setting of preceding vigorous physical activity
    - Clinical: sudden onset of multiple, tender, erythematous nodules on the soles ≫ palms
    - Ddx includes the 'pseudomonas hot-foot syndrome,' panniculitis (e.g. erythema nodosum), pernio and vasculitis (e.g. polyarteritis nodosa)
 l. Infectious disease (e.g. cellulitis, abscesses)
 m. Tick bites

6

6.1.4 Eosinophilic

a. Eosinophilic cellulitis (Well's Syndrome)
   – Clinically can mimic cellulitis; responds to prednisone
   – Path: "Flame figures"=pink "flames" from eosinophil degranulation deposited on collagen (non-specific)
b. Eosinophilic annular erythema
   – Thought to be a possible annular subtype of Well's Syndrome
   – May present as a figurate erythema, *see also Vascular:Figurate Erythemas*
c. Eosinophilic fasciitis
   – Aka "Shulman's syndrome"
   – Rapid onset of "woody induration" of extremities with peripheral eosinophilia
   – "Groove sign"=vein depressions in indurated skin
   – Often precipitated by recent strenuous activity
d. Eosinophilia-myalgia syndrome
   – Caused by exposure to L-tryptophan
   – Related to Spanish toxic oil syndrome, a 1981 outbreak in Spain from consumption of contaminated colza oil that killed 600 people
e. Eosinophilic pustular folliculitis
   – Most commonly in Japanese males
   – Folliculitis rather than dermal eosinophilic process; *see also Acneiform Disease:Folliculitis*

Note: the above eosinophilic disorders historically respond to anti-inflammatory therapies such as prednisone but more recently mepolizumab (anti-IL-5) and dupilumab have worked well in the literatureas steroid-sparing agents

6.1.5 Mastocytic

– Mast cells stained by Giemsa, c-kit (CD117), toluidine blue, tryptase
   a. Mastocytosis
      =Solitary tan or yellow-tan plaque or nodules or brown macules (in UP)
      – Solitary nodule in child ddx=mastocytoma, Spitz nevus, JXG
      – Darier's sign=urtication after stroking lesion (pseudo-Darier's can be seen in leiomyomas, neuroblastoma)
      – Tends to spare face/scalp/palms/soles
      – Can see bullous mastocytosis
      – Initial lab work-up typically just CBC and tryptase
      – Tryptase may be elevated in systemic mastocytosis (>20); most common lab abnormality is alkaline phosphatase; also, urinary histamine or histamine metabolites

- c-kit proto-oncogene encodes KIT, a tyrosine kinase, which is the receptor for mast cell growth factor. Mutation leads to activation and mast cell hyperplasia.
- c-kit deactivating mutation causes piebaldism; KIT also important in initiation of melanoblast migration
- Systemically can have flushing, GI symptoms, skeletal lesions, bone marrow involvement (in adults), splenomegaly
- Treatment = antihistamines, cromolyn sodium, epinephrine in acute episodes, avoidance of mast cell degranulators (PROMS and others), imatinib (though may be ineffective in c-KIT D816V mutations)
- Mnemonic PROMS for medication triggers = polymyxin B, radiocontrast, opiates, muscle relaxants, salicylates/NSAIDs
  I. Solitary mastocytoma
     - In infants, usually self-resolves, benign
  II. Childhood mastocytosis
     - Work up with CBC, tryptase, evaluate history forsystemic symptoms (e.g. GI symptoms)
  III. Urticaria pigmentosa (UP)
     - Form of mastocytosis with brown macules, papules
     - Adults usually progress to systemic disease, rarely hematologic disease
  IV. Telangiectasia macularis eruptiva perstans (TMEP)
     - Mastocytosis presentation in adults, in < 1%
     - Red-brown telangiectatic macules with irregular borders
  V. Mast cell leukemia
     - Mean survival < 6 mo historically
     - IL-2 receptor (CD25) levels highly correlated with the severity of bone marrow pathology
b. Urticaria
   - See also Vascular: Urticaria
c. Other
   - Can see mast cells increased in neurofibromas

6.1.6 Plasmacytic

- Note: increased plasma cells may be normal in mucous membranes,scalp
a. Plasmacytoma
   - Localized proliferation/tumor of plasma cells in the skin, benign
   - See also Neoplastic: Lymphomas: Cutaneous B cell lymphomas
b. Zoon's balanitis (balanitis circumscripta plasmacellularis)
   - Moist red, discrete plaques on the uncircumcised glans penis, may have "kissing lesions" involving prepuce
   - Ddx: erosive LP, SCC (so must biopsy)

6

- Path: dense lichenoid with abundance of plasma cells, "lozenge-shaped" basal cell keratinocytes
- Tx: TCS, TCI is palliative, circumcision is curative

c. Apocrine neoplasms
- *See also Neoplastic: Adnexal Tumors*

I. Syringocystadenoma papilliferum

d. Nodular amyloidosis
- Form of AL primary cutaneous amyloidosis caused by local plasma cell dyscrasia
- May progress to systemic amyloidosis (~8% lifetime risk)
- *See also Dermal: Despositional: Amyloid*

e. Infections
- Syphilis, Lyme, leishmaniasis, granuloma inguinale, rhinoscleroma, chanchroid, HIV, deep fungal
- *See also Infectious Disease*

6.1.7 Mixed Cell Infiltrate

a. Granuloma faciale
- Different from pyoderma faciale (a severe form of rosacea)
- *See also Dermal: Inflammatory: Neutrophilic*

6.2 Neoplastic

- *See other section, Neoplastic*
    1. Keratinocyte neoplasms
    2. Melanocytic neoplasms
    3. Adnexal tumors
    4. Other epidermal neoplasms/hyperplasias
    5. Vascular tumors
    6. Spindle cell tumors
    7. Fatty tumors
    8. Cysts
    9. Lymphatic malformations
    10. Lymphomas
    11. Other malignant (including metastatic)
    12. Other benign
    13. Syndromes with multiple tumors or multiple types of tumors
    14. Paraneoplastic syndromes
    15. Skin diseases associated with monoclonal gammopathy

6.3 Depositional

Note: Calcium and urate deposition may be "rock" hard on palpation
Mnemonic for depositions: MACULE[1] = mucin, amyloid, calcium, urate, lipid, exogenous/extra (implanted, pigment, hyaline-like).

6.3.1 Amyloid

- Historically, the term "amyloid" was used to describe protein with characteristic microscopic and staining appearance. Research has shownthese "amyloid" proteins to be heterogeneous and of different etiologies.
- Can see "cobblestoning" of the skin
- Path: very subtle, cotton candy
- Stains: Congo red (apple-green birefringence), Thioflavin-T (stainsaltered keratin type best), Crystal violet, and others
- AA loses affinity for Congo red (and apple-green birefringence) after incubation in potassium permanganate, while AL does not (a way to distinguish)
- AL = always loves Congo red
  a. Macular amyloidosis
     - Amyloid protein = altered keratin
     - Pruritic dusky-brown or grayish "rippled" or reticulated macules symmetrically over upper back or arms – from scratching
     - Significant overlap with notalgia paresthetica = focal, intense pruritus over medial scapular borders; see well-defined hyperpigmented patch
     - Can be associated with MENIIa (also lichen amyloidosis)
  b. Lichen amyloidosis
     - Amyloid protein = altered keratin
     - Pruritic, red-brown hyperkeratotic papules on shins – from scratching
     - DDx LSC
  c. Nodular amyloidosis
     - Clinically see solitary yellow–red nodule or cluster of nodules, may be atrophic or bullous; typically on face/scalp, genitals, acral surfaces
     - Amyloid protein = AL (amyloid light chain)
     - Path = deposition of amyloid in dermis/subcutis
     - Amyloid protein produced by monoclonal population of local plasma cells
     - May be associated with Sjögren's syndrome
     - Patients with primary systemic amyloid may have identical cutaneous findings to nodular amyloid and may progress to systemic amyloidosis, so must work-up (CBC, SPEP/UPEP, TSH, CMP, ANA, ESR)
     - See also Dermal:Inflammatory:Plasmacytic

---

1   This mnemonic ("MACULE") is used with permission by Dr. Donald Rudikoff.

6

d. Primary systemic amyloidosis
  – Cutaneous amyloidosis secondary to underlying primary amyloidosis
  – Amyloid protein = AL (amyloid light chain), myeloma-associated amyloidosis is also AL
  – Pathognomonic pinched purpura, periorbital ecchymosis (raccoon sign)
  – Biopsy from rectal mucosa or abdominal fat pad will show amyloid deposits in 80–90%
  – Can get macroglossia, carpal tunnel syndrome, post-tussive purpura (vessels so fragile, hemorrhage after cough)
  – Can appear as waxy yellow papules on eyelids (ddx NXG, amyloid, xanthelasma, lipoid proteinosis)
e. Secondary systemic amyloidosis
  – Secondary to chronic inflammatory diseases, infectious and non-infectious such as TB, RA, leprosy
  – Amyloid protein = AA
f. Familial amyloidosis
  = These have been associated with mutations in pyrin/NOD
  I. Muckle-Wells syndrome
    – Amyloid protein = AA
    – Acute febrile inflammatory episodes with arthritis, urticaria, abdominal pain, multiorgan amyloid; autosomal dominant, also causes sensorineural deafness
  II. Familial Mediterranean fever
    – Amyloid protein = AA
    – Recurring febrile episodes of 1–2 days
g. Hemodialysis-associated amyloidosis
  – From reduced renal excretion of amyloid proteins, leading to deposition, especially in synovial membranes
  – Amyloid protein = β2-microglobulin

6.3.2 Calcium

- von Kossa stain for calcium
  a. Calcinosis cutis (deposition of calcium in skin)
    I. Dystrophic calcification
        Note: dystrophic calcification occurs when a primary disease (CTD, etc.) causes tissue damage that allows for calcification
        1. Connective tissue disease
            – *See also Connective Tissue Disease*
            – Most common:
                a. Juvenile dermatomyositis
                    – Seen in 30–70% of patients, including calcinosis universalis

    b. Limited scleroderma/CREST
      – Usually on hands, UEs, at sites of trauma
  2. Genetic disorders/genodermatoses
    a. Pseudoxanthoma elasticum (PXE)
      – *See also Connective Tissue Disease: Non- autoimmune connective tissue disease*
    b. Ehlers-Danlos syndromes
      – *See also Connective Tissue Disease: Non- autoimmune connective tissue disease*
    c. Werner syndrome
      – *See also Vascular: Other Erythema*
    d. Rothmund-Thomson syndrome
      – *See also Vascular: Other Erythema*
  3. Lobular panniculitis
    – Pancreatic fat necrosis, lupus profundus
  4. Other
    – Infections (parasites superficially), neoplasms (pilomatricoma), trauma, pseudogout (rhomboid- shaped positively birefringent calcium pyrophosphate crystals)

II. Metastatic calcification
Note: metastatic calcification occurs when there are electrolyte abnormalities (elevated Ca or Phos) from any source (excluding iatrogenic) that lead to deposition of calcium systemically.
  1. Chronic renal failure
    Causes impaired Phos clearance; unable to make 1,25-vitamin D_3 (from 25-vitamin D_3), cannot absorb Ca; thus become hypocalcemic and secondarily hyperparathyroid
    a. Calciphylaxis (aka calcific uremic arteriolopathy)
      – Almost always in chronic renal failure, but non-uremic calciphylaxis has been reported
      – Typically Ca × Phos > 70 mg^2/dl^2 (nl = 30 s, elevated alkaline phosphatase, hyperparathyroidism, but has been reported without these
      – Progressive vascular calcification and ischemic necrosis of skin and soft tissues (ddx retiform purpura)
      – *See also Vascular: Purpura: Palpable Purpura/ Vasculitis: Vasculopathy*
      – Extremely painful
      – Tx = normalization of Ca-Phos by dialysis, phosphate binders, parathyroidectomy, IV and even intralesional sodium thiosulfate (which is a calcium chelator)
      – Mortality primarily from secondary infection/sepsis
    b. Benign nodular calcification of renal disease
  2. Milk-alkali syndrome
    – From excessive Ca or antacid intake

   3. Hypervitaminosis D
   4. Others: hyperparathyroidism, neoplasms, sarcoidosis, familial tumoral calcinosis
  III. Idiopathic calcification
    1. Idiopathic calcified nodules of scrotum (scrotal calcinosis)
    2. Subepidermal calcified nodule
    3. Tumoral calcinosis (sporadic)
    4. Milia-like calcinosis
     – Can see in Down's syndrome
  IV. Iatrogenic calcification
    – From IV calcium chloride, gluconate, and phosphate
    – Can see transiently after liver transplant
 b. Osteoma cutis (ossification/bone formation in skin)
  – From calcium hydroxyapatite
  I. Acquired
    1. Miliary osteoma cutis
     Can be from acne
  II. Inherited
    – From intramembranous ossification (except FOP)
     1. Albright's hereditary osteodystrophy
      – Two types: pseudohypoparathyroidism and pseudopseudohypoparathyroidism
      – Mutation in GNAS (G protein for cyclic AMP)
      Note: McCune-Albright syndrome = precocious puberty and CALMs, see activation of GNAS,characteristic shortened 4th and 5th digits, polyostotic fibrous dysplasia
     2. Progressive osseous heteroplasia (POH)
      – Seen in infants
     3. Plate-like osteoma cutis (POC)
     4. Fibrodysplasia ossificans progressiva (FOP)
      – Endochondral bone formation

6.3.3 Urate

a. Gout
 – Path: palisaded granuloma around urate, "feathery"
 – Negatively birefringent needle-shaped urate crystal deposition
 – Ddx pseudogout (calcium pyrophosphate crystals = positively birefringent)
 I. Acute gouty arthritis
 II. Chronic tophaceous gout
   – On big toe = podagra
   – Tophi = cutaneous deposits of monosodium urate, extremely firm on palpation, ddx calcinosis cutis, rheumatoid nodule, xanthoma

6.3.4 **Mucin**

- Mucin = protein-hyaluronic acid complex (mucopolysaccharides) normally produced in small amounts by fibroblasts
- Three main glucosaminoglycans (GAGs)=hyaluronic acid (mostimportant), chondroitin sulfate, dermatan sulfate
- Remember, hyaluronic acid as filler=Juvéderm, Restylane, others
- Path: blue-staining material between collagen bundles, or empty spacesin dermis
- Mucin stains = Alcian blue, colloidal iron, toluidine blue
  a. Scleromyxedema
     – Aka lichen myxedematosus (most use term for localized)
     – Aka papular mucinosis
     – A spectrum from localized to systemic disease
     – Systemic form usually associated with IgG-λ monoclonal gammopathy (levels do not correlate with disease severity), < 10% progress to multiple myeloma
     – *See also Neoplastic: Skin diseases associated with monoclonal gammopathy*
     – Small, firm, waxy papules and nodules; glabellar furrows (on leonine facies ddx – *see also Lists: Leonine Facies*)
     – Always rule out thyroid disease, SPEP, serum FLCs
     – Has been reported in assoc. with HIV, HCV, toxic oil syndrome, eosinophilia-myalgia syndrome (L-tryptophan)
     – Path=dermal fibromucinosis (increased fibroblasts and mucin)
     – Tx=IVIG now considered 1st line but also steroids, thalidomide, chemotherapy, auto stem-cell transplant
     – *See also Connective Tissue Disease: Sclerotic Disease: Other sclerodermoid conditions*
       I. Localized scleromyxedema
          1. Discrete papular lichen myxedematosus
          2. Acral persistent papular mucinosis
          3. Papular/cutaneous mucinosis of infancy
          4. Nodular lichen myxedematosus
          5. Self-healing papular mucinosis
  b. Scleredema adultorum of Buschke (scleredema)
     – Path: dermal mucinosis
     – *See also Connective Tissue Disease: Sclerotic Disease: Other sclerodermoid conditions*
     – Three types:
          1. Mostly in women, associated with *Strep*, resolves in months
          2. Mostly in women, associated with monoclonal gammopathy (mostly IgG reported), persistent
             – *See also Neoplastic: Skin diseases associated with monoclonal gammopathy*

3. Mostly men, associated with diabetes, persistent
   - Treatment of diabetes does not improve scleredema
   - Can have systemic involvement
c. Pretibial myxedema
   - Classic finding in hyperthyroidism (Graves)
   - Classically, waxy indurated nodules/plaques with *peau d'orange* appearance
   - Treatment of hyperthyroidism has no benefit, ILK can help, teprotumumab (IGF-1 blocker) works for nearly all manifestations but approved for eye disease
   - Note: Graves disease may also manifest with exophthalmos, thyroid acropachy (fingers/toes with swelling/clubbing) = new bone formation
d. Generalized myxedema
   - Can see in hypothyroidism (increased GAG deposition), in adultsor in children (cretinism)
e. Reticular erythematous mucinosis (REM)
   - A photo-aggravated plaque-like eruption on mid-chest/back of women, may be related to tumid lupus
f. Cutaneous lupus mucinosis
   - Tx: treat the underlying lupus
   - *See also Connective Tissue Disease: Lupus*
g. Follicular mucinosis/ alopecia mucinosa
   - Deposition of mucin in hair follicle; primary form in children that is benign and secondary form in adults that can be associated with folliculotropic MF, *see also Neoplastic: Lymphomas*
h. Digital mucous cyst (digital myxoid cyst)
   = Mucin deposition on acral surface, may cause nail dystrophy
i. Mucocele
   – = Mucin deposition on mucous membrane
   Path: collection of mucin surrounded by giant cells ± salivary glands
j. Myxoma/angiomyxoma
   - When multiple, may be a part of Carney complex(NAME/LAMB syndrome)
   - *See also Neoplastic: Syndromes with multiple tumors or multiple types of tumors and Neoplastic: Other Benign*

6.3.5 Lipid

a. Xanthoma/ xanthelasma (on the eyelids)
   - Path: "Foam cells," macrophages that have phagocytosed lipids in cytoplasm
   - *See also Dermal: Inflammatory: Granulomatous/Histiocytic*
      I. Eruptive xanthomas
         - Usually on extensor arms, hands, and on buttocks

- In hyperlipidemias type 1,4,5
- Associated with elevated triglycerides, or abrupt increase in TGs
- Can Koebnerize
    II. Tuberous xanthoma
- In hyperlipidemias type 2,3
- Type III = "broad beta disease"
    III. Tendinous xanthoma
- In hyperlipidemias type 2,3
- Usually on Achilles heel or extensor tendons
- Almost always with underlying lipid disorder
    IV. Verruciform xanthoma
- Usually occur in mouth > anogenital, periorificial
- Seen in CHILD syndrome (NSDHL gene)
- Path: on low power, looks like verruca; but on higher power, see foamy cells
- *See also Keratotic Disease: Ichthyoses: Genodermatoses with ichthyosis*
    V. Plane xanthoma/ xanthelasma
- In normolipemic patient, could be from multiple myeloma, Castleman's, CML (from monoclonal IgG binding LDL, enhancing phagocytosis)
- Dysbetalipoproteinemia (type III) may produce palmar xanthomas
- Type II may produce interdigital plane xanthomas
- On the palmar creases, called xanthoma striatum palmare
- *See also: Neoplasms/Tumors: Skin diseases associated with monoclonal gammopathy*
    VI. Xanthoma disseminatum
- Non-Langerhans cell histiocytosis, normolipemic
- Eruption of hundreds of xanthomas over the body
- Triad: diabetes insipidus, cutaneous xanthomas, mucous membrane xanthomas
- *See also Dermal: Inflammatory: Granulomatous/Histiocytic: Histiocytoses: Non-Langerhans cell histiocytoses*

6.3.6 Pigment Deposition

▬ *See also Pigmentary Disorders: Hyperpigmented conditions*
    a. Ochronosis
        I. Exogenous ochronosis
- Commonly from hydroquinone, phenol, anti-malarials
        II. Intrinsic ochronosis (alkaptonuria)
- Defect in homogentisic acid oxidase leads to accumulation of homogentisic acid (intermediate in tyrosine/phenylalanine metabolism), especially in cartilage– Premature arthritis (multiple joint replacements) from deposition in cartilage

6

     – Intervertebral disc calcifications, renal calculi and failure
     – Urine that turns dark on standing and alkalinization
     – Blue sclera, blue ear cartilage (from deposition)
     – Path: "banana bodies"
b. Hemochromatosis (iron deposition)
   – Aka "Bronze diabetes"
   – May see hyperpigmentation clinically
   – *See also Nutritional Disease*
c. Argyria (silver deposition)
   – Blue-gray discoloration
   – From topical application of silver sulfadiazine or from systemic ingestion of silver (old school health supplement)
   – Path: peri-eccrine deposition of silver salts
d. Tattoo (pigment deposition)
   Note: in tattoos, consider pigment reactions and sarcoid.
   – Red: Mercury/Cinnabar (mnemonic: red planet) [most contact sensitive], some tattoo artists changing to cadmium
   – Yellow: Cadmium (mnemonic: yellow taxi cad) [most photosensitive, mnemonic: yellow = sun]
   – Green: Chromium
   – Blue: Cobalt (mnemonic: cobalt blue)
   – Purple: Manganese (mnemonic: sounds like magenta purple)
   – Black: Carbon (mnemonic: black like carbon in coal)
   – White: Titanium (mnemonic: like titanium dioxide in white sunscreen)
   Note: amalgam tattoos are mercury > other metals
e. Drug-induced pigmentary deposition
    I. Minocycline
      – Blue pigment indicates iron on path
      Type 1: blue-black at sites of acne, inflammation; Path = iron in dermis.
      Type 2: blue-grey on normal skin; anterior legs; Path = melanin and iron in dermis/subcutis.
      Type 3: diffuse muddy brown on sun-exposed areas; Path = increased basal layer melanin, dermal melanophages, no iron.
    II. Amiodarone
      – Slate-gray photodistributed pigmentation
    III. Other medications
      – Clofazimine (lipofuscin), diltiazem, imipramine

6.3.7 Hyaline-Like Material Deposition

Mnemonic: LACE
a. Lipoid proteinosis
   – Aka Urbach-Wieth disease, or hyalinosis cutis et mucosae
   – Defect in ECM1, autosomal recessive

- Can present initially with hoarse voice or cry
- Path: "free-floating desmosomes" = desmosomes in intercellular space because of ECM1 role inadhesion
- "String of pearls" = beads of papules around eyelid margins (moniliform blepharosis)
- Can have warty plaques on knees/elbows
- Pathognomonic radiographic finding = bilateral, intracranial sickle/bean-shaped calcifications within temporal lobes (hippocampus)

b. Amyloidosis
- Hard to distinguish the other LACE depositions from amyloid – macular and lichen amyloid limited to papillary dermis, nodular amyloid in dermis/subcutis
- *See also Dermal: Depositional: Amyloid*

c. Colloid milium
- Translucent yellow papules on chronic sun-exposed sites; a papule of solar elastosis
- Ddx Favre–Racouchot syndrome

d. Erythropoietic protoporphyria (EPP)
- Defect in ferrochelatase
- *See also Dermal: Depositional: Porphyrias*

6.3.8 Implantable Depositions

a. Silicone
b. Fillers
- Includes collagen
c. Tattoo pigment
- *See also Dermal: Depositional: Pigment Deposition*

6.3.9 Porphyrias

How to work-up porphyrias:
1. If presented with erosions/blistering on sun-exposed areas, check uro-and co-proporphyrins (seen in PCT). If negative, check medication history (pseudoporphyria). Stool porphyrins will distinguish PCT (negative) versus VP or HCP (positive)
2. If presented with immediate burning/erythema on sun-exposed areas, check serum erythrocyte protoporphyrin (EPP). If negative, consider solar urticaria, hydroa vacciniforme (PMLE), xeroderma pigmentosum
3. CEP and HEP present at birth with severe cutaneous photosensitivity

Historical: some people wonder if myths about vampires and werewolves could be from people with porphyrias

a. Non-acute porphyrias

    I. Porphyria cutanea tarda (PCT)
- Cell poor subepidermal blisters on sun-exposed areas
- Deficiency of uroporphyrinogen decarboxylase
- Diagnose by acidifying urine and using Wood's lamp (or any UVA) to detect pink-red fluorescence
- *See also Vesiculobullous: Subepidermal Blisters*

    II. Pseudoporphyria (pseudo PCT)
- Clinical and histologically indistinguishable from PCT, but cannot detect abnormalities in porphyrin metabolism
- Commonly see in chronic renal failure, and with medications (NSAIDs especially naproxen, furosemide, antibiotics)
- *See also Vesiculobullous: Subepidermal Blisters*

    III. Erythropoietic protoporphyria (EPP)
- Defect in ferrochelatase, accumulate protoporphyrin IX
- No porphyrins in urine (Mnemonic: no pee in EPP) – only in serum
- Acute photosensitivity episodes that start in childhood
- Episodes = intense burning of sun-exposed skin, esp. on nose/cheeks/ dorsal hands - > erythema, edema, andpetechiae
- Build-up of protoporphyrins, can lead to cholestasis/gallstones, liver failure
- *See also Dermal: Depositional: Hyaline-like material deposition*

    IV. Congenital erythropoietic porphyria (aka Günther disease) (CEP)
- Defect in uroporphyrinogen III synthase
- Shortly after birth, severe cutaneous photosensitivity, blistering, followed by scarring and deformation, especially of hands
- "Vampire-like" photosensitivity?

    V. Hepatoerythropoietic porphyria (HEP)
- Same defect as PCT, but recessive form, and presents like CEP

b. Acute porphyrias

    I. Acute intermittent porphyria (AIP)
- Presents in puberty, no skin manifestations justneuropsychiatric episodes with abdominal pain
- Defect in porphobilinogen (PBG) deaminase, accumulate PBG (porphrobilinogen)

    II. Variegate porphyria (aka South African porphyria) (VP)
- Defect in protoporphyrin oxidase, accumulate protoporphyrinogen IX
- Cutaneous and neuropsychiatric findings (think of it as PCT + AIP)
- Concentration of protoporphyrin usually higher than coproporphyrin, can be detected in stool, even between attacks
- Attacks can be provoked by medications: especially barbiturates and sulfa drugs (Mnemonic = BEGS for alcohol (barbiturates, estrogen, griseofulvin, sulfa drugs, alcohol))
- Stool porphyrins positive (compared to PCT)

III. Hereditary coproporphyria (HCP)
  – Similar to variegate porphyria
  – Extremely rare
  – Coproporphyrin > > protoporphyrin in stool versus ariegate porphyria (high protoporphyrin in stool); urinecoproporphyrin only elevated with attacks
  – Of note, if treating porphyria with HCQ, must dose once or twice-weekly, otherwise can risk fulminant and fatal hepatic injury

6.3.10 Storage Disorders

a. Lysosomal storage disorders
  – These can be associated with multiple Mongolian spots (dermal melanocytosis)
  I. Mucopolysaccharidoses
    – Lysosomes unable to break down GAGs
    1. Hurler syndrome
      – Deficient in α-1-iduronidase, builds up dermatansulfate/ heparan sulfate
      – Corneal clouding, coarse facies
    2. Hunter syndrome
      – Deficient in iduronidate 2-sulfatase, builds updermatan sulfate/ heparan sulfate (GAG metabolism defect)
      – Retinal degeneration (no corneal clouding), coarse facies, mental retardation
      – Distinctive skin-colored to white papules over scapulae (pebbling)
      – Can have extensive dermal melanocytosis
      – X-linked recessive
b. Lipid storage disorders
  I. Gaucher disease
    – Deficiency of β-glucosidase (aka glucocerebrosidase)
    – Different types may have yellow–brown pigmentation, severe ichthyosis
  II. Niemann-Pick disease
    – Deficiency of sphingomyelinase
    – Can have cherry red spot on retina
  III. Fabry disease
    – Deficiency in α-galactosidase, X-linked recessive
    – Can be associated with angiokeratoma corporis diffusum
    – "Maltese cross" of birefringent lipid globules on polarizing microscopy of urine
    – Earliest symptom = paresthesias, pain
    – Associated with cardiovascular disease
  IV. Farber's disease
  V. Tay-Sachs disease

    – Deficiency in beta-hexosaminidase A
    – Can have cherry red spot on retina
c. Glycoprotein storage disorders

6.4 Subcutaneous/Panniculitis

- Clinically, with subcutaneous disease, bound down, may be difficult to get fingers around; pathology necessary to distinguish types
- Often not clear-cut septal or lobular

6.4.1 Mostly Septal Panniculitis

- Note: septal panniculitis can look like Cheerios in your bowl of cereal; i.e. minimal disruption of lobule appearance (the Cheerios)
  a. Mostly septal panniculitis without vasculitis
      I. Erythema nodosum
          – By far, most common panniculitis
          – May present with fever, arthralgia, fatigue, V/D
          – Etiologies: Idiopathic, *Strep* (#1 infectious cause), Meds (OCPs, abx), infections (especially TB, *Yersinia*, deep fungal), malignancy, IBD, sarcoidosis (Löfgren's)
          – Will not ulcerate
          – Classically on anterior shins
          – Path: early lesions with edema, hemorrhage, and neutrophils
          – "Miescher's radial granulomas" = clustered macrophages around small vessels, plasma cells and eosinophils
     II. Morphea/ scleroderma, "deep morphea"
          – *See also Connective Tissue* Disease:Sclerotic Disease
    III. Necrobiosis lipoidica (NLD)
          – *See also Dermal: Inflammatory: Granulomatous/Histiocytic*
     IV. Granuloma annulare – subcutaneous type
          – *See also Dermal: Inflammatory: Granulomatous/Histiocytic*
      V. Necrobiotic xanthogranuloma (NXG)
          – *See also Dermal: Inflammatory: Granulomatous/Histiocytic: Histiocytoses: Non-Langerhans cell histiocytoses*
     VI. Rheumatoid nodule
          – *See also Connective Tissue Disease*
  b. Mostly septal panniculitis with vasculitis
      I. Polyarteritis nodosa (PAN)
          – Involves small-medium vessels (arteries)
          – Can ulcerate
          – *See also Vascular: Purpura: Palpable Purpura/ Vasculitis: Medium Vessel Vasculitis*

II. Superficial thrombophlebitis
 – Involves large vessels (veins)
 1. Mondor disease
  = Cord/superficial thrombophlebitis often from breast/axillary procedures; axillary web syndrome is variant.
 2. Migratory thrombophlebitis (Trousseau's sign)
  Associated with pancreatic carcinoma
 3. Non-venereal sclerosing lymphangitis of the penis
  – Typically presents as ephemeral tender "cord-like" structure or nodule on the distal
  – penile shaft
  – Associated with recent vigorous sexual
  – activity/masturbation
  – Benign, though reasonable to r/o STIs

6.4.2 Mostly Lobular Panniculitis

Note: lobular panniculitis may look like oil on top of chicken soup; i.e. the lobules are disturbed with large distorted shapes like oil on soup
 a. Mostly lobular panniculitis without vasculitis
 I. Lupus profundus
  – Distribution often upper trunk/hips/face/upper arms, usually not symmetric; trauma may be precipitating factor
  – Similar panniculitis may be seen in dermatomyositis
  – Path: distinctive "hyaline necrosis" of fat lobules, lymphoid follicles; in more than half epidermis and dermis have changes of DLE
  – *See also Connective Tissue Disease*
 II. Pancreatic panniculitis
  – Classically affects lower extremities, especially knees and ankles; thighs, buttocks; clinical = subcutaneous erythematous nodules that may spontaneously ulcerate and exude oily brown material
  – Most often described in acute pancreatitis, chronic pancreatitis, pancreatic cancer (especially acinar cell carcinoma)
  – Etiology thought to be from pancreatic enzymes, especially lipase, but does not fully explain
  – Path: lobular panniculitis with intense necrosis/liquefaction, leaving "ghost adipocytes"
  – Dystrophic calcification may occur in ghost adipocytes by saponification (pancreatic enzyme breakdown of fat followed by calcium deposition)
 III. Traumatic
 1. Cold panniculitis
  – Can see in children, particularly on cheeks/chin from popsicles (popsicle panniculitis)

    2. Equestrian panniculitis
- Primarily in female horse-back riders, on the thighs and buttocks

IV. α-1-antitrypsin deficiency
- Recurrent episodes of painful/tender/ulcerative nodules; often precipitated by trauma
- Distribution often flanks/buttocks, resolves with atrophic scars
- Associated with liver cirrhosis, COPD
- Path = severe necrosis of fat lobules
- Tx includes dapsone, replacement of α-1-antitrypsin

V. Lipodermatosclerosis/ Sclerosing panniculitis
- Classically presents with bound down plaques on lower medial legs ("Upside-down champagne bottle" pattern)
- Associated with chronic venous insufficiency, arterial ischemia
- Path: "Arabesque pattern" (this term is supposed to make you think of a ballet dancer's extended wispy undulating leg while postured on the other leg) = lipomembranous changes of thickened, undulating membranes in fat; fat necrosis in lobular pattern
- Tx includes TCS, ILK, danazol and pentoxifylline

VI. Sarcoidosis
- Don't confuse the naked granulomas with the lymphoid follicles of lupus profundus!
- *See also* Dermal: *Inflammatory: Granulomatous/Histiocytic*

VII. Cytophagic histiocytic panniculitis
- Associated with hemophagocytic syndrome– Erythophagocytosis = phagocytosis of RBCs ≫ lymphocytes, nuclear debris (this is similar toemperipolesis of lymphocytes in Rosai-Dorfman disease)
- These enlarged and distended histiocytes called "bean-bag cells"

    1. Subcutaneous panniculitis-like T-cell lymphoma (SPTCL)
- Not a panniculitis, but always keep in the back ofyour mind (a mimic)
- This is an aggressive lymphoma that can clinically and histologically mimic panniculitis
- Associated with latent EBV infection
- *See also Neoplastic: Lymphomas*

VIII. Calciphylaxis
- *See also Vascular: Purpura: PalpablePurpura/Vasculitis: Vasculopathy andDermal: Depositional: Calcium*

IX. Oxalosis
- *See also Vascular: Purpura: PalpablePurpura/Vasculitis: Vasculopathy*

b. Mostly lobular panniculitis with vasculitis

I. Erythema induratum of Bazin/ nodular vasculitis
- Classically on posterior calves
- Some say 'erythema induratum' if evidence of TB, nodular vasculitis if not
- Will ulcerate

- This basically represents a vasculitis that causes a lobular ischemia and fat necrosis
- Path: lobular panniculitis with vasculitis, fat necrosis; neuts/lymphs/histiocytes with giant cells/granulomas
- Tissue culture for TB invariably negative, but some TB DNA studies have been positive (PCR)
- *See also Infectious Disease:Mycobateria:TypicalMycobacteria:Tuberculosis:Tuberculid eruptions*

II. Lucio phenomenon
- *See also Infectious Disease:Mycobateria:TypicalMycobacteria:Leprosy:Reactions*

III. Erythema nodosum leprosum
- *See also Infectious Disease:Mycobateria:TypicalMycobacteria:Leprosy:Reactions*

6.4.3 Other

a. Lipodystrophy
   I. HIV–associated lipodystrophy
      - Associated with protease inhibitors (indinavir), but NRTIs independently associated as well
      - Poly-L-lactic acid filler (Sculptra) approved for treatment
b. Panniculitides in childrenNote: Path shows "needle-shaped clefts" within lipocytes, hard to differentiate the 3 on path; cold panniculitis in children does not have needle-shaped clefts
   - These can all be considered mostly lobular panniculitides.
   I. Sclerema neonatorum
      - In severely ill premature neonates
      - More rapid onset, minimal inflammation compared to other two
      - Not really seen in the developed world anymore
   II. Subcutaneous fat necrosis of the newborn
      - Full-term infants, first 2–3 weeks of life
      - More inflammatory (unlike sclerema neonatorum)
      - May develop hypercalcemia (follow for 6 months)
      - Could be associated with birth trauma, cocaine use or other drugs (calcium channel blockers) in mother
   III. Post-steroid panniculitis
      - Following rapid withdrawal of steroids in kids
c. Foreign body/facticial panniculitis
d. Infectious panniculitis
   - Any neutrophilic lobular panniculitis should be cultured to rule out infectious cause
   - Ddx includes deep fungal, TB, atypical mycobacteria

Neoplastic

Contents

© The Author(s), under exclusive license to Springer Nature Switzerland AG 2024
J. Lipoff and D. Ruiz Dasilva, *Dermatology Simplified*,
https://doi.org/10.1007/978-3-031-66739-8_7

7

Abstract

Cutaneous neoplasms are either growths of cells normally in the skin or growths of cells that have abnormally migrated to the skin. Most neoplastic diseases fall under the dermal reaction pattern, but since it is such a large category, it is separated into its own section. Here neoplasms and tumors are divided by the type of proliferation.

Keywords

Skin neoplasms · Skin tumors

7.1 Keratinocyte Neoplasms

– Normally occurring cells of the epidermis include: keratinocytes, melanocytes, Langerhans cells, neuroendocrine cells
  1. Benign keratinocyte neoplasms/hyperplasias
     a. Seborrheic keratosis
        – Path: flat-topped papillomatous epidermis, horned pseudocysts
        – *See also Keratotic Disease: Hyperkeratotic Eruptions*
     b. Benign lichenoid keratosis
        – Aka lichen planus-like keratosis (LPLK)
        – *See also Keratotic Disease: Hyperkeratotic Eruptions*
     c. Epidermal nevi
        – *See also Keratotic Disease: Hyperkeratotic Eruptions*
     d. Warts
        – HPV-induced keratinocyte proliferations including verruca vulgaris and condyloma acuminata
        – *See also Infectious Disease: Viral: DNA Viruses: Papovavirus*
     e. Warty dyskeratoma
        – Papule of focal acantholytic dermatosis
        – *See also Vesiculobullous Disease: Intraepidermal Blisters*
     f. Clear cell acanthoma/Pale cell acanthoma
        – On path, can appear very similar to psoriasis, except cells notably pale (from glycogen), and clinically it is usually a solitary
     g. Chondrodermatitis nodularis helicis (CNH)
        – Chronic tender ulcerated nodule on helix of ear, ddx BCC and SCC
        – From pressure/friction, not a neoplasm
        – *See also Keratotic Disease: Lichen Simplex*

2. Premalignant keratinocyte neoplasms
   a. Actinic keratosis (AK)
      – Aka solar keratosis
      – Path: partial-thickness keratinocyte atypia (starting at basement membrane), parakeratosis that spares areas over adnexae
      – For each AK, apparently a 0.1–20% chance of progression to SCC
      – On lips, can see actinic cheilitis/cheilosis (lower > upper lip)
   b. Bowenoid papulosis
      – May represent an intermediate between condyloma and SCCIS
      – Papular HPV lesions most commonly on the penis that may have malignant potential
      – Most associated with HPV-16, 18
   c. Leukoplakia
      – Cannot be removed (unlike thrush)
      – Associated with tobacco (smoked and chewed) and alcohol
      – This is different from oral hairy leukoplakia, which is caused by EBV, but has no malignant potential, and may be a sign of HIV infection
      – One type seen in dyskeratosis congenita, *see also Vascular: Regional Erythema: Telangiectasia: Genodermatoses with early aging, telangiectasia, sun sensitivity*
3. Malignant keratinocyte neoplasms
   – Note: Collectively, squamous cell carcinomas and basal cell carcinomas are referred to as non-melanoma skin cancers (NMSCs). Others have used the term "keratinocyte carcinoma," which may be a more specific and accurate term.
   Note: in transplant/immunosuppressed patients, see increase in skin cancers estimated at: SCC (65X), BCC (5X), and MM (3X); SCC, by far, accounts for most. In HIV, skin cancer risk is increased, but at a much lower factor.
   a. Basal cell carcinoma (BCC)
      – BCC is the most common cause of skin cancer in Caucasians and East Asians; most common cancer of all organs overall
      – Clinically, may see pearly papule, ulcer with "rolled borders," dermoscopy with "arborizing vessels"
      – Gene most frequently mutated = PTCH (on Chr 9q) – PTCH's product = Patched, the transmembrane sonic hedgehog (Shh) receptor; normally hedgehog regulates Patched, which inhibits Smoothened (SMO, a proto-oncogene). Thus, Patched inactivation mutation and Smoothened activation mutations would constitutively activate expression, causing BCCs.
      – Other mutated relevant genes may include p53, MCR1
      – Path = basaloid growth, nuclear debris, mucinous stroma, peripheral palisading clefting/retraction; ddx trichoepithelioma, MAC
      – Metastases in < 0.55%
      – Surgical excision of BCCs: < 2 cm = 3-4 mm margin, ≥ 2 cm = 6 mm margin or Mohs surgery

- Evidence says imiquimod and 5-FU may be used as monotherapy (or combination) for superficial or nodular BCC; limit these topicals to low-risk areas, and not for other types of BCC
- Types:
  I. Superficial/Superficial multifocal
  II. Nodular
  III. Pigmented
  IV. Sclerosing
    - Aka morpheaform or sclerodermiform
    - Clinically may resemble a scar
    - Considered a more aggressive form of BCC; may extend farther histologically than is appreciable clinically
  V. Fibroepithelioma of Pinkus
    - Large tumor in lumbosacral area; may appear tag-like
    - Path: thin strands of anastamosing basal cells
  VI. Infundibulocystic
    - Controversial if different from basaloid follicular hamartoma
  VII. Syndromes that cause BCCs
    - *See also Neoplastic:Syndromes with multiple tumors or multiple types of tumors*
    1. BCC nevus syndrome
       - Aka Gorlin's syndrome/Gorlin-Goltz/nevoid BCC syndrome
       - Multiple BCCs at young age, othertumors, congenital abnormalities including odontogenic keratocysts of the jaw, calcification of falx cerebri, palmar pits, ovarian fibromas (4–24% of women)
       - Can be associated with medulloblastoma
       - PTCH (Patched) gene mutation, autosomal dominant
    2. Bazex-Dupré-Christol syndrome
       Note: do not confuse with acrokeratosis paraneoplastica (also called Bazex syndrome)
       - Genodermatosis of follicular atrophoderma and the early onset of multiple BCCs, may have hypohidrosis
       - X-linked dominant
    3. Rombo syndrome
       - Similar to Bazex, but with KP-like lesions of cheeks that can form honeycombed, worm-eaten appearance (atrophoderma vermiculatum)
       - Hypotrichosis but not hypohidrosis (mnemonic Rambo must sweat), blepharitis, milia (break down into atrophoderma), peripheral vasodilation with cyanosis, BCCs
    4. Multiple Hereditary Infundibulocystic BCC Syndrome
       - Several cases reported
  b. Squamous cell carcinoma (SCC)
    - Primary risk factors: UV, HPV, immunosuppression

- Most common mutation = p53 (Chr 17). Others include CDKN2A and PTCH
- Can occur at sites of chronic trauma/ulcers, scars (Marjolin's ulcer), chronic inflammation (e.g. lichen planus, lichen sclerosis, discoid lupus), radiation, or chemical exposure
- Arsenic is a well-defined cause of SCC; may see palmoplantar arsenical keratoses, multiple tumors as clue
- SCC is the most common cause of skin cancer in African- Americans and Asian Indians; may be more aggressive
- High-risk SCC generally defined as > 2 cm diameter, > 6 mm thickness, recurrent, poor differentiation, presence of perineural invasion, certain high-risk locations (ear/near parotid gland, nose, lip, perianal, genital), immunosuppression (especially with organ transplant), lymphovascular invasion
- Metastatic risk for SCC estimated at 0–10%
- Path = full-thickness keratinocyte atypia with invasion
- Surgical excision of SCCs: generally, low-risk = 3-4 mm margin, high risk = 6 mm margin or Mohs surgery

c. Squamous cell carcinoma in situ (SCCIS)
- Path = full-thickness keratinocyte atypia, confined by basement membrane; parakeratosis; may have loss of polarity (meaning that the superficial and deeper epidermis can no longer be distinguished), loss of proper maturation
- Evidence says topical 5-FU may be used as monotherapy (but not FDA approved); limit topicals to low-risk areas, and not for invasive SCC
  I. Bowen's disease
    - Some use the term "Bowen's" to refer only to SCCIS on the penis, and others use the term Bowen's as synonymous with all SCCIS
  II. Erythroplasia of Queyrat
    = Bowen's disease on the glans penis
  III. Erythroplakia
    - Like erythroplasia of Queyrat, but in the mouth

d. Keratoacanthoma (KA)
- Clinical: cutaneous horn or crateriform nodule, Path: keratin-filled crater/keratotic plug surrounded by proliferation of atypical keratinocytes/mitoses
- Usually considered a form of SCC or benign with a small risk of progression to invasive SCC
- Typical history = sudden onset (weeks)
- Should regress on own, but usually treated as SCC given inability to predict behavior of the tumor
  I. Muir-Torre syndrome
    - Subtype of hereditary nonpolyposis colorectal cancer (HNPCC) syndrome (aka Lynch syndrome), prone to colon, breast, GU cancers

7

– Sebaceous neoplasms (adenoma, epithelioma, or carcinoma), keratoacanthomas, and internal malignancies; sebaceous adenoma is a
unique hallmark (esp. off the head/neck)
– Mutations in MSH2, MLH1 (DNA mismatch repair gene) can be
identified in skin biopsy
– *See also Neoplastic/Tumors:Syndromes with multiple tumors or multiple types of tumors*

II. Ferguson-Smith syndrome
= Multiple spontaneously regressing KAs in sun-exposed areas,
autosomal dominant

III. Grzybowski syndrome
= Generalized eruptive KAs, thousands of papules resembling
milia

IV. Side effect of BRAF inhibitors
– Multiple eruptive keratoacanthomas and SCCs have been reported in association with BRAF inhibitors in treatment for
metastatic melanoma

e. Verrucous carcinoma
= A well-differentiated variant of SCC that is large, and pale and glassy
on pathology; not simply an SCC with a warty appearance
1. Giant condyloma acuminata (Buschke-Löwenstein tumor)
– Large, locally destructive verrucous plaque, usually on penis >
other anogenital
– May be associated with HPV-6,11
2. Oral Florid Papillomatosis (Ackerman Tumor)
– Warts in oral cavity, nasal sinuses
– May be promoted by smoking, radiation
3. Epithelioma Cuniculatum
– Verrucous carcinoma arising from a plantar wart on the foot
f. Adenoid SCC (pseudoglandular)
– May have acantholysis, so remember to consider acantholytic SCC in
ddx of herpes and acantholytic dermatoses (e.g. pemphigus)

7.2 Melanocytic Neoplasms

1. Benign melanocytic neoplasms
a. Common acquired melanocytic nevi
– Nests of melanocytes, predominantly in rete ridges
– On path: remember to evaluate size, symmetry, circumscription; need full
lesion (shave removal or excision)
I. Intradermal nevus
– Nest of melanocytes in dermis
– Clinically usually exophytic
– Clinical ddx acrochordon, neurofibroma

II. Compound nevus
  – Nests of melanocytes in epidermis and dermis
  – Path: center with melanocytes in dermis/junction, may have surrounding rim of junctional melanocytes = shouldering (creates fried egg appearance clinically)
III. Junctional nevus
  – Nests of melanocytes at D-E junction
  – Clinically macular
IV. Recurrent nevus
  – Recurrence after biopsy or excision, may look more concerning given altered appearance, but original path is key in determining plan
  – Path: melanocytic proliferation over a scar
V. Acral nevi
  – Benign dermoscopic patterns = parallel furrow (most common), lattice-like, and fibrillar patterns
  – Concerning dermoscopic patterns include parallel ridge and multi-component

b. Dysplastic/atypical nevus
  – Aka Clark's nevus
  – On path, these characteristics may be seen:
    1. Bridging of rete ridges
    2. Shouldering
    3. Lamellar fibroplasia (fibrosis around basement membrane)
    4. Slight atypia
  – Other atypical features include asymmetry, poor circumscription, Pagetoid spread
  – Though pathology is used to support this dx and grade the atypia, this is technically a clinical diagnosis and there is poor concordance between pathologists which makes diagnosis and management controversial
  – In general, dysplastic nevi are not considered premalignant lesions. They represent a patient risk factor for melanoma and are re-excised less because of concern that they will evolve into a melanoma and more because of concern that a melanoma diagnosis was missed
  – Typically, DNs are reported as having mild, moderate, or severe atypia; the risk of melanomas being misclassified as mild or moderate DNs appears to be extremely small to none. Severe DNs are uniformly re-excised (as they are borderline to MMIS). However, many are comfortable (and evidence supports) not re-excising mild and moderate DNs, especially if margins were clear on biopsy.
    I. "Dysplastic nevus syndrome"
      – Patients with multiple DNs with increased risk for MM; not a well-defined syndrome
    II. Familial atypical multiple mole melanoma (FAMMM) syndrome
      – An autosomal dominant disease, from mutation in CDKN2A (or p16) gene, or CDK4 gene
      – Predisposition to > 50 atypical nevi and multiple melanomas

– 70% will develop at least one melanoma, 30% will have multiple
– Increased risk for pancreatic cancer (20X), with lifetime risk of 15–20%

c. Congenital melanocytic nevus
  – Small < 1.5 cm, Medium = 1.5 cm–20 cm
  – Large/giant > 20 cm (or > 5% TBSA in prepubertal), can have "bathing trunk" distribution
  – Path: "congenital pattern" = wraps around adnexal structures
  – Increased risk of MM (primarily in large/giant), neurocutaneous melanosis (NCM) = syndrome of large congenital melanocytic nevi with meningeal melanosis or melanoma
  – Greatest risk for NCM in axial lesions with satellite nevi, screen with MRI
  – 50% with NCM get leptomeningeal MM

d. Spitz nevus
  – Aka "Benign juvenile melanoma;" appears concerning pathologically however behaves like a benign lesion
  – In kids, clinical ddx JXG, mastocytoma
  – Dermoscopy: starburst pattern
  – Path: circumscribed elongated nests (may look like bananas), separated from adjacent keratinocytes (clefting around nests), with Kamino bodies (pink globules)
  – Many Spitz have HRAS mutation associated
  – "Spitzoid features" of other nevi include: nests that are vertical, epithelioid appearance, spindle cells
  – Can observe in children, but always re-excise in adults

e. Pigmented spindle cell nevus of Reed
  – Classically a recently developed well-circumscribed black lesion on thigh of young woman (without other pigmented lesions on body)
  – Some classify this as a subtype of Spitz nevus
  – Path: fascicles of uniform, slender spindle cells with melanin

f. Deep penetrating nevus
  – Aka plexiform spindle cell nevus
  – Dark papule/nodule typically on head/neck in first few decades
  – Path: sharply demarcated wedge-shaped pigmented proliferation
  – Shares features with both Spitz nevi and blue nevi, and can mimic melanoma

g. Halo nevus
  – A nevus with a surrounding white halo, caused by an immune response to nevus cells (infiltrating lymphocytes onpath); repigments if remove nevus
  – No longer considered a high risk for melanoma marker (more akin to dysplastic nevi, inferring a slightly increased risk compared to baseline population)

h. Balloon cell nevus
  – Variant of nevus with predominance of altered, large melanocytes with vacuolated cytoplasm

  i. Becker's nevus/melanosis
- Unilateral, hyperpigmented patch, often with hypertrichosis
- On path, acanthosis, features of smooth muscle hamartoma, basilar hyperpigmentation; ddx accessory nipple (papillomatous)
- *See also Neoplastic:Spindle Cell Tumors:Smooth Muscle*

  j. Nevus spilus
= Speckled lentiginous nevus
- Can see in phakomatosis pigmentovascularis (with capillary malformation), phakomatosis pigmentokeratotica (with nevus sebaceus)

  k. Dermal melanocytosis

Note: Melanocytes may remain in dermis (stalled migration from neural crest during in utero development) most commonly in three areas: head/neck, lumbosacral, distal dorsal extremities

    I. "Mongolian spot"
- On lumbosacral
- Multiple can be associated with lysosomal storage diseases
- No longer considered an appropriate term to use given ethnic stereotyping

    II. Nevus of Ota
- Around eye
- Laser tx = q-switched Ruby or Alexandrite or pico

    III. Nevus of Ito
- On shoulder

    IV. Acquired dermal melanocytosis
- Not congenital; might represent reactivation of existing dermal melanocytes

    V. Blue nevus (dermal melanocytoma)
- GNAQ mutations may be associated

      1. Common blue nevus
- Path: el'ongated, wavy melanocytes, melanophages

      2. Cellular blue nevus
- Path: dendritic melanocytes associated with nests of spindle cells
- Atypical cellular blue nevi hard to distinguish from melanoma

  l. Lentigines (lentigo simplex)
- Increased number of melanocytes and melanin (but not a neoplastic proliferation)
- Essentially the same as café-au-lait macules, but < 5 mm
- Labial lentigo. path — mucosal, ectatic, broad rete ridges, basilar hyperpigmentation

Can be seen in many syndromes:

    I. Peutz-Jeghers syndrome
- Perioral and oral mucosal lentigines prominent
- Intestinal polyposis, risk of intussusception
- Mutation in STK11 (LKB1), a serine-threonine kinase
- Increased cancers (93% have cancer, 50% have died from cancer by age 57!), especially GI cancers, breast, ovarian

7

II. Laugier-Hunziker syndrome
 – Only lentigines, melanonychia, no other findings or risks
III. LEOPARD syndrome
 – Lentigines, Electrocardiographic conduction defects, Ocular hypertelorism, Pulmonary stenosis, Abnormalities of genitalia, Retardation of growth and Deafness (need lentigines and 2 ≥ other for dx)
 – Autosomal dominant, PTPN11 gene; defect in same gene causes Noonan syndrome
IV. Carney complex
 – Aka LAMB/NAME syndrome
 = Lentigines, Atrial myxoma, Mucocutaneous myxoma, Blue nevi
 = Nevi, Atrial myxoma, Myxoid neurofibroma, Ephelides
 – Essentially 3 main components: 1. Myxomas (skin, heart, breast), 2. Lentigines (spotty skin pigmentation), 3. Endocrine tumors/abnormalities
 – Associated with PRKAR1A gene mutation (tumor suppressor gene that encodes a cAMP-dependent kinase important in many endocrine processes), autosomal dominant—Less common components include large-cell calcifying Sertoli cell tumor of the testis (sexual precocity), psammomatous melanotic schwannoma, epithelioid blue nevus. Also, growth hormone-producing pituitary adenomas.
V. Cronkhite-Canada syndrome
 – Polyposis associated with lentigines of buccal mucosa, face, acral sites; nail dystrophy, alopecia
 – Usually in older men
m. Café-au-lait macules (CALMs)
 – Essentially the same as lentigines, but > 5 mm
 – Path: increased melanin/melanosomes, but not increased melanocytes
  I. Neurofibromatosis – types I and II
   – "Coast of California"-type CALMs
   – Axillary freckling "Crowe's sign"
   – Dx criteria for NF require ≥ 6 CALMS of 5 mm (prepubertal), 1.5 cm (postpubertal)
   – *See also Neoplastic:Syndromes with Multiple Tumors or Multiple Types of Tumors*
  II. McCune-Albright syndrome
   – Precocious puberty and CALMs
   – "Coast of Maine"-like CALMs
n. Solar lentigines (liver spots/solar lentigo)
 – See in older patients; may be precursors for macular seborrheic keratoses
 – From UV exposure
 – Path: club-shaped rete ridges with pigmentation, solar elastosis
o. Ephelides (freckles)
 – Only in sun-exposed areas, can see in kids

2. Malignant melanocytic neoplasms
   a. Melanoma (MM)
      – Melanoma represents less than 2% of skin cancers, but accounts for 2nd most skin cancer deaths behind SCC (about 8–10,000/year, slight decrease in last few years attributable to introduction of PD-1 inhibitors)
      – Sixth most common cancer diagnosis in US and the most common cancer in Caucasian women age 25–29
      – Path: atypical features as described in dysplastic nevi, neoplastic proliferation of melanocytes beyond nests, Pagetoid spread, artifactual splitting in epidermis from lack of cellular adhesions (desmosomes) with melanocyte infiltrate, regression
      – Risk factors include: exposure to sun (intense intermittent sun exposure appears more significant rather than total sun exposure), use of sunbeds/tanning beds, skin phenotype/pigmentation (Fitzpatrick skin type), number of melanocytic nevi and dysplastic nevi, family history of melanoma, personal history of melanoma
      – Despite association of melanoma with ultraviolet radiation (exemplified by xeroderma pigmentosum with defects in nucleotide excision repair), it is not clear how UVR causes melanoma; melanomas lack the UVB signature mutations seen in NMSCs. It is clear, however, that melanoma can occur without sun exposure.
      – Most melanomas occur de novo; less than 1/4 in association with nevi; dysplastic nevi no more likely to develop MM than other common nevi
      – Breslow depth (from top of granular layer to deepest point) relates to prognosis; Clark level was another measure of depth that was found to be poorly reproducible and thus has fallen out of favor
      – Hutchinson's sign = melanonychia with pigment on proximal nail fold, suggestive of melanoma
      – 2018 AJCC criteria (T/N/M staging):
      Tis = MMIS
      T1 <1mm thickness
         a: without ulceration and <0.8/mm
         b: <0.8/mm with ulceration or 0.8–1.0 mm regardless of ulceration
      T2 >1.0–2.0 mm thickness
         a: without ulceration
         b: with ulceration
      T3 >2.0–4.0 mm thickness
         a. without ulceration
         b: with ulceration
      T4 >4.0 mm thickness
         a: without ulceration
         b: with ulceration
      N1 a: Clinically occult, b: Clinically detected
      Staging:
         Stage 0 = Tis, N0, M0
         Stage IA = T1a, T1b; IB = T2a

Stage IIA = T2b, T3a; IIB = T3b, T4a; IIC = T4b
Stage III = any T, N>N0, M0
Stage IV = any T, any N, M1

- Increased LDH signifies poorer prognosis
- In-transit metastases are defined as lesions > 2 cm from primary tumor, but not to the nodes
- Satellite lesions are lesions within 2 cm of primary tumor; local recurrence typically defined as lesion within 2 cm of surgical scar
- Sentinel lymph node biopsy is standard of care since informs staging, but no mortality benefit to patients found; generally considered in stage III, IV, and even in any tumor with Breslow depth > 0.8 mm
- The primary difference in the updated AJCC8 is removing of mitosis from criteria (although most experts still feel that mitosis of 2 or more per HPF is very prognostically important)
- CDKN2A (Chr 9p) is the most common gene mutated in familial melanoma
- CDKN2A = tumor suppressor, encodes p14 and p16 which allow p53 and Rb respectively to function
- Most common gene mutation = BRAF, associated more with sun-protected area MM; codes for a kinase, BRAF, and also associated with papillary thyroid carcinoma and colorectal carcinoma; 90% of BRAF mutations are V600E (glutamic acid for valine)
- Majority of melanomas have BRAF (60%) or NRAS (20%) mutations (would not expect in same tumor)
- Increased c-KIT mutations in MM from mucosal, acral, and chronically sun-damaged skin; imatinib (Gleevec) is potential therapy
- Gene expression profiling (GEP) has been developed and clinically tested over the last several years to aid in diagnosis and prognosis of MM. There is a 23-GEP and a 35-GEP (numbers refer to number of genes tested) that helps determine if an atypical melanocytic lesion is more likely to be benign or malignant (this is a test ordered by a pathologist on existing tissue block when rendering diagnosis). There is also a 31-GEP test that helps determine a prognosis and need for SLNB on invasive MM (best used in at least 0.3 mm depth). This is typically requested by the clinician who performed the biopsy
- Patients with history of MM should have GYN, ophtho, and dental f/u (for screening of areas where melanoma may occur that dermatologists may not evaluate well)
- "Melanoma of unknown primary" is another important and rare entity in which metastatic MM is identified in an organ system outside of the mucocutaneous system in a patient who does not have a concerning lesion on skin exam (presumably the index tumor was wiped away by the immune system/regression)
- Treatment for metastatic melanoma: Historically, standard chemotherapy included dacarbazine (DTIC) and IL-2 despite response rates of only 15–25%

– Modern treatments include:

(1) BRAF inhibitors: sorafenib (nonselective, and not very efficacious in trials), vemurafenib, inhibits BRAF with V600E mutation (these may increase keratoacanthoma-type SCCs, however)

(2) Immunotherapy: Ipilimumab, a monoclonal antibody against cytotoxic T-lymphocyte antigen 4 (CTLA-4), and Pembrolizumab/Nivolumab/Atezolizumab (PD-1/PD-L1) potentiates T-cell anti-tumor response. Best response from combo of these mechanisms, but also higher side effect profile

(3) Imatinib (Gleevec) – potential for patients with c-KIT mutation (acral and mucosal)

(4) MEK inhibitors in combination with BRAF inhibitors; also (*see also Basic Science:Genes in Melanoma*)

(5) Newest focus has been on immunotherapy targeting LAG-3 (Relatlimab) as well as combination therapies with many comparative trials in the pipeline to determine most efficacious regimens

– NSAIDs/ASA may decrease melanoma incidence

– Melanoma appears to occur more frequently on L > R (perhaps from sitting in car on driver's side?)

– Important immunohistochemistry stains:

S100 = sensitive, not specific

– Stains melanocytes, dendritic cells, neuralcells, adipocytes, sweat glands, breast epithelium

– Good for desmoplastic MM

HMB-45 = specific, not sensitive

– Stains only superficial

– Poor staining in spindle cell/desmoplasticMM

– Gradient pattern might help ddx MM vs. Spitz

Melan-A/MART-1 = current standard

– Most sensitive/specific marker for demonstrating melanocytes

Surgical margins by depth (in general):

MMIS = 0.5 cm

MM < 1mm = 1 cm

MM < 1-2 mm = 2 cm

MM > 2mm = 2 cm

I. Superficial spreading
 – 60–70% of melanomas

II. Nodular
 – No radial growth phase, 15–30%

III. Acral lentiginous
 – 5–10%
 – Noted in darker skin patients, not because increased incidence, but all other types decreased incidence

IV. Lentigo maligna melanoma
 – 5–15%, slow growing on sun-exposed skin, usually MMIS

  V. Amelanotic
      – Ddx pyogenic granuloma, BCC, SCC, purple plums
      – May have worse prognosis, but also often with delays in di-
        agnosis
  VI. Desmoplastic/Spindle cell melanoma
      – May have tendency to locally recur due to neurotropism
  VII. Ocular
      – Melanocytes found in the posterior uveal tract; posterior
        uveal chamber MM can metastasize to liver (hematogenous
        spread)
  VIII. Mucosal
    IX. Melanoma in situ
      – Includes lentigo maligna

Note: Diagnosis of MMIS and MM has dramatically increased in the last couple of decades, without any corresponding impact on melanoma mortality; thus, it follows that melanoma is likely overdiagnosed, meaning lesions called melanoma are not necessarily all life-threatening; however, the challenge remains that we must treat all the same, because we don't know which are necessarily more concerning.

7.3 Adnexal Tumors

Note: some tumors appear to have either eccrine or apocrine derivation (may be
   controversial), but this is generally not clinically relevant
1. Eccrine
   – Primary function of eccrine glands is thermoregulation; also electrolyte balance
   – Ketoconazole, griseofulvin, and chemotherapeutic agents may be secreted in
     sweat
   – Eccrine sweat = 99% water plus electrolytes, secreted by merocrine (eccrine)
     secretion
   – Innervated by sympathetic postganglionic innervation, but functionally cho-
     linergic (neurotransmitter = acetylcholine)
   a. Poroma
      – A papule or nodule, often on palms/soles, can be on scalp
      – Clinical ddx: pyogenic granuloma, amelanotic melanoma
      – Path: downward growth of blue basaloid cells with ducts
      – Three variants:
         I. Eccrine poroma (both epidermal and dermal)
         II. Hidroacanthoma simplex (epidermal)
         III. Dermal duct tumor (dermal)
         IV. Porocarcinoma
   b. Syringoma
      – Typically around eyes, but can be on abdomen/thighs/genitals
      – Path: multiple small ducts in fibrous stroma, nests may resemble com-
        mas or tadpoles; "paisley tie ddx"
      – Can be eruptive in Down syndrome

Variants include:
  I. Clear cell syringoma
    – May be associated with diabetes
  II. Chondroid syringoma (aka mixed tumor)
    – Tubular/epithelial layers, mucoid stroma, Alcian blue (+)
    – Can see ghost cells (pink), but no basaloid cells, ddx pilomatricoma
c. Eccrine hidrocystoma
  – Glistening papule, typically infraorbital, *see also Neoplastic:Cysts*
d. Eccrine spiradenoma
  – In the painful tumor ddx
  – Actually thought to be apocrine-derived by most now
e. Clear cell hidradenoma (nodular hidradenoma)
f. Eccrine carcinoma
g. Other eccrine disorders
  I. Hyperhidrosis
    – Treatment = antiperspirants (aluminum chloride hexahydrate), topical and systemic anticholinergics (glycopyrrolate), iontophoresis, neurotoxins (Botox), and last resort = surgical nerve ablation
      1. Frey's syndrome (auriculotemporal syndrome or gustatory sweating)
        – Common after parotid surgery or trauma
  II. Hypohidrosis
    1. Hypohidrotic ectodermal dysplasia (HED)
      – Aka anhidrotic ectodermal dysplasia, Christ-Siemens-Touraine syndrome
      – Thin, sparse, or absent hair, missing or peg-shaped teeth, inability to sweat correctly
      – Primarily X-linked recessive
      – *See also Alopecia:Non-scarring alopecia:Ectodermal dysplasias*
  III. Bromhidrosis
    – Eccrine sweat is odorless; however, maceration can allow bacterial colonization, and apocrine sweat can be decomposed by bacteria
      1. Trimethylaminuria (TMA)
        – Known for causing "fishy"-odor
        – Inherited deficiency of FMO3 (flavin-containing monooxygenase-3)
        – Tx = avoid eggs, kidney, liver, fish in diet
  IV. Chromhidrosis (colored sweat)
    – No effective tx outside of reducing sweat
  V. Miliaria
    – *See also Vesiculobullous:Other*
  VI. Uremic frost
    – Rarely, see uric acid deposits on skin in ESRD
2. Apocrine
  – Apocrine gland variants: Moll's glands on the eyelids, cerumen producing glands of inner ear, milk-producing apocrine glands

– Apocrine glands secrete via decapitation secretion
– Apocrine tumors can be associated with increased plasma cells
a. Cylindroma
  – Clinical: "turban tumors"
  – Path: "jigsaw puzzle," well-circumscribed pieces, two cell populations, glassy rim
    I. Brooke-Spiegler syndrome
      – Mutation in CYLD (a tumor suppressor), which encodes a deubiquitinating enzyme (a protease), which inhibits the NF-κB pathway
      – Cylindromas, trichoepitheliomas, and spiradenomas
      – *See also Neoplastic:Syndromes with Multiple Tumors or Multiple Types of Tumors*
b. Spiradenoma
  – Related to cylindromas; can see in Brooke-Spiegler
  – Path: Round "blue balls" in the dermis, but not as well circumscribed as jigsaw of cylindroma; 3 cell types = 1. pale, 2. dark, and 3. lymphocytes (this may be why it is painful)
c. Hidradenoma (hidradenoma papilliferum)
  – Seen in vulvar and perianal areas
  – Path = partially cystic with papillary and glandular areas, no epidermal connection
d. Apocrine adenoma
    I. Syringocystadenoma papilliferum
      – Presents as warty papule/plaque, may ooze serosanguinous fluid
      – Almost exclusively on head/neck, 1/3 occur in nevus sebaceus
      – Path = irregular papillary projections protrude into invagination of surface epithelium; stroma with plasma cell infiltrate, often an epidermal connection
e. Apocrine hidrocystoma
  – Clinical: glistening cystic papule, typically on the eyelid, *see also Neoplastic:Cysts*
  – Path = dilated apocrine gland on eyelid skin, shows decapitation secretion, lined by two layers of cells
f. Microcystic adnexal carcinoma (MAC)
  – Most commonly occurs on the upper lip, locally aggressive
  – Path: poorly circumscribed, deeply infiltrative (subcutaneous to even muscle) with perineural invasion
g. Extramammary Paget's disease
  – Most commonly in groin, perianal, scrotum, vulva
  – 10–25% associated with cutaneous malignancy
  – Path = atypical cells with abundant pale cytoplasm, can see Pagetoid spread. CK7 and CK20 staining helpful (CK7 more in primary cutaneous vs. CK20 more with internal malignancy)
  – Regardless of staining pattern, need complete malignancy workup with endoscopy, imagining, etc.

- Treatment for primary cutaneous is with Mohs±imiquimod; for malignancy-associated need oncology management
  - h. Syringoma (see eccrine)
  - i. Apocrine poroma
  - j. Apocrine carcinoma
3. Sebaceous
   - Remember association with Muir-Torre; in particular, the sebaceous adenoma is a unique hallmark (especially off the head/neck)
   - Note: nevus sebaceus is not a sebaceous neoplasm
   - Sebaceous gland variants:
     - Eyelids: Mebomian glands (inflamed = chalazion) Glands of Zeis (superficial margin, inflamed = hordeolum/stye); Mnemonic: Mebomian almost rhymes with chalazion, Zeis almost with stye.
     - Areolae: Montgomery tubercles
     - Vermillion, buccal mucosa: Fordyce spots
     - Genitalia: Tyson's glands
       - a. Sebaceous hyperplasia
         - Yellow delled papules on face/chest
         - Path: large sebaceous lobules grouped around a central dilated duct (all connected to hair follicle)
       - b. Sebaceous adenoma
         - The hallmark lesion of Muir-Torre syndrome (MLH1, MSH2 defect)
         - Path: multiple sharply demarcated sebaceous lobules, separated and compressed connective tissue septa; classically, approximately half ofthe cells are mature sebocytes
       - c. Sebaceoma (sebaceous epithelioma)
         - On a spectrum with sebaceous adenoma (some controversy about how to distinguish), may be associated with Muir-Torre
         - Path: similar to sebaceous adenoma, classically with a majority of sebocytes undifferentiated/germinative and only scattered clusters of mature sebocytes
       - d. Sebaceous carcinoma
         - Classically on eyelid, though BCC more likely in this location
         - Path: may see Pagetoid spread
       - e. Muir-Torre syndrome
         - Sebaceous neoplasms (adenoma = defining, epithelioma, or carcinoma), keratoacanthomas, and internal malignancies
         - Defects in MLH1, MSH2 (DNA mismatch repair genes, which can be stained for by dermatopathologist)
         - See also Keratinocyte Neoplasms:Malignant Keratinocyte Neoplasms:- Keratoacanthoma and Neoplastic:Syndromes with Multiple Tumors or Multiple Types of Tumors
4. Hair Follicle
   - a. Trichofolliculoma
     = On head/neck, skin-colored papule, perhaps with dilated central umbilication with tuft of emerging vellus hairs

7

= A follicular hamartoma rather than a true neoplasm
- Path: "Mother follicle with her babies" – small follicles radiate from larger central follicle

b. Trichoepithelioma/trichoblastoma
- These terms have overlap; trichoblastoma usually meant to refer to larger, deeper, more nodular lesions
- May be solitary, multiple, or desmoplastic
- Papules usually in central part of face (often by nasolabial folds, ddx BCC)
- May be associated with cylindromas or spiradenomas
- Path: islands/cords of basaloid cells, some with abortive hair follicle differentiation (called papillary mesenchymal bodies), but no retraction (ddx BCC), dense fibroblast-rich stroma

   I. Epithelioma adenoides cysticum (Brooke's disease)
      = Multiple trichoepitheliomas
   II. Brooke-Spiegler syndrome
      - Associated with multiple cylindromas and trichoepitheliomas, CYLD mutations
      - *See also Neoplastic:Syndromes with Multiple Tumors or Multiple Types of Tumors*
   III. Desmoplastic trichoepithelioma
      - Annular lesion with raised border, depressed center
      - Path: small cords and islands of basaloid cells in a fibrous stroma; may have small cysts (only rarely seen in syringomas)
      - Ddx sclerosing BCC

c. Trichoadenoma
- Nodular lesion of face/buttocks
- Path: multiple horn cyst islands in dermis

d. Trichilemmoma
- Small solitary papules on face
- Considered old viral warts by some in past (Ackerman)
- Path: sharply circumscribed squamoid cells with glycogen vacuolization; thickened basement membrane, has differentiation toward the follicular outer sheath
- Multiple are associated with Cowden disease
- *See also Neoplastic:Syndromes with Multiple Tumors or Multiple Types of Tumors*

e. Pilomatricoma/pilomatrixoma
- Aka calcifying epithelioma of Malherbe
- Usually head/neck, upper extremities, in children/adolescents
- "Tent sign"=stretching of overlying skin gives a multifaceted, angulated appearance, likely due to calcification in the lesion
- "Teeter totter sign"=pressure on one side causes elevation on the other side
- Path: eosinophilic cornified matrical cells aka "ghost cells" or "shadow cells"

– β-catenin activation mutation (CTNBB1 gene), dystrophic calcification
– Can be associated with myotonic dystrophy (eruptive), Turner syndrome, and Rubinstein-Taybi syndrome
– May see pilomatricoma-like changes in EICs of Gardner's (APC inactivation causes β-catenin accumulation)

f. Fibrofolliculoma, trichodiscoma, perifollicular fibroma
= Not clinically distinctive (skin-colored papule on face, can appear as acrochordons)
– Characteristic of Birt-Hogg-Dubé syndrome

g. Nevus sebaceus (of Jadassohn)
– Aka organoid nevus
– Can develop neoplasms: #1 trichoblastomas; also BCC, syringocystadenoma papilliferum (formerly considered #1)
– Usually on scalp
– Can monitor but previously controversial if should be excised to prevent BCCs
– Path: papillated epidermis, apocrine glands deep, increase in all other adnexal structures, sebaceous glands not connected to follicles that directly connect to epidermal surface

h. Eruptive vellus hair cysts
– Small bluish papules typically on mid chest/sternum, rarely extremities; ddx steatocystoma multiplex, acne, *see also Neoplastic:Cysts*

i. Pilar cysts (trichilemmal cysts)
– Aka trichilemmal cyst
– From hair follicle ishthmus, no granular layer (since that is derived from infundibulum)

j. Proliferating pilar tumor
– Path: "Rolls and scrolls," all pink with no basaloid areas, ddx pilomatricoma but no ghost cells

k. Tumor of the follicular infundibulum
– May be variant of seborrheic keratosis
– Path: downward growth pattern, keratocysts (can be confused with fiboepithelioma of Pinkus), entrapped "windows" of dermis

l. Folliculosebaceous cystic hamartoma
– Path: hamartoma composed of follicular, sebaceous, and mesenchymal elements

7.4 Other Epidermal Neoplasms/Hyperplasias

1. Merkel Cell Carcinoma
– Rare, highly aggressive, primary cutaneous neuroendocrine tumor
– Clinical: firm red/purple nodule (purple plum), favors head/neck > buttocks, extremities; most often in older white patients
– This is what killed Jimmy Buffett

- Aka trabecular carcinoma
- Path – blue gray balls in dermis
- Merkel cells normally in basal layer
- Stains for cytokeratin 20 (CK20) in perinuclear dot pattern; TTF-1 negative (which is positive in metastatic small cell carcinoma, on the ddx)
- Neuron specific enolase (+), but not specific; also chromogranin, synaptophysin, epithelial membrane antigen (EMA) usually positive (neuro-endocrine markers)
- Linked to a virus, Merkel cell polyomavirus (MCV); there is an antibody test that can be used to track response to treatment and detect recurrence
- Full body PET/CT + SLNB recommended for staging (1/3 with occult LN disease at diagnosis)
- Treatment = excision with 3 cm margins (if possible) + XRT is standard of care but adjuvant immunotherapy (e.g. pembrolizumab) becoming nearly 1st line as well

2. NK cell carcinoma
   - CD-56 positive
3. Histiocytoses
   - Traditionally, proliferations of histiocytes are not considered neoplastic since they lack a monoclonal component, although malignant histocytoses are possible
   - *See also Dermal: Histiocytic: Histiocytoses*

7.5 Vascular Tumors

Note: Factor VIII stains endothelium; CD31, CD34 stain vascularproliferations
1. Hemangioma
   a. Infantile hemangioma (strawberry hemangioma)
      - Proliferative phase = months to 1 year
      - Involution phase = may start at age 1, continue for years
      - Can ulcerate
      - #1 risk factor = low birth weight, #2 = preterm birth
      - Associated with GLUT-1 positivity
      - Treatments = systemic corticosteroids (more historical), propranolol (and topical timolol), may especially have benefit in proliferative phase
      - Lumbosacral hemangiomas assoc. with anomaly in 1/3 (!)
      - "Beard" hemangiomas → r/o airway obstruction
        I. PHACES syndrome.
           - Posterior fossa malformation, Hemangiomas (mainly facial), Arterial, Cardiac, Eye, and Sternal abnormalities
           - Think: if hemangioma on face, r/o cardiac defects, CNS defects (e.g. Dandy-Walker malformation)

   – W/u for PHACES includes: MRI/MRA with and without contrast, cardiac echo, ophtho and neuro exams, airway exams for "beard" hemangiomas
 b. Congenital hemangiomas
   – These present fully grown at birth (intrauterine proliferation)
   – Unlike infantile hemangiomas, these are GLUT-1 negative
   I. Rapidly Involuting Congenital Hemangioma (RICH)
   II. Non-Involuting Congenital Hemangioma (NICH)
   III. Partially-Involuting Congenital Hemangioma (PICH)
 c. Cherry angioma
 d. Glomeruloid hemangioma
   This is specific for:
   I. POEMS syndrome
     – Polyneuropathy, Organomegaly, Endocrinopathy, Monoclonal gammopathy, Skin changes
     – Actually see more cherry angiomas then glomeruloid, though glomeruloid is specific
     – See increased expression of VEGF (explains hemangiomas)
     – Not associated with multiple myeloma
 e. Targetoid hemosiderotic hemangioma (hobnail hemangioma)
   – May arise from trauma to hemangioma
   – Path: superficial dilated vessels with hobnail nuclei, hemosiderin, vascular proliferating wrapping around vessels and adnexae
 f. Tufted angioma
   – Path = "cannonball distribution" of capillaries and vascular tufts with lymphatic-like spaces; GLUT-1 negative
   – Can be associated with Kasabach-Merritt
 g. Kaposiform hemangioendothelioma
   – Path: looks like infantile hemangioma with features of Kaposi's, GLUT-1 negative
   I. Kasabach-Merritt syndrome
   = Hemangioma with thrombocytopenia; rapidly enlarging vascular tumor (congenital Kaposiform hemangioendothelioma > tufted angioma) with consumptive coagulopathy
2. Pyogenic granuloma
   – Aka lobular capillary hemangioma
   – Classically on fingers/toes after trauma
   – Can be caused by trauma, pregnancy, drugs (retinoids, HIV protease inhibitors, indinavir, —e.g. methotrexate, OCPs, anti-EGFR)
3. Angiokeratoma
   – Can look like MM clinically
   – Path: hyperkeratosis, acanthosis, dilated papillary dermal vessels
   a. Solitary angiokeratoma
   b. Angiokeratoma of Fordyce
     – On scrotum and vulva

7

    c. Angiokeratoma corporis diffusum
- Assoc. with Fabry disease (α-galactosidase deficiency), accentuated in bathing trunk distribution
- Also assoc. with other inherited enzyme deficiencies including fucosidosis, sialidosis
- *See also Dermal: Depositional: Storage Diseases*

    d. Angiokeratoma of Mibelli
- Usually on dorsal/lateral fingers/toes in age 10–15

    e. Angiokeratoma circumscriptum
- Grouped papules, starting in infancy

    f. Acral pseudolymphomatous angiokeratoma of children (APACHE)
- Considered a type of pseudolymphoma

4. Venous lake
- Usually on lips (but in any photo area, including ears)

5. Angiolymphoid hyperplasia with eosinophilia (ALHE)
- Benign plaques/nodules on head/neck, esp. around the ears
- Ddx Kimura's disease (larger lymphoid follicles, usually on posterior neck), IgG4-related disease
- Tx: timolol, imiquimod, ILK, cryotherapy, excision, laser

6. Kimura's disease
- Until recently, thought to be a variant of ALHE
- Compared to ALHE, has larger lymphoid follicles, usually on posterior neck

7. Glomus tumor/glomangioma
- Often subungual
- Arise from the arterial component of the glomus body (aka Sucquet-Hoyer canal), an arteriovenous shunt; smooth muscle-derived
- On path, can appear like a hemangioma, but much more cellular

8. Kaposi's sarcoma
- Purple patches, plaques, nodules; tends to favor feet/legs, face, oropharynx (always look)
- Cultural references: in the movie, *Philadelphia*, Tom Hanks' character had a KS lesion on his face leading to his discriminatory firing. In the play and movie, *The Normal Heart*, the first cases of AIDS classically had KS on their feet.
- Path: irregular slit-like vascular spaces and vessels, spindle cells, inflammatory infiltrate (variable based on patch to plaque to nodule); Promontory sign = small vessel protruding into abnormal vascular space
- All types associated with HHV-8
- Viscerally, can involve the GI tract, lymphatics, lungs; generally, for every 5 cutaneous lesions, there will be 1 internal lesion
- Tx = if underlying HIV, HAART. Otherwise, can consider imiquimod, local destruction with cryotherapy, radiation, or excision
- With visceral involvement, consider systemic chemotherapy with oncology referral (liposomal doxorubicin, paclitaxel)

- KS may reappear during use of prednisone/immunosuppression in patients with a history of it, so use caution
  a. Classic
  b. HIV epidemic type
  c. African endemic type
  d. Immunosuppressed (non-HIV, iatrogenic) type
9. Bacillary angiomatosis
   - May resemble pyogenic granuloma or Kaposi's sarcoma clinically
   - Path: may look like pyogenic granuloma, but see organisms (purplish granular material), neutrophils
10. Acroangiodermatitis (aka pseudo-Kaposi's sarcoma)
    - A variant of stasis dermatitis, hyperplasia of existing vessels that may mimic Kaposi's
11. Intravascular papillary endothelial hyperplasia (aka Masson's tumor or pseudoangiosarcoma)
    - Unusual reaction pattern of organization of a thrombus within a vein
12. Angiosarcoma
    - Classic patients: elderly man with a scalp tumor, breast cancer survivor with lymphedema
    - Other classic associations: any lymphedema especially post-breast cancer and mastectomy (Stewart-Treves) and post-radiation
    - Path: ill-defined vascular spaces lined by atypical endothelial cells
    - CD31 and CD34 positive (vascular markers)
    a. Stewart-Treves syndrome
       = Angiosarcoma developing in long-standing chronic lymphedema
    b. Dabska tumor
       - Rare, low-grade angiosarcoma seen in children
13. Angiolipoma (see fatty tumors)
14. Angiofibroma (see spindle cell tumors)
15. Maffucci's syndrome
    = Multiple enchondromas of bone and multiple vascular tumors
    - Increased risk of chondrosarcoma
    - *See also Neoplastic:Syndromes with Multiple Tumors or Multiple Types of Tumors*
16. Vascular malformations
    a. Nevus flammeus (port wine stain)
       = Generic congenital vascular malformation
          I. Sturge-Weber syndrome
          II. Klippel-Trenaunay syndrome
          III. Phakomatosis pigmentovascularis
    b. Venous malformations (cavernous hemangiomas)
       I. Blue rubber bleb nevus syndrome
          - In the painful tumor ddx (not actually tumors)
          - Multiple compressible blue rubbery cavernous hemangiomas of skin, GI tract, others
          - May have local hyperhidrosis, Fe deficiency anemia from GI hemorrhage

17. Lymphangiomas (*see also Neoplastic: Lymphatic Malformations*)
18. Cutaneous endometriosis
    – Rare, classically in the umbilicus or inguinal area
    – Path: blue glandular cells in vascular stroma

7.6 Spindle Cell Tumors

– Spindle cells can represent fibroblasts, smooth muscle cells, neural cells, and other – e.g. can see spindle cells in vascular tumors
1. Fibrohistiocytic
   – Spindle cells individually and in fascicles/bundles (nondescript)
   a. Dermatofibroma
      – Aka benign fibrous histiocytoma (a formerly more general term)
      – Clinical: most commonly on legs, "dimple sign"
      – Path: nodular proliferation of spindled fibroblasts and histiocytes in the reticular dermis with hyperplasia and epidermal basal layer hyperpigmentation ("dirty fingers"), collagen trapping at edges; rete ridges not flat (as in scar)
      – CD34-, factor13a +, stromelysin3 + (in 60%) ("minus plus plus")
      – Can see multiple eruptive in autoimmune disease (SLE), immunosuppression (HIV)
      – Are they reactive or neoplastic? Unclear etiology
      – Variants = dermatofibroma with monster cells (or atypical cells) – Has large histiocyte-like cells; sclerosing hemangioma (aka hemosiderotic or aneurysmal), dermatomyofibroma
         I. Dermatomyofibroma
            – Path: east–west spindle cells, proliferation spares adnexal structures, + corkscrew nuclei
   b. Dermatofibrosarcoma protuberans (DFSP)
      – Clinical: may appear as indurated plaque with superimposed nodules (or multiple protuberances), in purple plum ddx; typically in young to middle-aged adults
      – Path: storiform pattern (like woven yarn) of fascicles (or honeycombing), extends into fat; only mild atypia (unlike atypical fibroxanthoma)
      – CD34 +, factor13a-, stromelysin3- (+ in 10%) ("plus minus minus")
      – t(17;22) translocation reported in~90% resulting in COL1A1-PDGF-β fusion
      – Tx = Mohs = treatment of choice; also, wide local excision of 3 cm deep to fascia. May use radiation as adjuvant therapy to decrease recurrence. Also may use imatinib (Gleevec) for unresectable cases.
      – Local invasion, rare reports of lung metastases
      – Variant: Bednar tumor = pigmented variant of DFSP
   c. Scar
      – Hypertrophic scars do not overgrow wound edge

– Path: epidermis atrophic or normal; in dermis, loss of rete ridge pattern, fibroblasts and collagen bundles often parallel to flattened D-E basement membrane, vertical vessels

d. Keloid
  – Overgrows wound edge (beyond original site of injury), like a neoplasm
  – Path: disordered collagen bundles (not parallel to basement membrane), pink "keloidal" collagen
  – TGF–β may induce
  – May see an increase tendency to keloid in Noonan syndrome, Rubinstein-Taybi, *see also Neoplastic:Lymphatic Malformation*
  – Tx: TCS, imiquimod, ILK, IL-5FU, cryotherapy, excision, XRT

  I. Fibromatoses
    1. Palmar fibromatosis (Dupuytren's disease)
    2. Plantar fibromatosis (Ledderhose's disease)
    3. Penile fibromatosis (Peyronie's disease)
    4. Knuckle pads (holoderma)
    5. Desmoid tumors (deep)
      – Can be associated with Gardner's (*see also Neoplastic:Syndromes with Multiple Tumors and Multiple Types of Tumors*)
      – Don't confuse with dermoid cyst (*see also Neoplastic:Cysts*)

  II. Polyfibromatosis syndrome
    – Syndrome of keloids, knuckle pads, Dupuytren's
    – Can be X-linked recessive

e. Infantile digital fibroma/inclusion body fibroma (Reye tumor)
  – Spares thumbs/big toe, occur in 1st year of life
  – Path: eosinophilic cytoplasmic inclusion bodies (actin)

f. Acquired digital fibrokeratoma/acral fibrokeratoma
  – Path: massive orthokeratosis, acral, thickened collagen parallel to long axis of lesion (ddx accessory digit withnerve bundles, traumatic neuroma, and accessory nipple with smooth muscle)

g. Giant cell tumor of the tendon sheath
  – Clinical: uncommon nodule of finger or acral skin, fixed to tendon sheath or fascia
  – Path: plump fibroblasts, osteoclast-like giant cells; in deep dermis (might not see epidermis)

h. Angiofibroma
  – More of a spindle cell tumor than a vascular tumor
  – Path: papule with concentrically oriented collagen around follicles or perpendicular to epidermis; mayhave a few dilated blood vessels, stellate fibroblasts
  – Most common types: fibrous papules (of the nose), adenoma sebaceum and Koenen tumors in TS, pearly penile papules (and equivalent in vulva)
  – Can see in tuberous sclerosis, MEN-I >> Birt-Hogg-Dubé, Cowden (in case reports only)

    I. Tuberous sclerosis
- – Adenoma sebaceum (see syndromes with multiple tumors)
- – Periungual fibroma (Koenen tumor) is a variant

i. Sclerotic fibroma
- – Associated with Cowden's
- – *See Neoplastic:Syndromes with Multiple Tumors or Multiple Types of Tumors*
- – Path: short parallel collagen bundles, like "plywood"

j. Nodular fasciitis
- – Aka pseudosarcomatous fasciitis
- – Rapidly growing subcutaneous nodule, solitary, 1 to 5 cm, classically in young adult (20s), most common on upper extremity
- – Path: spindle-shaped and stellate fibroblasts ("tissue-culture fibroblasts") in mucinous stroma, some mitoses; may have vascular proliferations

k. Atypical fibroxanthoma (AFX)
- = A low-grade sarcoma in the sun-damaged head and neck skin of elderly patients; may be a superficial form of PDS
- – Path: storiform (woven) spindle cell proliferation, cells with bizarre/haphazard nuclei (usually dx of exclusion)

l. Pleomorphic dermal sarcoma (PDS)
- – Some consider this simply a deep AFX; severely pleomorphic, bizarre cells; higher risk of neural, vascular invasion and metastasis
- – AFX, PDS on a spectrum of malignant biologic behavior with undifferentiated pleomorphic sarcoma which has highest morbidity/mortality

m. Epithelioid sarcoma
- – Rare nodule on acral sites, especially hand or finger of young adults; metastasizes in 50%
- – Atypical nodular proliferation of spindle cell to round epithelioid cells; stains for keratin (epithelial-like) and vimentin (sarcomatous), hence the name; CD34 may be +

2. Smooth muscle
- – Spindle cells in fascicles/bundles, box-car, perinuclear vacuolization
- – Spindle cells with cigar-shaped (boxy) nuclei suggests smooth muscle
- – In skin, find smooth muscle normally in arrector pili, vessels, areola, Dartos muscle of scrotum
- – Stains include SMA (smooth muscle actin) and vimentin

    a. Leiomyoma (smooth muscle tumor)
- – Arise from arrector pili muscles (may be painful in cold temp)
- – Spindle cell tumor, elongated nuclei, vacuolated cytoplasm

        I. Reed's syndrome (leiomyomatosis and renal cancer)
- – From deficiency in fumarate hydratase (causes fumarase deficiency)
- – See multiple cutaneous and uterine leiomyomas, renal cell carcinoma

    b. Angioleiomyoma
- – Leiomyoma arising from smooth muscle of vessel wall
- – May see large pink dermal tumor with dilated vessels

c. Smooth muscle hamartoma
  – Clinical and path overlap with Becker's nevus, may have pseudo-Darier's sign (piloerection upon palpation)
d. Becker's nevus/melanosis
  – *See also Neoplastic:Melanocytic Tumors:Benign Melanocytic Tumors*
e. Leiomyosarcoma
  – Stains: actin (+), mostly desmin (+), negative for keratin (vs. SCC), negative for S100 (vs. desmoplastic MM); sarcomas tend to be vimentin positive (carcinomas are negative)
  – DDx also includes AFX/PDS (some overlap), nodular fasciitis, nerve sheath tumors

3. Neural
  – S-shaped spindle cells, more tapered nuclei, fascicles
  – Stain S100(+) (just like melanocytes, Langerhans cells)
  – Main 3 types = neurofibromas, Schwannomas, and neuromas
  a. Neurofibroma
    – Clinical ddx: acrochordon, intradermal nevus
    – Path: non-encapsulated, spindle cells with wavy nuclei, pale myxoid "bubble gum" stroma, mast cells common
    I. Neurofibromatosis
      – *See also Neoplastic:Syndromes with Multiple Tumors or Multiple Types of Tumors*
    II. Plexiform neurofibroma
      – "Bag of worms," pathognomonic for NF1
      – Risk of transformation into malignant peripheral nerve sheath tumor so often excised (though medical management with selumetinib, a MEK inhibitor, can be used in inoperable cases)
  b. Neurilemmoma (schwannoma)
    – Derived from the nerve sheath, can be associated with NF2
    – Path: hypercellular areas (Antoni A with Verocay bodies = the arrangement of palisaded nuclei in double rows) alternating with hypocellular areas (Antoni B), which can be myxoid; almost always well encapsulated
    I. Psammomatous melanotic schwannoma
      – Seen in Carney complex
      – *See also Neoplastic:Syndromes with Multiple Tumors or Multiple Types of Tumors*
  c. Neuromas
    I. Traumatic neuroma
      – Regeneration/proliferation of nerve fibers following trauma, e.g. amputation
      – Path: randomly oriented nerve bundles, ddx accessory digit (on low power)
    II. Palisaded encapsulated neuroma
      – Hamartomatous proliferations of nerve fibers without apparent antecedent trauma

      – Path: well-circumscribed, but poorly encapsulated compared to schwannoma; more superficial palisading (may resemble schwannoma)

   III. Mucosal neuromas

      – Associated with MEN-IIB syndrome

      – *See also Neoplastic:Syndromes with Multiple Tumors or Multiple Types of Tumors*

  d. Accessory digit

    – Path: acral skin with haphazardly arranged nerve bundles, ddx amputation neuroma/traumatic neuroma, acquired digital fibrokeratoma with dermal fibrosis, and accessory nipple with smooth muscle

  e. Granular cell tumor

    – Predilection for tongue (30%), 70% on head/neck

    – Multiple granular cell tumors reported in Noonan and LEOPARD syndromes (PTPN11 mutations), neurofibromatosis

    – Derived from Schwann cells

    – Path: pseudoepitheliomatous hyperplasia, granular cells

  f. Neurothekeoma (nerve sheath myxoma)

    – Path: sharply demarcated, encapsulated, divided into lobules by fibrous septae

    – Two types: hypocellular myxoid and cellular with little mucin

    – Favors head and neck

  g. Neuroblastoma

    – Third most common malignant neoplasm in children (rare in adults presenting as single cutaneous lesion)

    – Can present with blueberry muffin baby lesions (blue to violaceous papules/nodules); may have pseudo-Darier's sign (piloerection upon palpation), from release of catecholamines

    – Elevated serum/urine catecholamines

  h. Nasal glioma

    – In infants on nasal root, ddx dermoid cyst,encephalocele

  i. Neuroendocrine carcinoma (Merkel cell carcinoma)

    – *See also Neoplastic:Other Epidermal Tumors*

  j. Neural mechanoreceptors

    I. Meissner's corpuscles

      = Finger-like projections in dermal papillae

      = Sense light touch

    II. Pacinian corpuscles

      = Onion-shaped structures of concentric layers of tissue in the deeper dermis

      = Sense deep pressure

4. Other spindle cell tumors

  a. Melanocytic neoplasms

    – *See also Neoplastic:Melanocytic Neoplasms*

    I. Desmoplastic melanoma (spindle cell melanoma)

    II. Pigmented spindle cell nevus of Reed (a type of Spitz nevus)

III. Blue nevi
  b. Keratinocytic neoplasms
    – *See also Neoplastic:Keratinocytic Neoplasms*
      I. Spindle cell squamous cell carcinoma

7.7 Fatty Tumors

1. Lipoma
  – No septae seen in lobules of fat (clue that this is not just fat)
  a. Lipoma types
    I. Angiolipoma
      – The only lipoma type with normal cytogenetics
      – Path: fibrin thrombi in blood vessels (may explain why can be a painful tumor)
    II. Spindle cell lipoma
      – Classically on back/neck/shoulder
    III. Pleomorphic lipoma
      – Path: floret giant cells (overlapping hyperchromatic nuclei)
    Multiple lipomas can be seen in several syndromes:
    – *See also Neoplastic:Syndromes with Multiple Tumors or Multiple Types of Tumors*
  b. Dercum's disease (adiposa dolorosa)
    = Multiple painful lipomas, see in postmenopausal women
      Mostly on thighs, inner arms, abdomen
  c. Benign symmetric lipomatosis (Madelung disease or Leaunois-Bensaude's)
    – Symmetric fat deposits in head/neck/shoulders
  d. Benign familial lipomatosis
    – Multiple discrete, mobile lipomas mostly on forearms/thighs, spares neck/shoulders
  e. Proteus syndrome
    – Multiple lipomas, epidermal nevi, plantar cerebriform lesions, vascular malformations, macrodactyly
  f. Gardner syndrome
  g. Bannayan-Riley-Ruvalcaba syndrome
  h. MEN Type I
    – Tuberous sclerosis-like clinical appearance, can have lipomas
2. Nevus lipomatosis superficialis
  – "Michelin tire," mostly on buttocks or thighs
  – On path, ddx Goltz syndrome (fat comes up to epidermis)
  – In kids/young adults, adipose tissue in superficial dermis
  a. Michelin tire baby syndrome
    – Phenotype of generalized nevus lipomatosis superficialis or smooth muscle hamartomas as large linear masses along skin folds

Compare with:

b. Goltz syndrome (focal dermal hypoplasia)
  – Defect in PORCN gene, thought to be important for palmitoylation and secretion of Wnt protein, a key regulator of skin/bone development; X-linked – Clinically, Blaschkoid punctate, cribriform atrophy with telangiectasia, ice pick depressions; coloboma (in eye)
  – Osteopathia striata – vertical striations in metaphysis of long bones
  – Lobster claw deformity; syndactyly (attached toes), oligodactyly (missing toes)
  – Don't confuse with Gorlin-Goltz (BCC Nevus syndrome)

3. Lipoblastoma
  – Immature fat cells, usually before age 3, tends to be on extremities

4. Piezogenic pedal papules
  – Painful herniations of fat through dermis of heels/wrists

5. Hibernoma
  – Lipoma of immature brown fat
  – Path: "Mulberry cells"

6. Liposarcoma
  – Five histopathologic subtypes: well-differentiated, myxoid, round cell, pleomorphic, dedifferentiated

7.8 Cysts

A true cyst is a cavity with an epithelium, whereas a pseudocyst is a cavity that lacks such a lining

1. True cysts
  a. Cysts with stratified squamous epithelium
    I. Epidermal inclusion cyst (EIC)
      – Aka epidermoid cyst, sebaceous cyst (misnomer since not of sebaceous origin)
      – From hair follicle infundibulum, + granular layer
      – Associated with Gardner syndrome/FAP
      – Milia are small epidermoid cysts
      – *See also Acneiform Disease:Follicular Cysts*
    II. Pilar cyst
      – Aka trichilemmal cyst
      – From hair follicle isthmus, no granular layer (since that is derived from infundibulum)
      – May appear in families in autosomal dominant inheritance
    III. Eruptive vellus hair cysts
      – Small bluish papules typically on mid chest/sternum, rarely extremities; ddx steatocystoma multiplex, acne
      – Tend to be familial, appear in childhood

      – *See also Neoplastic:Adnexal Tumors* and *Acneiform Disease:Follicular Cysts*

      – Path: multiple vellus hair shafts in cyst

  IV. Steatocystoma

      – Cystic papules with oily, yellow liquid

      – May be triggered by puberty, ddx eruptive vellus hair cysts, acne

      – Has granular layer and thin eosinophilic, crenulated "shark tooth" cuticle of keratin, may have sebaceous glands connecting to the cyst wall

      – *See also Neoplastic:Adnexal Tumors* and *Acneiform Disease:Follicular Cysts*

      1. Steatocystoma multiplex

        – Autosomal dominant, keratin 17 mutation

        – Can be associated with eruptive vellus hair cysts, pachyonychia congenita type 2 (K6b, K17 mutations), natal teeth

  V. Dermoid cyst

      – Common around eyes (usually lateral), face

      – Multiple types of adnexal glands in cyst wall, sebaceous glands open directly into cavity

      – Do not confuse with desmoid tumor (*see also Neoplastic:Spindle Cell Tumors*)

      – Ddx nasal glioma, encephalocele

  VI. Ear pits (preauricular cysts)

      – Congenital defect from defective fusion in first two branchial arches

      – Common (up to 1% of people), with deafness, can be associated with renal and other abnormalities

  VII. Cystic acne

      – *See also Acneiform Disease:Acne*

b. Cysts with non-squamous epithelium

  I. Eccrine hidrocystoma

      – Glistening papule, typically infraorbital

      – *See also Neoplastic:Adnexal Tumors:Eccrine*

  II. Apocrine hidrocystoma

      – Glistening papule, typically on eyelid

      – Path shows decapitation secretion

      – *See also Neoplastic:Adnexal Tumors:Apocrine*

  III. Bronchogenic cyst

      – Cyst contains keratin, surrounded by lymphocytic infiltrate

      – Lined by respiratory mucosa (cilia), smooth muscle, goblet cells; may see nearby cartilage

      – Usually in suprasternal notch

  IV. Thyroglossal duct cyst

      – Median/midline neck

      – Number one congenital abnormality of the neck

      – No smooth muscle

7

    V. Branchial cleft cyst
      – Derived from second branchial cleft
      – On lateral neck
    VI. Cutaneous ciliated cyst
      – Classically on lower extremities of young women
      – Cuboidal/columnar epithelium with cilia, but no goblet cells (ddx bronchogenic cyst)
    VII. Median raphe cyst
      – On ventral penis or glans
  c. Sinuses
    I. Dental sinus
      – Related to intraoral dental abscess
      – Classically lesion on cheek with retraction in a patient with a history of poor dentition/tooth infections
      – Check X-ray, may need tooth extraction/antibiotics
    II. Follicular occlusion tetrad
      – *See also Acnieform Disease: Acne*
        1. Hidradenitis suppurativa
        2. Acne conglobata
        3. Dissecting cellulitis
        4. Pilonidal sinus
    III. Cutaneous Crohn's disease
      – *See also Dermal: Granulomatous/Histiocytic*
    IV. Infectious disease presenting with cutaneous sinus tracts
      – *See also Infectious Disease: Bacterial and Infectious Disease: Fungal*
        1. Mycetoma
        2. Actinomycosis
        3. Nocardiosis
2. Pseudocysts (cysts with no epithelium)
  a. Mucocele
    – Arise from disruption of minor salivary glands
  b. Digital mucous cyst
    – Path: acral skin with collection of mucin
    – Impinges upon proximal nail matrix, causes nail dystrophy
    – Can be drained, destroyed (cryo, cautery), or excised
  c. Pseudocyst of the auricle

7.9 Lymphatic Malformations

1. Lymphedema (acquired or congenital)
  – With lymphedema, remember risk of angiosarcoma (Stewart-Treves)
  a. Elephantiasis nostra verrucosa (cutis)
    = Verrucous cobblestone plaques from chronic lymphedema of any cause

  – Often associated with chronic tinea pedis, secondarily infected by GAS →cellulitis →lymphangitis →fibrosis of lymphatics (can't drain well); ultimately from repeated cellulitis/fibrosis
  – Path: verrucous hyperplasia over fibrosed lymphatics
 b. Filiarial elephantiasis
  – *See also Infectious Disease: Parasites*
 c. Podoconiosis
  = Endemic non-filarial elephantiasis
  – Caused by abnormal inflammatory reaction to irritant soils (red clay) from volcanic deposits, appears to have genetic predispositions
  – Tends to be bilateral, but asymmetric
  – Common in tropics, where people are not wearing shoes
 d. Noonan syndrome
  – May have lymphedema at birth, as well as other lymphatic abnormalities such as cystic hygroma
  – Associated with short stature, webbed neck, CV defects, mental retardation
  – Often due to PTPN11 mutation (nonreceptor protein tyrosine phosphatase) of the Ras/MAPK pathway; defect in same gene causes LEOPARD syndrome
  – Associated with increased granular cell tumors
  – Increase in follicular keratoses, lentigines, keloids
 e. Turner syndrome
  – Short stature, broad chest with widely spaced nipples, amenorrhea, sterility, lymphedema, neck webbing, coarctation aorta
  – From XO karyotype
 f. Milroy syndrome
  – From autosomal dominant defect in VEGFR3
  – Typically lymphedema limited to the legs
2. Lymphangiomas
 a. Lymphangioma circumscriptum (superficial lymphangioma)
  – Persistent, multiple clusters of translucent vesicles that usually contain clear lymph fluid (like "frog spawn"); can be red from hemorrhage
  – Can have warty appearance (and in genital area, can be misdiagnosed)
  – Tx with CO_2 laser ablation, excision or destruction; some newer evidence for topical sirolimus
 b. Cavernous lymphangioma (deep lymphangioma)
 c. Cystic hygroma (deep lymphangioma)

7.10 Lymphomas

Note: Most cutaneous lymphomas are T-cell derived (~75%) versus B-cell lymphomas (~25%)
 T-cell markers: CD2, CD3, CD4, CD5, CD6, CD7, CD8

B-cell markers: CD20, CD79a, PAX-5
1. Primary cutaneous T-cell lymphomas (CTCLs)
   a. Mycosis fungoides (MF)
      – Note: MF is the most common of the CTCLs (the terms are not synonymous, although since MF is so common, occasionally MF and CTCL are used interchangeably)
      – Typically a chronic, indolent disease in middle aged to elderly patients
      – Clinical: papulosquamous/eczematous/erythrodermic patches/plaques/tumors; perhaps "smudgy" (not well demarcated) borders with superficial atrophy, can see poikiloderma (poikiloderma vasculare atrophicans), ddx eczema, psoriasis; may resemble PLEVA/PLC, folliculitis, vitiligo, pigmented purpuric dermatosis; one of the great imitators and has even been identified in "normal skin" biopsy of chronic pruritus patients
      – Classically limited to non-sun exposed areas, may favor the buttocks/bathing suit distribution
      – Etiology: thought to be caused by chronic antigenic stimulation leading to a clonal expansion of T helper memory cells
      – Path: band-like lymphocytic infiltrate with epidermotropism, "Pautrier's microabscesses" (intraepidermal nests of atypical cells—this is specific, but seen only in minority of cases); lymphocytes may have cerebriform nuclei
      – Atypical T-cells classically are CD4, CD45RO positive, CD8 negative, CD26 negative, and may show loss of pan-T-cell surfaceantigens such as CD2, CD3, CD5 and/or CD7
      – T-cell monoclonality: in CTCLs, may see alpha/beta or gamma/delta T-cell receptor (TCR) gene rearrangements. In MF, expect in~50% patch, 73% plaque, 83–100% tumors, but may also see in 25–65%benign inflammatory disorders
      – Work-up: diagnosis may require multiple skin biopsies for H&E to capture classic pathology, TCR gene rearrangement positivity may be suggestive but not specific, blood flow cytometry and TCR gene rearrangement may also be suggestive. With B symptoms (fever, night sweats, weight loss), lymphadenopathy, or for full staging, check LDH and consider full body CT or PET/CT
      – Staging:
      IA = <10% BSA skin involvement
      IB = >10% BSA skin involvement
      IIA = any skin involvement, lymphadenopathy
      IIB = one or more tumors 1 cm or larger, ± lymphadenopathy
      III = erythroderma, ± lymphadenopathy
      IVA = erythroderma, lymph node metastasis, cancerous lymphocytes in blood
      IVB = erythroderma, visceral organ metastases, ± lymph node metastasis

Classically stages described clinically as:
    Note: all of these clinical stages may be concurrent
    Patch stage = flat patches, may be atrophic
    Plaque stage = thickened plaque lesions, ddx psoriasis
    Tumor stage = nodules and tumors

Variants of MF =

I. Sézary syndrome
  – Note: pronounced [Sez uh ree]
  = An aggressive leukemic variant of MF
  – Defined as diffuse lymphadenopathy, erythroderma, Sézary cells(malignant T cells) in peripheral blood (>1000/cubic millimeter, CD3+/CD4+/CD26- of >30% or CD3+/CD4-/CD7- of >40%)
  – Death from opportunistic infection

II. Large cell transformation of MF
  – Represents conversion of relatively indolent MF to more aggressive malignancy
  – Path: Large T-cell lymphocytes (>25% diagnostic); these stain with CD30

III. Granulomatous slack skin
  = Rare form of MF, can be associated with Hodgkin's
  – Tends to affect axillae, groin

IV. Hypopigmented mycosis fungoides
  – Tends to occur in darker skin types (African-Americans)
  – Can see loss of CD4, retained CD8
  – Relatively better prognosis

V. Localized pagetoid reticulosis (localized MF)
  – Aka Woringer-Kolopp disease
  – A solitary variant of MF, typically on extremity; most cases occur in adolescents
  – Ddx acral pseudolymphomatous angiokeratoma of children (APACHE), a pseudolymphoma

VI. Folliculotropic MF
  – Usually affects head and neck
  – May be associated with a mucinous degeneration of the hair follicle (follicular mucinosis or alopecia mucinosa), *see also Dermal:Depositional:Mucin*
  – May cause hair loss of eyebrows especially
  – Generally more aggressive than typical MF and tends to be very itchy

VII. Syringotropic MF
  – A form of MF with atypical lymphocytes tropic to eccrine glands

Treatments:
  – For early stage disease (IA-IIA = topical steroids, phototherapy (PUVA and NBUVB), bexarotene, topical chemotherapy (mechlorethamine and carmustine), MTX
  – For advanced MF and Sézary syndrome = total skin electron beam therapy, bexarotene, extracorporeal photopheresis, brentuximab, mogamulizumab, HDAC inhibitors (vorinostat, romidepsin), interferons, and other systemic chemotherapy.

7

- Note: topical steroids should be avoided prior to biopsy as may delay diagnosis; if suspicion high and patient already on TCS, should instruct them to not treat a lesion for a few weeks then biopsy
  b. CD30 positive T-cell lymphomas
  I. Primary anaplastic large cell lymphoma (ALCL)
    - Can sometimes be histologically indistinguishable from LyP, CD30+
  II. Lymphomatoid papulosis (LyP)
    - Perhaps 5–20% associated with lymphoma, excellent prognosis; controversy on whether this is just a lymphoproliferative disease and not truly lymphoma-associated
    - Types A and C are CD30+
    - Nicknamed "evil PLEVA" given clinical overlap with PLEVA, but distinct disease from PLEVA and PLC, which are considered on a spectrum; see also Papulosquamous: Other
    - CD30 positive (excludes PLEVA/PLC), like anaplastic large cell lymphoma (ALCL), Hodgkin's
    - May be assoc. with MF, ALCL, Hodgkin's
  c. Other primary cutaneous T-cell lymphomas
  I. Adult T-cell leukemia/lymphoma (ATLL)
    - Abnormal CD25 positive cells
    - Associated with HTLV-1; typically presents with impressive hypercalcemia
  II. Subcutaneous panniculitis-like T-cell lymphoma (SPTCL)
    - Aggressive; associated with EBV
    - See also Dermal: Subcutaneous/Panniculitis
  III. Extranodal NK/T-cell lymphoma, nasal type
    - Aggressive; associated with EBV
    - Most common in nasal cavity/nasopharynx, but on skin may present as midfacial destructive tumor; previously referred to as "lethal midline granuloma"
    - Often invades vessels (angiocentric), causing vascular destruction, thrombosis, and necrosis
  IV. Aggressive epidermotropic cytotoxic CD8+ T-cell lymphoma
    - An aggressive variant, very poor survival; can mimic Mucha Haberman disease (severe form of PLEVA)
  V. Cutaneous γ/δ T-cell lymphoma
    - Typically aggressive, fatal disease, resistant to multiagent chemotherapy
2. Primary cutaneous B-cell lymphomas
  - Note: Borrelia is thought to play a role in at least a minority of cases of primary cutaneous B-cell lymphomas
  - The diffuse large types carry an intermediate prognosis, whereas the follicle center and marginal zone types are typically indolent

- Tx = local excision (for indolent localized), intralesional or systemic interferon-α-2a or rituximab, or XRT and for severe disseminated disease the most common regimen is rituximab + CHOP chemotherapy

a. Primary cutaneous diffuse large B-cell lymphoma, leg type
  - Large round cells, Bcl-2 +, MUM1/IRF-4 +
  - Worst prognosis
  - While typically on the legs, tumors with the same features can occur in other areas of the body, despite name

b. Primary cutaneous diffuse large B-cell lymphoma, other
  - Includes B-cell lymphoblastic lymphoma, which presents in children/ young adults as tumors on head and neck

c. Primary cutaneous marginal zone B-cell lymphoma
  - Closely related to MALT lymphomas of the GI tract
  - More indolent
  - Can arise in areas affected by acrodermatitis chronica atrophicans (suggesting a stronger link to *Borrelia*) than the other types of B-cell lymphoma

d. Primary cutaneous follicle center lymphoma
  - Common sites = scalp, forehead, back
  - Favorable prognosis

e. Multiple myeloma
  - Plasma cell malignancy
  - Rarely involves the skin
  - Can be associated with primary systemic amyloidosis (AL), necrobiotic xanthogranuloma, plane xanthoma/xanthelasma, leukocytoclastic vasculitis, scleromyxedema
  - Clinically, can be associated with nasal spicules
  - *See also: Neoplams/Tumors: Skin diseases associated with monoclonal gammopathy*

f. Plasmacytoma
  - Localized proliferation/tumor of plasma cells in the skin, benign
  - *See also Dermal: Inflammatory: Plasmacytic*

3. NK cell lymphoma
  - CD-56 positive

4. Pseudolymphoma (lymphocytoma cutis or cutaneous lymphoid hyperplasia)
  - Benign mimicker clinically/histologically of lymphoma
  - Idiopathic, caused by drugs, insect bites, infections (Lyme)
  - Includes lymphomatoid drug eruption, lymphomatoid contact dermatitis, arthropod-induced pseudolymphoma, actinic reticuloid, lymphocytoma cutis, acral pseudolymphomatous angiokeratoma of children (APACHE)
  - Follows normal anatomical structures, mixed cell types, polyclonal (unlike lymphoma → no regard for anatomy, often destroys structures; monotypic, often atypical morphology, monoclonal); is "top heavy" rather than more monomorphic, "bottom heavy" infiltrate of lymphoma
  - *See also Dermal: Inflammatory: Lymphocytic*

7

7.11 Other Malignant (Including Metastatic)

1. Leukemia cutis
   – Clinical: papules, nodules, plaques
   – Most commonly from acute monocytic leukemia and acute myelomonocytic leukemia
   – Leukemia can be associated with Sweet syndrome, pyoderma gangrenosum, vasculitis, urticarial
   a. Chloroma
      = Greenish tumor of leukemia cutis, from myeloperoxidase
      – Most commonly from AML
   b. Blastic plasmacytoid dendritic cell neoplasm (BPDCN)
      – Can be difficult to distinguish from myeloid leukemia, and can precede clinically detectable leukemia (an "aleukemic leukemia"), very poor survival
2. Lymphoma cutis
   – Both systemic T-cell and B-cell lymphomas can involve the skin
   – *See also Neoplastic:Lymphomas*
3. Metastatic carcinoma
   – Path: "Indian filing," often pleomorphic undifferentiated cells, easily crushed/friable (crush artifact)
   Most common cutaneous metastases in men:
   1. Melanoma
   2. SCC of head/neck
   3. Lung cancer
   Most common cutaneous metastases in women:
   1. Breast cancer
   2. Melanoma
   3. Ovarian cancer
1. Specific types of breast cancer skin metastases
   a. Carcinoma en cuirasse
      – Sclerotic metastases, "cuirasse" means armor that covers the torso in French
   b. Carcinoma erysipeloides (inflammatory breast cancer)
      – Named because resembles cellulitis
   c. Carcinoma telangiectoides
      – Telangiectatic patch, may resemble lymphangioma circumscriptum
   d. Alopecia neoplastica
      – Scalp nodules with alopecia
   e. Paget's disease
      – Associated with ductal carcinoma of breast, usually by direct extension, but can be metastatic, must involve nipple
      – Weeping "erosive" dermatitis on nipple with extension to areola
      – Can look like unilateral nipple eczema, can be indurated
      – 100% associated with breast carcinoma
      – Biopsy must be of nipple for dx

– Pagetoid spread = single cells spread in epidermis/adnexae; ddx = MM, SCC/SCCIS, sebaceous carcinoma, Paget's, extramammary Paget's
– Preserved basal layer ("crushed basal layer") in Paget's usually helps distinguish from MM; CK7+, PAS+, Alcian blue+, mucicarmine+

Most common on scalp:
– Breast, lung, stomach, pancreas, kidney

Note: recognize renal cell carcinoma metastases by clear cells with lots of blood

Most common in kids:
– Neuroblastoma, rhabdomyosarcoma, leukemia

4. Extramammary Paget's
   – In groin/axillae, can be associated with malignancies (in 25%); usually anogenital, but can be anywhere with apocrine glands
   – Plaque with erosions and scale giving "strawberries and cream" appearance

5. Aggressive digital papillary adenocarcinoma
   – Path: papillated deep dermal tumor
   – Can metastasize to lungs
   – Tx = wide excision/amputation

7. Adenoid cystic carcinoma
   – Path = "cribriform" pattern
   – Salivary gland derived

7.12 Other Benign

1. Acrochordon
   – *See also Keratotic Disease: Papillomatous Epidermal Eruptions*

2. Connective tissue nevi
   – Includes collagenomas and elastomas
   a. Buschke-Ollendorff syndrome
      – Aka dermatofibrosis lenticularis disseminata
      – Connective tissue nevi (soft yellow-skin colored papules)
      – Osteopoikilosis = small sclerotic opacities in bones, typically in carpal bones, phylanges
      – From defect in LEMD3, nuclear envelope

3. Myxomas
   – Connective tissue tumors with mucin
   – Can see in association with Carney complex, *see also Neoplastic: Syndromes with multiple tumors or multiple types of tumors*

4. Nipple adenoma

5. Accessory nipple (polythelia)

6. Accessory digit
   – *See also Neoplastic: Spindle Cell Tumors: Neural*

7. Accessory tragus
   – Path: polypoid with dermal vellus hairs

7

    a. Goldenhar syndrome (oculo-auriculo-vertebral syndrome)
-     – Congenital abnormality of 1st branchial arch
-     – Ear abnormalities including accessory tragi, Arnold-Chiari type I malformation
-     – Can see limbal dermoids, coloboma, "tag" like tragi

8. Congenital cartilaginous rests of the neck
   - – Aka "wattles" or cervical accessory tragi

7.13 Syndromes with Multiple Tumors or Multiple Types of Tumors

- Hamartoma: benign malformation/hyperplasia of elemental tissue from a given location where that tissue would normally occur.
- Phakoma: a hamartomatous finding in a phakomatosis. This includes retinal-hamartomas, Lisch nodules, shagreen patches, neurofibromas, etc.
- Phakomatosis: Ectodermal genetic diseases affecting the CNS along with other ectodermal tissues (skin and retina).
- Choristoma: benign neoplasm of "normal" (non-malignant) tissue in an ectopic location.
- Note: several syndromes may be associated with GI polyposis: Peutz-Jeghers syndrome, Cronkhite-Canada syndrome, BCC nevus syndrome, Cowden disease, Bannayan-Riley-Ruvalcaba syndrome, Gardner syndrome

1. Tuberous sclerosis
   - Aka Bourneville disease, epiloia (epilepsy, low intelligence, adenoma sebaceum); only 29% have all 3 of triad, 6% have none
   - Cutaneous features:
     Angiofibromas (70–80%) = adenoma sebaceum, fibrous plaque of forehead
     Hypomelanotic macules (polygonal, ash leaf/lance ovate, confetti macules)
     Shagreen patch (collagenomas), notably on lower back
     Periungual fibromas (Koenen tumors)
   - Other features:
     Retinal hamartomas (phakomas)
     Enamel pits (>90%)
     Gingival fibromas
     Multiple bilateral renal angiomyolipomas
     Lymphangiomyomatosis (LAM) (in adult women)
     Seizures (70–95%), astrocytomas, cortical tubers, mental retardation
     Cardiac rhabdomyoma (80%)—r/o with Echo
     - Work-up: if >?3 ash leaf macules (no defined criteria), full derm exam, head CT/MRI, renal ultrasound, EKG
     - Can do EEG, behavioral tests, Chest CT in adult women, Echo
     - Defect: mutations in TSC1 – hamartin (Chr 9), TSC2 – tuberin (Chr 16); hamartin and tuberin together form tumor suppression complex.

This complex usually inhibits mTOR (mammalian target of rapamycin), which promotes tumor growth.
  – Immediately adjacent to TSC2 on Chr 16 is PKD1, mutated in polycystic kidney disease, so may see concurrently
  – Autosomal dominant, though 2/3 from spontaneous mutations
  – Ddx MEN type I (facial angiofibromas)
  – Rapamycin/sirolimus (systemic and topical), which inhibits mTOR, has been shown to successfully treat features of tuberous sclerosis
2. Neurofibromatosis
  a. Neurofibromatosis type I
    – Aka von Recklinghausen's disease
    – Dx requires ≥ 2 criteria:
      1. Café-au-lait macules (CALMs): Dx criteria for NF require ≥ 6 CALMs of 5 mm (prepubertal) or 1.5 cm (postpubertal)
      2. Two or more neurofibromas (appear in adolescence)
      3. Axillary/inguinal freckling "Crowe's sign"
      4. Optic gliomas
      5. Two or more Lisch nodules (iris hamartomas)
      6. Osseous lesion (e.g. sphenoid dysplasia, bowing of tibia)
      7. First degree relative with NF1
    – NF1 caused by mutations in neurofibromin on Chr 17; autosomal dominant, 50% from spontaneous mutations; segmental variants cause by mosaicism
    – Neurofibromin is a tumor suppressor gene that modulates Ras
    – NF1 diagnostic criteria are less sensitive for children; Crowe's sign is the most specific of the criteria
    – Neurofibromas are derived from Schwann cells, typically appear in puberty
    – Lesser known findings include blue-red and pseudoatrophic macules
    – Plexiform neurofibromas are usually congenital; 8–12% of NF1 patients will develop a malignant peripheral nerve sheath tumor, and these usually arise from preexisting plexiform neurofibromas
    – Plexiform neurofibromas usually described as "bag of worms"
    – Most common bone finding is scoliosis, but also macrocephaly, osteopenia/osteoporosis, sphenoid wing dysplasia (sphenoid bone dysplasia [posterior orbital wall] → pulsating exophthalmos), long bone dysplasia (e.g. bowing of tibia)
    – Purported association between JXG, NF1, and juvenile myelomonocytic leukemia (JMML aka juvenile CML), though there is still some debate (higher risk in all NF1 patients)
    – NF1 patients are known to have learning disabilities; some study into whether statins could improve cognitive deficits of children with NF- no success as of yet
    – Risk of HTN from 3 things: pheochromocytoma, renal HTN (renal artery stenosis), essential HTN

  – Tumor risk: malignant peripheral nerve sheath tumors (3–15%), pheochromocytoma (1%), optic glioma (10–15%), JMML, breast cancer
b. Neurofibromatosis type II
  – Bilateral acoustic neuromas (schwannomas), usually no neurofibromas cutaneously, may see a few hairy schwannomas
  – Merlin (schwannomin) – Chr 22
c. Other neurofibromatosis types
  I.   NF3 = mixed
  II. NF4 = variant
  III. NF5 = segmental
  IV. NF6 = CALMs only
  V.   NF7 = late onset
  VI. NF-NOS = not otherwise specified
d. NF1-like syndrome (Legius syndrome)
  – May have Crowe's sign and CALMs
  – From mutations in SPRED1
3. Basal cell carcinoma nevus syndrome
  – Aka Gorlin's syndrome/Gorlin-Goltz/nevoid-BCC syndrome—Multiple BCCs at young age, other tumors, congenital abnormalities including odontogenic pseudocysts of the jaw, calcification of the falx cerebri, palmar pits
  – Can be associated with medulloblastoma
  – PTCH gene, autosomal dominant
  – Different than Goltz syndrome (focal dermal hypoplasia)
  – Tx with sonic hedgehog inhibitor, vismodegib or sonedigib, is a newer therapeutic option given immense BCC burden from young age and surgical fatigue
4. Cowden disease (multiple hamartoma syndrome)
  – Autosomal dominant, PTEN gene, multiple hamartomatous tumors of ectodermal, mesodermal and endodermal origin
  – Trichilemmomas, acral keratoses, oral papillomas and sclerotic fibromas (can appear as skin tags), angiofibromas; high-arched palate
  – Mnemonic: in COWden, can have trichilemMOOmas
  – Associated with breast and thyroid especially (follicular) carcinomas
  – Can have GI polyposis
  – Can be associated with dysplastic cerebellar gangliocytoma (Lhermitte-Duclos disease)
5. Bannayan-Riley-Ruvalcaba Syndrome
  – Shares many features with Cowden disease
  – May have penile lentigines (on the "banana")
  – PTEN gene mutation
6. Proteus Syndrome
  – Body asymmetry, linear epidermal nevi, and vascular malformations, palmoplantar cerebriform hyperplasia, lipomas
  – May have association with PTEN gene mutation (controversial)

- Cultural note: it is thought that Joseph Merrick, "the elephant man," whose life was the inspiration for a play and movie, may have had Proteus syndrome, or perhaps a combination of Proteus syndrome and neurofibromatosis type I.

7. Birt-Hogg-Dubé Syndrome
   - Multiple skin tags = fibrofolliculomas, trichodiscomas, perifollicular fibromas, acrochordons (actually just look like tags, but are the aforementioned); can have angiofibromas
   - Folliculin, tumor suppressor protein (FLCN gene mutation)
   - Associated with spontaneous pneumothorax, renal cell carcinoma (especially chromophobe and hybrid oncocytic carcinomas)

8. Brooke-Spiegler syndrome
   - Mutation in CYLD, which encodes a deubiquitinating enzyme, which inhibits the NF-κB pathway
   - Spiradenomas, cylindromas, trichoblastomas

9. Muir-Torre syndrome
   - Subtype of hereditary nonpolyposis colorectal cancer (HNPCC) syndrome (aka Lynch syndrome), prone to colon, breast, GU cancers
   - Sebaceous neoplasms (adenoma, epithelioma, or carcinoma), keratoacanthomas, and internal malignancies; sebaceous adenoma is a unique hallmark
   - MSH2, MLH1 (DNA mismatch repair gene), can be stained for in biopsy tissue
   - *See also Neoplastic:Keratinocyte Neoplasms*

10. Gardner syndrome
    - Epidermoid cysts, osteomas, desmoid tumors, congenital hypertrophy of retinal pigment epithelium (CHRPE), may have lipomas
    - Mnemonic = "chirping bird in the grass (sod)" = CHRPE in the SOD (sebaceous cyst, osteomas, desmoid tumors)
    - Multiple adenomatous polyps of colon, associated with FAP (familial adenomatous polyposis)
    - APC (adenomatous polyposis coli) gene, Chr 5, autosomal dominant
    - Usually treated with prophylactic colectomy

11. Multiple endocrine neoplasia (MEN) syndromes
    a. MEN Type 1 (Wermer)
       - Multiple facial angiofibromas, collagenomas, lipomas
       - 3Ps: Pituitary, parathyroid, pancreas
       - Some overlap with tuberous sclerosis (angiofibromas, collagenomas)
       - MEN1 (MENIN) gene; menin is a nuclear protein
    b. MEN Type 2A (Sipple)
       - RET gene; RET is a tyrosine kinase receptor (proto-oncogene)
       - Parathyroid, Thyroid (medullary carcinoma),Pheochromocytoma
       - Can be associated with macular/lichen amyloid
    c. MEN Type 2B
       - RET gene

– Multiple mucosal neuromas
– Thyroid (medullary carcinoma) - check calcitonin, Adrenal
– Clinically, patients are Marfanoid (75%); can have megacolon
12. Carney complex
   – Aka LAMB/NAME syndrome
   = Lentigines, Atrial myxoma, Mucocutaneous myxoma, Blue nevi
   = Nevi, Atrial myxoma, Myxoid neurofibroma, Ephelides
   – PRKAR1A gene, encodes protein kinase/tumor suppressor
   – Essentially 3 main components: 1. Myxomas, 2. Lentigines, 3. Endocrine tumors
   – Growth hormone-producing pituitary adenomas; and testicular Sertoli cell tumors; psammomatous melanotic schwannoma
13. Reed's syndrome (leiomyomatosis and renal cancer)
   – From deficiency in fumarate hydratase (causes fumarase deficiency)
   – See multiple cutaneous and uterine leiomyomas, renal cell carcinoma
14. Maffucci's syndrome
   – Multiple enchondromas, risk of chondrosarcoma

7.14 Paraneoplastic Syndromes

Paraneoplastic syndrome = manifestation of neoplasm wherein no neoplastic component is found (reactive to presence of neoplasm)
– This is a list of specific paraneoplastic phenomena, but always consider underlying malignancy in erythroderma, generalized pruritus, urticarial, vasculitis
   1. Leser-Trélat sign
      – Sudden increased size/number of seborrheic keratosis; controversial if this really exists
      – Associated with gastric or colonic adenocarcinoma, breast carcinoma, and lymphoma
      – May be associated with malignant acanthosis nigricans
   2. Acanthosis nigricans
      – May have sudden onset, associated with stomach, other GI cancers
      – "Tripe palms" = acanthosis nigricans on hands
   3. Erythema gyratum repens
      – Associated with lung carcinoma
   4. Hypertrichosis lanuginosa acquisita
      – Sudden growth of lanugo hairs
      – Associated with colorectal cancer, bronchial cancer, cervical cancer
      – There is also an inherited autosomal dominant form, see also Alopecia: Other hair disorders
   5. Necrolytic migratory erythema
      – Associated with glucagonoma (glucagonoma syndrome)
      – Also pseudoglucagonoma syndrome from liver disease, malabsorption syndromes

6. Bazex syndrome (acrokeratosis paraneoplastica)
   – Do not confuse with Bazex syndrome (BCC syndrome)
   – Associated with carcinoma, usually upper airway "aerodigestive"
7. Sweet syndrome
   – Associated with AML
8. Pyoderma gangrenosum (vesiculobullous type)
   – Associated with AML
9. Paraneoplastic pemphigus
   – Most associated with non-Hodgkin's lymphoma (40%), CLL (30%), Castleman's disease (10%), also thymoma (especially in kids)
10. Dermatomyositis
    – Most common in women: ovarian/breast cancer, men: GI, lung cancer
11. Necrobiotic xanthogranuloma
    – Associated with paraproteinemia (>80% of cases, most often IgG with κ light chains), multiple myeloma in a minority
12. Trousseau syndrome (migratory thrombophlebitis)
    – Associated with pancreatic carcinoma
13. Pachydermoperiostosis
    – Aka primary hypertrophic osteoarthropathy
    – Associated with lung carcinoma
14. Cutis verticis gyrata
    = Cerebriform folding of the skin of the scalp
    – Can be paraneoplastic in metastatic carcinoma
15. Pityriasis rotunda
    – Circular scaly patches, may be associated with malnutrition, malignancy,mycobacterial infections
16. Multicentric reticulohistiocytosis (MRH)
    – Periungual "coral bead" papules/nodules, arthritis mutilans (can be like RA)
    – No consistent association, but often seen with malignancy (in 28%, bronchial, breast, stomach and cervical carcinomas)
    – *See also Dermal:Granulomatous/Histiocytic:Histiocytoses*

7.15 Skin Diseases Associated with Monoclonal Gammopathy

Note: Plasma cell dyscrasia = clonal proliferation of plasma cells (includes myeloma)
   – Monoclonal gammopathy = usually IgG > IgA >> IgD, IgM, includes amyloidosis
   – IgA monoclonal gammopathies seem associated with neutrophilic entities
   – Paraproteinemia and monoclonal gammopathy are synonymous
   1. Diseases caused by infiltration/extension of monoclonal gammopathy
      a. Waldenström macroglobulinemia cutis (IgM storage papules)
      b. Primary systemic amyloidosis (AL)

7

    c. Cryoglobulinemia (types I and II)
       = Monoclonal IgM or IgG
    d. Plasmacytoma
    e. POEMS syndrome (including osteosclerotic myeloma)
       = Polyneuropathy, Organomegaly, Endocrinopathy, Monoclonal gammopathy, Skin changes
       – Major criteria: Monoclonal gammopathy (IgA or IgG, λ type), Polyneuropathy (need one)
       – Skin changes include diffuse hyperpigmentation, glomeruloid hemangiomas (actually more cherry angiomas), hypertrichosis
       – See increased expression of VEGF (causes angiomas)
       – Can have overlap with Castleman's disease
       – Not associated with multiple myeloma
2. Diseases only associated with monoclonal gammopathy
    a. Scleromyxedema (papular mucinosis)
       – Associated with monoclonal gammopathy (classically IgG-λ)
    b. Scleredema (adultorum of Buschke)
       – Mostly IgG monoclonal gammopathy reported in one type
    c. Necrobiotic xanthogranuloma (NXG)
       – Associated with paraproteinemia (>80% of cases, most often IgG with κ light chains), multiple myeloma in a minority
    d. Plane xanthoma
       – In normolipemic patient, could be from multiple myeloma, Castleman's, CML (from monoclonal IgG binding LDL, enhancing phagocytosis); may see "diffuse" plane xanthomas
    e. Schnitzler's syndrome
       – Chronic non-pruritic urticaria, FUO, disabling bone pain, hyperostosis, monoclonal IgM κ gammopathy – can progress to neoplasm (Waldenström's)
    f. Neutrophilic dermatoses (weaker association)
       – Can be associated with IgA monoclonal gammopathy
          I. Sweet's syndrome
          II. Pyoderma gangrenosum
          III. Subcorneal pustular dermatosis (Sneddon-Wilkinson disease)
          IV. Erythema elevatum diutinum
    g. Acquired cutis laxa
       – From inflammatory disease, ID (Borrelia), plasma cell dyscrasias, medicines (penicillamine)
    h. TEMPI syndrome
       = Telangiectasias, Elevated erythropoietin level and erythropoiesis, Monoclonal gammopathy, Perinephric-fluid collections, and Intrapulmonary shunting
       – Associated with IgG-κ gammopathy
       – *See also Vascular: Regional erythema: Telangiectasia*

3. Cutaneous signs of monoclonal gammopathy
    a. Purpura
        – Especially periorbital, axillary
    b. Nasal spicules
        – Associated with multiple myeloma, amyloid

Acneiform Disease

Contents

© The Author(s), under exclusive license to Springer Nature Switzerland AG 2024
J. Lipoff and D. Ruiz Dasilva, *Dermatology Simplified*,
https://doi.org/10.1007/978-3-031-66739-8_8

8

Abstract

Acneiform disease includes conditions on the spectrum of acne and folliculitis as well as conditions that may resemble acne clinically, such as rosacea.

Keywords

Acne · Rosacea · Acneiform eruptions

8.1 Acne

1. Acne vulgaris
   - Common inflammatory skin disease, most often in puberty
   - Morphologies include comedonal, papular, pustular, nodulocystic
   - Pathophysiology related to:
     1. Increased sebum production
     2. Abnormal follicular epidermal turnover/keratinization
     3. Overgrowth of bacteria (gram positive diphtheroid anaerobe *Propionobacterium acnes*)
     4. Inflammatory response (to foreign body)
   - Typical therapeutic ladder:
     1. Benzoyl peroxide in conjunction with topical antibiotic (clindamycin, erythromycin or minocycline) and topical retinoid (for comedones); topical anti-androgen (clascoterone)
     2. Systemic antibiotic (tetracyclines) or anti-androgens (females)
     3. Systemic retinoid (isotretinoin)
   - Androgenic hormones have significant influence on acne; with suspected strong hormonal component (e.g. acne flares monthly localizing more on jawline, chin), consider oral contraceptives and spironolactone
   - The role of diet in acne is controversial, but no strong evidence for diet connection outside of potentially dairy (skim milk) and high glycemic diets being possible triggers
2. Follicular occlusion tetrad
   - These four diseases are thought to be closely related and may co-exist; the primary pathophysiology involves occlusion and rupture of hair follicles with associated inflammation
   - This spectrum may be associated with inflammatory bowel disease, pyoderma gangrenosum, acne syndromes
   - a. Hidradenitis suppurativa
     - Aka "acne inversa"
     - Clinically may see sinus tracts and nodules, "double comedones"

- Localizes typically to intertriginous areas (axillae, inguinal folds, inframammary and buttocks)
- Previously, thought to be a primarily apocrine disease given the typically apocrine gland bearing affected areas, but now thought that apocrine glands are only secondarily inflamed and fibrosed
- Associated with smoking, obesity, Down syndrome
- Treatments include intralesional steroids, topical and systemic antibiotics, isotretinoin (often not effective), anti-TNF biologics (adalimumab approved, infliximab often used for severe cases), secukinumab (IL-17 inhibitor) recently approved, surgery; other biologics and JAKi may be on the horizon

b. Acne conglobata
  - Unusually severe nodulocystic acne with sinuses and scarring
c. Dissecting cellulitis
  - Aka perifolliculitis capitis abscedens et suffodiens
  - Clinically presents as draining cystic nodules on the scalp
  - May have overlap with folliculitis decalvans, which is more typically a flat and boggy scalp plaque
  - *See also Alopecia:Scarring alopecia*
d. Pilonidal sinus
  - Involves gluteal cleft

3. Acne syndromes
  a. Acne fulminans
    - Severe nodulocystic acne with variable systemic manifestations (fevers, arthralgias, hepatosplenomegaly), may have osteoclastic lesions, especially of the clavicle
  b. SAPHO syndrome
    - Syndrome of *s*ynovitis, *a*cne conglobata, *p*ustulosis (often palmoplantar), *h*yperostosis, *o*steitis
    - Can be associated with Sweet's
  c. PAPA syndrome
    - Sterile *p*yogenic *a*rthritis, *p*yoderma gangrenosum, and *a*cne
    - Has been associated with pyrin/nod defects
  d. PASH and PAPASH syndromes
    - Pyoderma gangrenosum, acne, and suppurative hidradenitis (PASH) and pyogenic arthritis, pyoderma gangrenosum, acne, and suppurative hidradenitis (PAPASH)

4. Other types of acne
  a. Neonatal acne/neonatal cephalic pustulosis
    - No open or closed comedones seen
    - Onset usually first 2–3 weeks of life, resolves on own with no scarring within weeks, therapy not necessary
    - Associated with *Malassezia sympodialis*
  b. Infantile acne
    - Usually begins at 3–6 months, may be associated with precocious secretion of gonadal androgens

8

           – Can persist; treated with topical retinoid/ benzoyl peroxide
- c. Drug-induced acne
  - – Usually from corticosteroids ("steroid acne"), but also lithium, androgens, phenytoin, ACTH, INH, EGFR inhibitors
  - – Can see abrupt eruption of monomorphic papules/pustules without comedones
  - – Would also include halogenoderma (includes iododerma) as a potential drug-induced acneiform eruption
  - – *See also Vascular: Toxic Erythema: Drug Eruptions*
- d. Chloracne
  - = Occupational acne caused by exposure to chlorinated aromatic hydrocarbons (dioxins), such as Agent Orange (herbicide/defoliant used in Vietnam War). Famous case: Ukranian president Viktor Yuschenko poisoned.
  - – Particularly seen behind ears and over the malar crescent
- e. Acne excoriée (de jeunes filles)
  - – Picking at one's face with history of mild acne
- f. Acne aestivalis (Mallorca acne)
  - – Monomophous eruption of red papules on the face from UVA light (similar to PMLE), no comedones
- g. Trichostasis spinulosa
  - – Small dark follicular papules on the nose; from clusters of vellus hairs embedded within hair follicles; may be variant of comedones
- h. Favre–Racouchot syndrome
  - = Nodular elastosis with cysts and comedones
  - – Associated with UV and smoking
- i. Solid facial edema
  - – Aka Morbihan disease
  - = Soft tissue edema associated ± acne leading to midline facial distortion
  - – Has also been associated with rosacea and Melkersson-Rosenthal syndrome
- j. Tropical acne
  - – Acneiform eruption from extreme heat or occupational exposure
- k. Acne mechanica
  - – Caused by repeated rubbing under occlusion
  - I. Fiddler's neck

8.2 Rosacea

- ▬ Aka acne rosacea; rosacea is considered a distinct entity from acne with different pathophysiology, though may respond to similar therapeutics
- ▬ Rosacea is classically recognized by central erythema of the face with stinging/burning sensations; however, different types may have different clinical morphologies

- Classic triggers include sunlight, alcohol, caffeine, spicy foods, emotions, hot drinks
- Pathophysiology of rosacea is unclear, but it is thought to reflect a vascular dysregulation
- Has been associated with increased levels of toll-like receptor 2, and increased expression of cathelicidin, LL-37, and kallikrein 5
- *Demodex folliculorum* is implicated in etiology
- Treated topically with metronidazole, azelaic acid, sodium sulfacetamide, even retinoids, permethrin, ivermectin; systemically with oral antibiotics (since etiology unclear, why these work is also unclear), ivermectin, isotretinoin; also pulsed dye laser
  1. Classic types of rosacea
     a. Erythematotelangiectatic
     b. Papulopustular
     c. Phymatous (including rhinophyma)
     d. Ocular (including blepharoconjunctivitis)
  2. Pyoderma faciale/rosacea fulminans
     – A more severe inflammatory form of rosacea
     – Some use former term to mean more localized, latter term for whole face
     – Presents as eruption of inflamed papules and yellow pustules in the centrofacial region
  3. Perioral/periorificial dermatitis
     – May be within rosacea spectrum, but also can be caused by topical steroid use; classically spares vermillion border of lips
     – Includes periorificial dermatitis of childhood
     – Often effectively treated with oral tetracyclines and topical calcineurin inhibitors
  4. Granulomatous rosacea
     – Clinically consistent with rosacea, but with lesions with granulomatous clinical morphology (red-brown/orange papules) and pathology
     – *See also Dermal:Inflammatory:Granulomatous/histiocytic*
  5. Lupus miliaris disseminatus faciei
     – Aka acne agminata
     – Granulomatous eruption on face; some consider a form of rosacea
     – Previously thought to be a tuberculid reaction

Note on treatment: It is important to be conservative when starting systemic retinoids for severe nodulocystic acne or rosacea fulminans. Isotretinoin can lead to a marked flare with high risk scarring potential. Consider using systemic corticosteroids for a week to a month or so to mitigate this risk and start the retinoid at low dose e.g. 10 mg of isotretinoin daily or every other day. There is also evidence that H1 antihistamines may help mitigate this risk.

8

8.3 Folliculitis

8.3.1 Superficial Folliculitis

a. Bacterial
     I. Impetigo of Bockhart (*Staph*)
     II. Gram negative folliculitis
     III. Hot tub folliculitis (*Pseudomonas*)
b. Fungal
     I. Dermatophytes
         1. Tinea barbae (*T. mentagrophytes* and *T. verrucosum*)
         2. Tinea capitis (especially *T. tonsurans* and *M. canis*)
     II. *Candida*
     III. Pityrosporum
c. Viral
     I. Herpes simplex (HSV)
d. Eosinophilic pustular folliculitis (EPF)
     – Three types
     I. HIV-associated EPF
     – Presents as pruritic papules on chest/back/face; can mimic acne
     II. Ofuji's disease
     – Seen primarily in Asians/Japanese
     III. Eosinophilic pustulosis of infancy
     – Ddx erythema toxicum neonatorum
e. Demodex folliculitis
f. Other non-infectious
     I. Disseminate and recurrent infundibulofolliculitis (DRIF)
     – Aka Hitch and Lund disease
     – Numerous monomorphic follicular papules on chest
     – Can appear like lichen spinulosus
     – Ddx juxtaclavicular beaded lines, an entity perhaps related to sebaceous hyperplasia
     II. Irritant/frictional

8.3.2 Deep Folliculitis

a. Infectious
     I. Furunculosis
     – Aka boils or follicular abscesses
     – From *Staph* and *Strep* primarily
     – Primary treatment is incision and drainage; may also use systemic antibiotics
     – *See also Infectious disease: Bacterial: Staph and Strep*

II. Sycosis barbae (*Staph*/mycotic/herpetic)
- Homophone with "psychosis"
- Localizes to the beard area
III. Majocchi's granuloma (deep dermatophyte folliculitis)
T. rubrum
- Often on legs, with topical steroid use

8.3.3 Pseudofolliculitis

= From in-grown hairs
a. Pseudofolliculitis barbae (PFB)
- Often treated with topical antibiotics for presumed associated folliculitis, TCS for inflammatory component and retinoid for follicular hyperkeratinization; also treated with gentle shaving practices
b. Acne keloidalis/Acne keloidalis nuchae (AKN)
- May represent a scarring reaction to pseudofolliculitis; treated same as above + ILK
- *See also Alopecia:Scarring alopecia*

8.4 Follicular Cysts

- *See also Neoplastic:Cysts*
1. Milia
= Benign, keratin-filled cysts (small epidermoid cysts); do not confuse with miliaria (from obstruction of sweat gland ducts)
a. Primary milia
- From vellus hair follicles
b. Secondary milia
- From damage to pilosebaceous unit (as in subepidermal blistering diseases)
2. Epidermal inclusion cysts
- Aka epidermoid cysts or sebaceous cyst (misnomer) or infundibular cyst (from the infundibulum)
- Associated with Gardner syndrome/FAP
- Has granular layer
3. Pilar cysts
- Aka trichilemmal cysts, sometimes autosomal dominant
- Derived from the outer root sheath trichilemma of the hair follicle
- Lacks granular layer
4. Foreign body granulomatous reaction to ruptured follicular cyst (ruptured cyst/keratin granuloma)
5. Eruptive vellus hair cysts
- Small bluish papules typically on mid chest/sternum, rarely extremities
- *See also Neoplastic:Cysts*

8

6. Steatocystoma/steatocystoma multiplex
   – Cystic papules with oily, yellow liquid
   – *See also Neoplastic: Cysts*

8.5 Newer Therapies for Acne

1. Topical retinoids
   – Many developed recently with PAD (polyaphron dispersion) technology which essentially encapsulates active molecules allowing for uniform drug delivery in a moisturizing vehicle with superior tolerability
   – Tretinoin/BPO (Twyneo), tretinoin lotion (Altreno), tazarotene foam (Fabior), trifarotene (Aklief), tazarotene lotion (Arazlo); all of these apparently have lower irritation compared to say generic tazarotene cream with frequent irritation; regardless, these newer formulations are all more expensive perhaps making it more cost effective to start with tretinoin
2. Topical antibiotic
   – Minocycline foam (Amzeeq) is delivered in a moisturizing foam vehicle; greasy nature and yellow discoloration/residue limits patient adherence
3. Topical anti-androgen
   – Clascoterone (Winlevi) is new as a topical hormonal therapy—not exactly topical spironolactone (which can be compounded, but not very effective); can use in both males and females; best when used in combination with other therapies (relatively low efficacy as monotherapy), reported low risk of adrenal suppression
4. Systemics—newer oral antibiotics and retinoids
   – Sarecycline (Seysara) is a narrow spectrum tetracycline efficacious against *P. acnes* while limiting effect on the gut microbiome and overall antibiotic resistance; also weight based with once daily dosing, purportedly less photosensitivity and GI distress—however, these are more expensive making it more cost effective to start with doxycycline/minocycline
   – Isotretinoin (Absorica LD) is a new generation isotretinoin with increased absorption regardless of fat-rich meal consumption (vitamin A is a fat-soluble vitamin, similarly isotretinoin is best absorbed with fat), but probably more cost effective to start with other isotretinoins
   – *See also: High Yield Topics: Medications*

Alopecia

Contents

9

Abstract

This section focuses on diseases that cause hair loss or hair abnormalities. Clinically, scarring alopecia is suggested by loss of hair follicle ostia and smooth, shiny patches of skin between tufts of hair (like doll's hairs). Non-scarring alopecias typically retain hair follicles despite loss of hair. With time, however, even non-scarring alopecias may show loss of follicular ostia. On pathology, scarring alopecias may show changes from minimal inflammation to perifollicular fibrosis and ultimately true follicular scars. The hair cycle consists of: anagen/growth phase (~2–6 years), catagen/transition phase (~3 weeks), telogen/release phase (~3 months); mnemonic: rule of 3s, 3 yrs (anagen), 3 wks (catagen), 3 mos (telogen).

Keywords

Alopecia · Scarring alopecia · Non-scarring alopecia

9.1 Scarring Alopecia

9.1.1 Inflammatory Scarring Alopecia

a. Lymphoid scarring alopecia
  I. Discoid lupus (DLE)
    – Classically hyperkeratotic plaques with follicular plugging and scarring alopecia; typically on face, scalp, conchal bowls of ears
    – "Carpet tack sign" = horny plugs on undersurface when scale removed (non-specific)
    – "Lupus hairs" = short, fragile frontal hairs
    – *See also Connective Tissue Disease: Lupus*
  II. Lichen planopilaris (LPP)
    – Classically scarring alopecia with perifollicular scaling
    – Frontal fibrosing alopecia = appears to be a pattern of LPP, mostly in postmenopausal women
    – Graham-Little-Piccardi-Lasseur Syndrome = LPP, KP, axillary/genital non-scarring alopecia
    – Recent interest in treating LPP with JAKi, with many promising case reports
    – *See also Papulosquamous: Lichenoid: Lichen Planus*
  III. Central centrifugal cicatricial alopecia (CCCA)
    – Aka follicular degeneration syndrome
    – Aka "Hot comb" alopecia

- Classically associated with history of chemical treatments, relaxing, perms, hot combs although no strong evidence to support these associations and many patients with no definitive trigger; recent evidence of genetic predisposition

b. Neutrophilic scarring alopecia
  I. Folliculitis decalvans
    - Flat and boggy plaques of alopecia, can become pseudopelade
    - Usually treat with antibiotics, steroids; in recalcitrant cases, can use dapsone, isotretinoin, TNFi, apremilast, JAKi
    - Some may use term almost interchangeably with dissecting cellulitis
  II. Dissecting cellulitis
    - Aka perifolliculitis capitis abscedens et suffodiens
    - Terrible name: not dissecting, not a cellulitis
    - Part of the follicular occlusion tetrad, *see also Acneiform Disease*
    - Clinically more separate nodules/cysts in scalp with associated alopecia, can become pseudopelade
    - Some may use term almost interchangeably with folliculitis decalvans
    - Treatment with tetracyclines, isotretinoin, TNFi, IL17i, IL23i

c. Mixed infiltrate scarring alopecia
  I. Acne keloidalis nuchae
    - Exact etiology unclear, but may represent a scarring reaction to ingrown hairs (pseudofolliculitis), *see also Acneiform Disease*
    - Name is at least partially a misnomer—it is not caused by acne and lesions are not keloidal (on pathology), though it does classically appear on the posterior neck
    - Commonly seen in African-American patients with short curly hairs and short haircuts (which all predisposes to pseudofolliculitis)
    - Treatment with tetracyclines, TCS, topical retinoids, BPO, ILK

d. Pseudopelade of Brocq
  = End stage of scarring alopecia, tufted doll's hairs, "footprints in the snow"

9.1.2 Non-inflammatory Scarring Alopecia

a. Trauma
b. Traction alopecia
  - Sometimes non-inflammatory, sometimes inflammatory
  - Typically non-scarring initially, but may become scarring
c. Aplasia cutis congenita (ACC)
  - A focal congenital loss of skin/hair in newborns, may evaluate with imaging/MRI (don't want to risk biopsy)
  - "Hair collar sign" = a collar of hair seen around the skin defect
  - Ddx nevus sebaceus
  I. Adams-Oliver syndrome
    = ACC with cutis marmorata telangiectatica congenita
  II. Bart's syndrome
    = ACC with epidermolysis bullosa

9

9.2 Non-scarring Alopecia

9.2.1 Non-inflammatory Non-scarring Alopecia

a. Androgenic/androgenetic alopecia
   – Norwood classification describes the stages of male pattern hair loss
   Path: small superficial hair follicles (normally deep in fat)
   I. Male pattern – vertex and bitemporal/frontal scalp
   II. Female pattern – central thinning on crown; usually not frontal (which is more likely from traction)
b. Telogen effluvium
   – Early/excessive loss of club hairs, associated with stressor (pregnancy, surgery, illness, diets, seasonal variation, emotional trauma etc.) – 2–4 months later
   – Can have a chronic form, saw increase during COVID-19 pandemic
   – > 25% telogen hairs is diagnostic
c. Traction alopecia
   – From tight braids or curlers, initially reversible, but eventually can have permanent loss of hair follicles
d. Trichotillomania
   – Bizarrely shaped focal patches of alopecia, but never complete patches as in alopecia areata, which it can mimic
   – Either from absent-minded twirler or psych patient (classically with OCD)
   – Can be associated with prurigo, dermatitis artefacta
   – If swallowing hair, can develop trichobezoar (hairball in stomach, which can cause obstruction)
   – Path: on vertical section, pigmented hair casts
   – Treatment may be directed at underlying disorder (e.g. antipsychotics, SSRI) or n-acetylcysteine supplementation
e. Anagen effluvium
   – From chemotherapy
   – Starts 7–14 days after chemo initiated, most apparent 1–2 months after
   – Caused by narrowed, weakened hair shaft, easily broken
   – Can also be associated with pemphigus
f. Nutritional alopecia
   – Can see alopecia in iron, vitamin D, zinc deficiencies
g. Acquired progressive kinking of the hair
   – Term for acquired curled, frizzy hair in frontotemporal or vertex region; common in young men, assoc. with thinning
h. Temporal triangular alopecia (congenital triangular alopecia)
   – Normal number of follicles, but vellus hairs rather than terminal hairs in b/l temporal areas
   – Aka Brauer nevus

9.2.2 Inflammatory Non-scarring Alopecia

a. Alopecia areata
   – Round patches of non-scarring alopecia with "exclamation point hairs" (broad distally, thin proximally) along periphery
   – Nail findings may include regular/geometric nail pitting, trachyonychia
   – Can be associated with autoimmune thyroid disease, vitiligo, atopy
   – Path: lymphs around anagen hair bulb (does not affect bulge, where the stem cells are, so can regrow), "swarm of bees"
   Patterns:
   I.   Localized alopecia areata
       1. Ophiasis pattern
          – Alopecia around periphery (O-shaped)
       2. Sisaipho pattern: (ophiasis spelled backwards)
          – Alopecia of central scalp only (mnemonic: bald like Cicero)
   II. Diffuse alopecia areata – otherwise diffusely on scalp
   III. Alopecia totalis – entire scalp
   IV. Alopecia universalis – entire body
b. Secondary syphilis
   – Classically, "moth-eaten alopecia"
   – Path: histiocytes/plasma cells, can appear identical to alopecia areata
c. Other infectious
   – Tinea capitis, kerion, HSV/VZV
   – Path: neutrophils
   – *See also Infectious Disease*
d. Alopecia mucinosa/follicular mucinosis
   – In adults, can be associated with folliculotropic MF, *see also Neoplastic:Lymphomas and Dermal:Depositional:Mucin*
   – May also be associated with scarring alopecia
e. Psoriatic alopecia
   – Psoriasis will not directly cause hair loss from scalp involvement; however, "psoriatic alopecia" is a rare non-scarring or scarring alopecia that may be associated with TNF inhibitors

9.3 Genodermatoses Associated with Alopecia

1. Loose anagen syndrome
   – Anagen hairs can be pulled from root with little effort
   – Usually in blonde girls, improves with age
   – Cuticle folds back like "rumpled sock"
2. Short anagen syndrome
   – Hairs simply do not grow that long because of shortened anagen (but they do not come out easily)

9

3. Atrichia with papular lesions
   = Autosomal recessive disorder, presents in infancy
   – Sparse initial hair shed, leading to alopecia by age 1, and later papules (follicular cysts); ddx alopecia universalis
4. Ectodermal dysplasias
   Note: these all have defects in ectodermal layer derived tissues (skin, hair, nails)
   a. Hidrotic ectodermal dysplasia (Clouston syndrome)
      – Progressive alopecia associated with PPK and nail changes; normal sweating and teeth
      – Autosomal dominant, defect in connexin 30
   b. Hypohidrotic ectodermal dysplasia (HED)
      – Aka anhidrotic ectodermal dysplasia, Christ-Siemens-Touraine syndrome
      – Thin, sparse, or absent hair, missing or peg -shaped teeth, inability to sweat correctly
      – Primarily X-linked recessive, defect in EDA (ectodysplasin A) and also NEMO
   c. Naegeli-Franceschetti-Jadassohn syndrome (NFJS)
      – Hyperpigmenation of abdomen, periocular, perioral primarily; dental abnormalities, palmoplantar hyperkeratosis with absent or hypoplastic fingerprints
      – Defect in keratin 14
   d. Dermatopathia pigmentosa reticularis
      – Defect in keratin 14, may be variant of NFJS
   e. Hay-Wells syndrome
      – Coarse/sparse hair, ankyloblepharon (fibrous bands fusing upper and lower eyelids together), cleft palate
      – Associated with mutation in p63, autosomal dominant

9.4 Hair Shaft Abnormalities

9.4.1 Structural Abnormalities with Increased Hair Fragility

a. Trichorrhexis nodosa
   – Most common structural hair abnormality, may be congenital or acquired (repeated trauma)
b. Trichorrhexis invaginata aka "bamboo hair"
   I. Netherton syndrome
      – Mutation in SPINK5, encodes LEKTI, a serine protease inhibitor → increased pruritus (like allergens, eczema, *Staph* infections cause)
      – Ichthyosis linearis circumflexa = "double edged scale"

c. Monilethrix aka beaded hair
- Short, fragile, brittle hairs after a few months of normal hairs
- Think of in a patient with alopecia and KP (follicular hyperkeratosis)
- Defect in keratins 81 and 86 (aka hair keratins 1 and 6), autosomal recessive form with dsg4 defect
d. Trichoschisis due to trichothidystrophy
= A clean transverse break through the hair
e. Trichothiodystrophy
- Autosomal recessive, sulfur-deficient brittle hair
- "Tiger-tail banding" on hairs
- DNA-repair gene mutations
- Severe neurologic and developmental abnormalities
- PIBIDS = photosensitivity, ichthyosis, brittle hair, infertility, developmental delay, short stature
- May have same genes mutated as in xeroderma pigmentosum/ Cockayne syndrome
f. "Bubble hair"
- In young women, localized uneven, fragile hairs
- From traumatic hair care, like malfunctioning hair dryer
g. Pili torti aka twisted hair
I. Menkes kinky hair
- ATP7A, defect in copper transport
- X-linked recessive
- Classic finding of pili torti, but can also see monilethrix, trichorrhexis nodosa
- *See also Nutritional Disease*
h. Trichonodosis aka knotted hair
i. Pohl-Pinkus constriction
- Caused by systemic illness, like Beau's lines in nails
j. Trichomalacia
= Deformed hair shaft; may see in trichotillomania

9.4.2 Structural Abnormalities Without Hair Fragility

a. Pili annulati aka ringed hair
- Has bright and dark bands from air-filled cavities within the hair (dark regions)
b. Pili trianguli et canaliculi aka spun-glass hair (uncombable hair)
- Thought to be from abnormal keratinization of inner root sheath
c. Woolly hair
Think: rule out heart defect!
I. Naxos disease
- Plakoglobin defect, autosomal recessive
- PPK, woolly hair, R ventricular cardiomyopathy

9

– Mnemonic: N and P are on R side of alphabet (Naxos, plakoglobin, R ventricular cardiomyopathy)

II. Carvajal disease
  – Desmoplakin defect, autosomal recessive
  – PPK, woolly hair, L ventricular cardiomyopathy
  – Mnemonic: C and D are on L side of alphabet (Carvajal, desmoplakin L, ventricular cardiomyopathy)

9.5 Excess Hair Growth

1. Hirsutism
  = Presence in women of terminal hairs in a male pattern
  – Most often associated with polycystic ovarian syndrome (PCOS), but also in endocrinopathies or peri-menopausal hormonal changes
  – May evaluate for cause with DHEA-S (elevated suggests adrenal origin) and free testosterone
2. Hypertrichosis
  = Simply an increase in amount of hair
    I. Hypertrichosis lanuginosa
      = A generalized overgrowth of hair
      – Can arise in childhood as an congenital autosomal dominant disor-der (for an exaggerated cultural reference, think the Addams family's Cousin Itt) or as an acquired paraneoplastic syndrome
      – *See also Neoplastic: Paraneoplastic syndromes*
3. "H" syndrome
  = Recently described autosomal recessive genodermatosis consisting of many findings that start with the letter H: hyperpigmentation, hypertrichosis, hepatosplenomegaly, heart anomalies, hearing loss, hypogonadism, low height, and occasionally, hyperglycemia
  – Defect in nuceloside transporter hENT3 (*SLC29A3* gene)

9.6 Treatments

– Alopecia may be difficult to treat, and in many cases incurable however there are some well established treatments that can help stabilize hair loss, strengthen existing hair and even regrow lost hair on a case-by-case basis
  1. Topicals:
    a. Minoxidil 5% is a mainstay of nearly any alopecia tx and is OTC; used once daily in females, twice daily in males (do not recommend the 2% women's formula, as this is less effective. We generally recommend all pa-tients only the men's 5% minoxidil which is cheaper than women's 5% minoxidil and by all accounts the same formulation)

b. Finasteride or dutasteride (androgen blockers) can be compounded with or without minoxidil and tretinoin (to help boost penetration); note efficacy may be lower than systemic equivalents and less studied

c. TCS or TCI can be adjunctive treatment in any inflammatory alopecia

d. Compounded topical metformin has been reported for CCCA

2. Systemics:

a. Low dose oral minoxidil (1.25–5 mg daily) has become markedly popular for any alopecia given marked safety, tolerability and efficacy; note potential mild orthostasis in those with low BP, ankle edema, and hirsutism (note: unlikely but reported pericardial effusion)

b. Spironolactone (anti-androgen) in higher doses of 100–200 mg daily effective in AGA; best used in premenopausal females

c. Oral finasteride or dutasteride (blocks both 5-alpha reductase I & II) effective for AGA in males and females; use in females typically limited to postmenopausal though can use in younger if counseled about potential birth defects; dutasteride also known as a effective 1st line tx for lichen planopilaris/FFA. Note: questionable association with increased risk for breast cancer.

d. Immune modulators/anti-inflammatories such as naltrexone, pioglitazone, hydroxychloroquine, tetracyclines have been used in scarring alopecia

e. Traditional immunosuppressants such as systemic corticosteroids, MMF, MTX, AZA, cyclosporine have been used in scarring alopecia and AA

f. JAK inhibitors are now approved for moderate to severe AA (baricitinib in 18 + and ritlecitinib in 12 +); these drugs have also been used off label for scarring/inflammatory alopecia with success

3. Injectables

a. ILK is a mainstay of tx for alopecia areata and scarring alopecia (2.5–10 mg/cc)

b. Platelet rich plasma (PRP) has limited evidence of efficacy in AGA and other alopecias, though it has become a popular option. This procedure involves drawing a patient's blood and using a centrifuge to isolate the PRP component then inject it into the scalp in the same manner as ILK. Expense and relative lack of efficacy compared to the systemic agents limit its use (especially as monotherapy).

4. Hair transplantation

a. Techniques and technology have evolved over the last decade to lead to better outcomes

b. Particularly useful in AGA however many will also use in scarring alopecia if process has been burnt out or halted with medical management

Connective Tissue Disease

Contents

10

Abstract

The term connective tissue disease (and sometimes collagen vascular disease) refers to the autoimmune spectra of lupus erythematosus, rheumatoid arthritis, dermatomyositis, Sjögren's, and scleroderma. This category reviews all of these entities, but also includes other diseases that affect the connective tissues with relevance to dermatology. A number of non-specific clinical findings may suggest the possibility of autoimmune connective tissue disease. These include: Raynaud's phenomenon, non-scarring alopecia, livedo reticularis, pericuticular erythema, telangiectasias, palpable purpura (leukocytoclastic vasculitis) (strongest association with lupus and rheumatoid arthritis).

Keywords

Lupus · Dermatomyositis · Connective tissue disease · Collagen vascular disease

10.1 Lupus Erythematosus (LE)

- Lupus is a heterogeneous autoimmune disease associated with deposition of immune complexes; the manifestations can be understood as autoantibody immune complexes depositing in the small blood vessels of the skin, brain, kidneys, joints and other organs; it is not entirely clear why only certain organs and certain people are affected by these autoantibodies
- Clinically can appear as erythematous dermal plaques, papulosquamous and rarely vesiculobullous lesions
- Path (classic): interface dermatitis/vacuolar change, superficial and deep perivascular lymphs with mucin
- Lupus is difficult to classify and has many clinical presentations in the skin; here cutaneous presentations of lupus are divided into acute, subacute, and chronic clinical findings along with specific lupus types.
- The name "lupus" comes from the "wolf-like" or lupine facial rash
- Labs to rule out SLE should be ordered at diagnosis and can be checked yearly for screening purposes (CBC, CMP, U/A w/ micro, ANA, dsDNA, SSA, SSB, U1RNP, anti-smith, APLA, complements)

1. Acute
   Clinical findings: malar erythema "butterfly rash," diffuse erythema, bullae
   Types:
   a. Systemic lupus erythematosus (SLE)
      – Per the 11 ARA criteria, $\geq 4/11 = $ SLE; these were designed for defining SLE for clinical studies. This may not be sensitive enough for all patients.

- The 11 ARA Criteria:
- 4 skin findings: malar, discoid, oral ulcers, photosensitivity (photosensitivity not well defined)
- 2 types of antibodies: ANA (99% sensitive) and anti-Smith (or anti-dsDNA) (specific)
- 5 systems: Heme (hemolytic anemia, leukopenia, or thrombocytopenia), Renal (proteinuria or cell casts), Neuro (seizures or psychosis), Rheum (arthritis), and Cards/Pulm (pericarditis/pleuritis)
- SLICC criteria now more widely used: ≥4 criteria (at least one clinical and one lab) OR biopsy proven lupus nephritis with positive ANA or dsDNA
- Clinical: acute and chronic cutaneous lupus erythematosus (ACLE, CCLE), oral or nasal ulcers, non-scarring alopecia, arthritis, serositis, renal (proteinuria or cell casts), neuro (seizures or psychosis), hemolytic anemia, leukopenia, thrombocytopenia
- Lab: ANA, dsDNA, anti-smith, antiphospholipid ab, low complement, direct Coomb's test
- Classically the malar erythema of SLE should involve the nasal bridge and spare the nasolabial folds, which would be shaded by the nasal alae; if biopsy-proven, really is specific for SLE
- Lupus band test = DIF shows DEJ IgG deposits in normal skin of SLE; an old non-specific test, not often used (when done on sun protected area has higher specificity, when done on sun exposed area has higher sensitivity)
- Smoking may exacerbate lupus, and increase risk for lupus. Also, smoking may inhibit effectiveness of antimalarials in lupus.
b. Drug-induced systemic lupus
- Presents with joint pains, usually no skin findings
- Resolves in days to months
- Most common: hydralazine (5%), procainamide (15–25% of patients taking the drug!!), quinidine, TNF antagonists
- Has been reported with minocycline (assoc. with + ANA)
- Anti-histone Ab in 95%- this is positive in 50% of SLE
c. Bullous SLE
- Subepidermal blistering manifestation of SLE (not a part of any other form); may overlap with epidermolysis bullosa acquisita
- If biopsy-proven, really is specific for SLE
- *See also Vesiculobullous: Subepidermal blisters: Neutrophilic*
2. Subacute
Clinical findings: annular (and polycyclic), papulosquamous
Types:
a. Subacute cutaneous lupus (SCLE)
- Strong anti-Ro association, tend to be ANA positive
- About half may meet criteria for SLE
- Can develop Sjögren's; 10–15% may develop internal disease (nephritis)

  – Drug-induced by HCTZ (#1), terbinafine (most reported), Ca channel blockers, NSAIDs, griseofulvin, PPIs

b. Neonatal lupus erythematosus
  – Rash typically periorbital
  – Risk of third degree heart block (15–30%) and thrombocytopenia (5–10%)
  – Check for Ro (most common in 95%), La, anti-U1-RNP
  – Mother usually asymptomatic (50%), usually Ro positive
  – 25% risk of next child developing
  – Ro binds to fetal cardiac myocytes (injures conducting system)
  – Anti-U1-RNP associated with lower risk of heart block
  – Systemic steroids or IVIG does not decrease risk for subsequent child but HCQ does

3. Chronic
  Types: discoid, panniculitis, hypertrophic/lichenoid
  Note: Chronic LE is typically associated with scarring
  a. Discoid lupus (DLE)
    – Only 5% progress to SLE, but ~20% of patients with SLE have DLE
    – Early lesions can appear psoriasiform
    – For biopsy, select old lesion for more characteristic path
    – "Carpet tack sign" = horny plugs on undersurface when scale removed (non-specific)
    – *See also Alopecia:Scarring alopecia*
  b. Lupus profundus (panniculitis)
    – *See also Dermal:Panniculitis:Mostly lobular panniculitis without vasculitis*

4. Other
  a. Lupus erythematosus tumidus (tumid lupus)
    – Non-scarring
    – May overlap with Jessner's benign lymphocytic infiltrate and cutaneous lymphoid hyperplasia
    – On face/trunk, annular plaques (?urticarial plaques) with no secondary changes (e.g. no scale)
    – Could be independent entity, but often seen in lupus pts
    – On path, lymphocytic, absence of DEJ/interface involvement, but has mucin deposition
  b. Lichen planus-lupus overlap syndrome
    – Controversial, lesions with overlapping features of LP and LE; may not have positive ANA
  c. Rowell syndrome
    – Overlap of erythema multiforme and lupus; may just represent LE patients developing EM
  d. SLE pernio (Chilblain lupus)
    – Red/dusky purple plaques on fingers/toes brought on by or exacerbated by cold in the context of SLE (unlike perniosis)

5. Treatments
   a. Topicals - TCS, TCI, PDE4-inhibitors, topical JAKi have all been used with variable success as monotherapy (strict photoprotection is also key!)
   b. Systemics - systemic steroids, HCQ (gold standard 1st line, evidence that it decreases progression from CLE to SLE), chloroquine (if not responding to HCQ), MTX, MMF, acitretin, oral JAKi (deucravacitinib, baricitinib, upadacitinib with most evidence), finally thalidomide/lenalidomide, IVIG or rituximab (in most recalcitrant cases)

10.2 Dermatomyositis

Clinical signs:
   Most classic:
   – Heliotrope rash (periocular violaceous erythema)
   – Gottron's papules = papulosquamous pink to violaceous papules over MCPs, DIPs, PIPs, sparing between joints
Other common signs:
   – Gottron's sign = pink/red/purple atrophic or scaly papules/plaques/patches over extensor knuckles, knees, elbows (can mimic psoriasis)
   – Shawl sign = erythema and scale ± poikiloderma over shoulders, upper back
   – Periungual telangiectasias and cuticular changes (Samitz sign)
   – Central face erythema
   – "Mechanic's hands" = can be associated with anti-synthetase (Jo-1)
   – Proximal muscle weakness (e.g. cannot lift arms, stand up from chair)
   – Scalp erythema, intense pruritus
   – Holster sign = pink, violaceous erythema on the lateral thighs
   – Rare manifestation: flagellate erythema (ddx bleomycin toxicity, Shiitake-mushroom dermatitis)
Like other connective tissue diseases, skin involvement may be photodistributed or photoaccentuated

Amyopathic dermatomyositis (dermatomyositis sine myositis) = cases without clinical muscle involvement or muscle enzyme changes) which may represent up to 20–30%; these cases are still at risk for interstitial lung disease and malignancy association so dermatology recognition/management is key

- Ddx periocular rash: heliotrope rash, contact dermatitis, trichinosis
- Papulosquamous extensor surface eruption may resemble psoriasis
- Check for elevated CK and aldolase (muscle enzymes)
- Drug induced dermatomyositis is rare, but notably hydroxyurea can cause a poikiloderma of the dorsal hands that is similar; also, statins

Important: r/o underlying malignancy (especially likely if age > 50); routine screening + CT of chest/abdomen/pelvis, intravaginal ultrasound, prostate exam, colonoscopy in any adult; highest risk in the first 2-3 year after diagnosis
- Antibody associations:

anti-Jo-1 = aka, anti-synthetase, predicts more lung involvement
anti-Mi-2 = predicts benign course, less lung involvement
anti-Ku = DM/scleroderma overlap
anti-SRP = anti-signal-recognition particle, cardiac disease
anti-CADM-140 (MDA-5) = clinically amyopathic dermatomyositis (CADM), associated with severe, rapidly progressive lung involvement
anti-p155/140 (TIF1-γ) = associated with malignancy
anti-p140 (NXP-2) = juvenile dermatomyositis, in adults associated with malignancy and lower extremity edema

1. Juvenile dermatomyositis
   - Compared to adult form, more associated with dystrophic calcification (calcinosis cutis) and vasculopathy
   - Calcinosis is a good prognostic factor
2. Adult dermatomyositis
   - Compared to juvenile form, more associated with malignancy and interstitial lung disease
   - Must r/o paraneoplastic syndrome; in women: especially ovarian/breast cancer, men: GI, lung cancer
3. Treatments
   - Systemic steroids + TCS initially then transition to steroid sparing regimen. HCQ or chloroquine ± quinacrine (1st line), MTX vs. MMF (2nd line), JAKi vs. IVIG (3rd line). JAKi works relatively better in dermato compared to lupus. Also, case reports of apremilast, ustekinumab, and lenabasum.

10.3 Sclerotic Disease

10.3.1 Scleroderma/Systemic Sclerosis

a. Morphea (formerly known as localized scleroderma)
   - Melorheostosis = thickening/sclerosis of bones, usually in 1st big toe (pronounced [Mallory ostosis])
   - May have "lilac border" indicative of activity
   - Three forms: plaque, linear, generalized
   - Classically not associated with Raynaud's or systemic disease; if present, consider possibility of systemic sclerosis
     Forms of linear morphea (associated with high ANA titers, thought to be same condition on a spectrum):

    I. En coup de sabre
- Aka frontoparietal linear morphea
- Named since can look like a sword's blow

    II. Parry-Romberg syndrome
- Progressive hemi-facial atrophy
- May be associated with seizures (from meningeal involvement), ipsilateral brain lesions, L > R, Female > Male
- Associated with nerve paralysis, headaches (migraines)
- 5–15 year progression, then stabilizes

b. Limited cutaneous systemic sclerosis

    I. CREST syndrome
- A subset of limited cutaneous systemic sclerosis
- CREST = Calcinosis, Raynaud's, Esophageal dysmotility, Sclerodactyly, Telangiectasias (matted)
- Most common antibody association = anti-centromere

c. Diffuse cutaneous systemic sclerosis
- Aka generalized morphea by some
- No internal organ involvement

d. Progressive systemic sclerosis (scleroderma)
- May see CREST findings, plus tightened face, fixed "bird-like" facies, pursed lips, confetti depigmentation, loss of skin creases, digital ulceration, ventral pterygium
- Systemic involvement: interstitial lung disease, pulmonary HTN, esophageal dysmotility, cardiomyopathy, palpable tendon friction rubs (cracking/crepitus over tendon when flexing a joint), renal crisis, sicca syndrome
- May have early edematous phase (swelling of digits) and pitted scars from ulcerations from Raynaud's
- Anti-Scl-70 Ab
- #1 mortality = lung disease (previously most common was scleroderma renal crisis, less given treatment with ACEIs)
- #1 morbidity = GI

e. Treatments
- Systemic steroids + TCS initially then transition to steroid sparing regimen. HCQ or CLQ ± quinacrine, MTX, MMF, JAKi, IVIG, lenabasum, bone marrow transplant in recalcitrant cases

10.3.2 Lichen Sclerosus (et Atrophicus)

- Aka LS et A, LS&A
- "Ivory white" plaques; most common on genitalia (85%), then back
- May have hourglass/figure eight configuration (perivulvar + perianal)
- Some consider extragenital LS on the morphea spectrum
- Can have Ab to ECM-1 (in 80%)
- Note: increased risk of SCC (50% penile SCC associated with LS&A)

10

– Path: hyperkeratosis, epidermal atrophy, hyalinized papillary dermis, may have follicular plugging; can look like LP early
– Tx = superpotent topical steroids (rare situation where okay to use on genitalia every day). Some alternate with TCI if well controlled. Can use MTX or MMF in recalcitrant cases
a. Balanitis xerotica obliterans (BXO)
    – In male genitalia, especially glans penis; can cause urethral meatal stenosis
b. Kraurosis vulvae
    – In female genitalia

10.3.3   **Other Sclerodermoid Conditions**

a. Scleromyxedema
    – *See also Dermal: Depositional: Mucin*
b. Scleredema
    – *See also Dermal: Depositional: Mucin*
c. Eosinophilic fasciitis
    – Aka "Shulman's syndrome"
    – Rapid onset of "woody induration" of extremities with peripheral eosinophilia
    – "Groove sign" or "dry river bed sign" = vein depressions in indurated skin
    – Often precipitated by recent strenuous activity
    – Tx: similar to above with prednisone, HCQ, and MTX
d. Nephrogenic systemic fibrosis (NSF)
    – Aka nephrogenic fibrosing dermopathy (NFD)
    – Associated with gadolinium-based contrast agents (GBCAs) in chronic renal disease patients on dialysis and renal transplant patients
    – Pathogenic mechanism unclear, but gadolinium deposition has been detected in disease; in addition, clonal T-cell populations may play role in pathogenesis
    – Clinical: thick, indurated plaques symmetric on extremities, yellow sclerotic plaques extracutaneously in sclera of eyes; typically spares the face
    – Path: like scleromyxedema (but history of renal disease and no monoclonal gammopathy), CD34 + (unlike morphea)
    – Ddx includes scleroderma and scleromyxedema
    – Tx: UVA1 therapy may be an option if transplant not possible
e. Chronic graft versus host disease (GVHD)
    – *See also Vascular: Toxic erythema: Other reactive toxic erythema*
f. Chronic radiation dermatitis
g. Eosinophilia-myalgia syndrome
    – *See also Dermal: Eosinophilic*
h. Sclerodermoid porphyria cutanea tarda
    – *See also Vesiculobullous: Subepidermal blisters*

i. Acrodermatitis chronica atrophicans
  – Associated with *Borrelia*, ddx morphea
j. Atrophoderma of Pasini and Pierini.
  – Brown atrophic plaques with "cliff-drop" borders, no surrounding erythema like may see in morphea
k. Phenylketonuria (PKU)
  – Characteristic edematous scleroderma-like changes of the extremities, sparing the hands and feet

10.4 Rheumatoid Arthritis

- Destructive inflammatory arthritis; may be indistinguishable from a type of psoriatic arthritis, especially when Rf seronegative
- Associated with rheumatoid factor (Rf), anti-CCP antibody; can be seronegative
- Can be associated with LCV
- Bywater's lesions = vasculitic lesions on fingers that may resemble septic emboli or traumatic lesions
1. Rheumatoid nodule
  – Classically by elbows
  – Path: palisaded granuloma around fibrin
  – Rheumatoid nodulosis = accelerated formation of nodules due to initiation of methotrexate
  – Tx is by excision
2. Still's disease/Juvenile rheumatoid arthritis (JRA)
  – Can present with evanescent salmon colored rash
  – A diagnosis of exclusion, but typically see very high ferritin
3. Rheumatoid arthritis neutrophilic dermatosis
  – *See also Dermal:Neutrophilic*

10.5 Sjögren's Syndrome

- Dry eyes, dry mouth (Sicca syndrome)
- Associated with anti-Ro and La, anti-α-fodrin
- Can be associated with subacute cutaneous lupus, nodular amyloidosis

10.6 Other Autoimmune Connective Tissue Disease

1. Raynaud's disease/syndrome
  = Red, white, and blue from vasospasm in fingers; white from vasoconstriction; then blue from cyanosis, and red from reflex vasodilatation
  a. Primary Raynaud's (idiopathic)

10

   b. Secondary Raynaud's
      I. Connective tissue disease
      II. Vibration syndrome
         – May see in jackhammer operators
      III. Polyvinyl chloride exposure
   Tx: Amlodipine vs. nifedipine (1st line), sildenafil (2nd line), pentoxifylline, prostaglandins, SSRIs, endothelin antagonists, botulinum toxin in recalcitrant cases
2. Relapsing polychondritis
   – On ears, recognized by only affecting cartilaginous areas (spares lobes)
   – Can also affect nose, trachea (leading to tracheal collapse) and asphyxia, aorta (leading to aortic insufficiency)
   – Can be associated with MAGIC syndrome (Mouth And Genital ulcers and Inflamed Cartilage = relapsing polychondritis + Behçet's)
3. Mixed connective tissue disease (MCTD)
   – Associated with anti-U1-RNP Ab
   – Different from overlap of two concurrent CTDs
4. Polymorphous light eruption (PMLE)
   – ANA, Ro, La positive in 10–40% (Ro correlates best of all Ab with photosensitivity)
   – *See also Dermal:Inflammatory:Lymphocytic*

10.7 Non-autoimmune Connective Tissue Disease

Note: Verhoeff-van Gieson stain—stains elastin black, collagen red

10.7.1 Inherited Non-autoimmune Connective Tissue Disease

– Note: A thru E can be associated with elastosis perforans serpiginosa
a. Marfan syndrome
   – Defect in fibrillin-1 (cutis laxa = fibulin, Birt-Hogg-Dubé = folliculin)
   – Ectopia lentis (upward, mnemonic: look up because Marfan is tall)
   – Ddx MEN Type 2B, which is typically Marfanoid
   – Cultural note: some speculate that President Abraham Lincoln had Marfan syndrome (or MEN-2B), though it is unknown
b. Ehlers-Danlos syndromes
   – From defects in various collagens
   – Gorlin sign: ability to touch nose with tongue (10% of people can do this; 50% of Ehlers-Danlos)
   Types I/II = Classic
      – Collagen V, Tenascin X
      – Hyperextensibility, easy bruising

Type III = Hypermobility
- COL3A1, Tenascin X

Type IV = Vascular
- Defect in α1-chain of type III collagen
- Worst form; risk of arterial, GI, or uterine rupture
- Translucent skin

Type VI = Kyphoscoliosis
- Ocular problems
- Defect in lysyl hydroxylase

Type VII = Arthrochalasia
- Congenital bilateral hip dislocation

c. Osteogenesis imperfecta
- Several types, usually from defects in type I collagen
- Fractures, blue sclera
- Think: Elijah Price/Mr. Glass from Unbreakable/Glass movies

d. Pseudoxanthoma elasticum (PXE)
- Discrete yellow papules in flexural areas (classically, the lateral neck and axillae), "plucked chicken skin"
- Inherited defect in ABCC6 (Chr 16), which encodes an ATP binding cassette transporter (defect may allow accumulation of substances with affinity for elastic fibers)
- Path: calcium deposits on altered/clumped squiggly elastic fibers (black on von Kossa stain)
- May affect eyes; retinopathy with angioid streaks caused by calcification of elastic tissue in Bruch's membrane of the retina
- Increased vascular disease

e. Cutis laxa
- "Bloodhound facies"
- Defect in fibulin 4 or 5 (Marfan = fibrillin)
- Also may be from inflammatory disease, ID (*Borrelia*), plasma cell dyscrasias, medicines (penicillamine)

f. Homocystinuria
- Marfanoid habitus, ectopia lentis (downward; mnemonic: look down at urine), mental retardation
- Cystathionine synthetase deficiency
- Risk: vascular events

g. Buschke-Ollendorff syndrome
- Aka dermatofibrosis lenticularis disseminata
- Connective tissue nevi (soft yellow-skin colored papules)
- Osteopoikilosis = small sclerotic opacities in bones, typically in carpal bones, phylanges
- From defect in LEMD3, nuclear envelope

10.7.2 Acquired Non-autoimmune Connective Tissue Disease

a. Anetoderma
   – Localized loss of elastic tissue
   – Can be caused by penicillamine (breaks collagen/elastin crosslinks)
   – "Button-hole" sign
b. Mid-dermal elastolysis
   = Selective loss of elastic tissue in the mid-dermis often in trunk/neck/arms
   – Clinical: well circumscribed area(s) of fine wrinkling
c. Pseudoxanthoma elasticum-like papillary dermal elastolysis
   – Acquired elastic tissue disorder
d. Acrodermatitis chronica atrophicans
   – From *Borrelia afzelii*
e. Scurvy (vitamin C deficiency)
f. Perforating diseases
   – Including elastosis perforans serpiginosa (EPS)
   – *See also Keratotic diseases: Perforating diseases*
g. Striae (stretch marks)
   – Can be caused by Cushing syndrome (including exogenous corticosteroids), puberty, pregnancy, Marfan's, Ehlers-Danlos, MASS syndrome (myopia/mitral valve prolapse, aortic enlargement, skin and skeletal findings; ddx Marfan's)
h. Solar elastosis
   – Degeneration of elastic tissue from sun damage
      a. Favre–Racouchot syndrome
         = Nodular elastosis with cysts and comedones
         – Associated with UV and smoking
      b. Colloid milium
i. Piezogenic pedal papules
   – Painful herniations of fat through dermis of heels/wrists

Infectious Disease

Contents

© The Author(s), under exclusive license to Springer Nature Switzerland AG 2024
J. Lipoff and D. Ruiz Dasilva, *Dermatology Simplified*,
https://doi.org/10.1007/978-3-031-66739-8_11

11

Abstract

Many types of infection can affect the skin. In this section, infectious skin diseases are categorized by the type of infectious agent. Some listed infectious diseases may not typically have skin findings, but are included for clarity in understanding the categories of infectious diseases.

Keywords

Skin infection · Bacterial infection · Viral infection · Fungal infection

11.1 **Bacterial**

11.1.1 **Gram Positive Bacteria**

11.1.1.1 *Staphylococcus* and *Streptococcus*

I. Local cutaneous infection
   A. Impetigo (*Staph* >> *Strep*)
      – Aka impetigo contagiosa
      – Can cause post-*Strep* glomerulonephritis (not rheumatic fever), a significant cause of pediatric renal failure secondary to impetiginized scabies in the developing world
         1. Bullous impetigo (*Staph*)
            – *Staph* exfoliative toxin A, from *Staph* group 2, phage 71 against dsg1
            – Can be considered a localized form of SSSS
         2. Non-bullous impetigo
            – *Strep* > *Staph*
   B. Ecthyma
      – Ulcerated form of non-bullous impetigo in which the early lesion extends into the dermis to produce a shallow ulcer
   C. Bacterial folliculitis
      – Aka Impetigo of Bockhart (*Staph*)
      – *See also Acneiform Disease: Folliculitis*
   D. Furunculosis (follicular abscesses)
      – Deep folliculitis at bulb, usually *Staph*
      – Furuncle involves one hair Follicle, carbuncle involves Combination of follicles
      – *See also Acneiform Disease: Folliculitis*

E. Cellulitis
  1. Erysipelas
    – Aka "St. Anthony's fire"
    – Most common cause = group A *Strep*
    – Painful, often on face, though more on lower extremities
F. Necrotizing fasciitis
  – Type 1: polymicrobial (including *Clostridium*)
  – Type 2: group A *Strep* (~ 10%)
    1. Fournier's gangrene
      = Necrotizing fasciitis of the perineum and groin
        DDx Meleney gangrene (progressive bacterial synergistic gangrene, may be associated with *Staph*)
G. Blistering distal dactylitis
  – Usually solitary on fat pad of finger
H. Felon (Staphylococcal whitlow)
  = Painful abscess on fingertip
I. Botryomycosis
  – Chronic granulomatous infection, mostly *Staph* but also *Pseudomonas*
  – Splendore-Hoeppli phenomenon = eosinophilic, pseudomycotic structures composed of necrotic debris and immunoglobulin
J. Lymphangitis
  – Ascending red streaks
K. Perianal *Strep* (perianal cellulitis)
II. Systemic infection
  A. Toxic shock syndrome
    1. *Staph*
      – From phage group 1, many types
      – TSST-1 (toxic shock syndrome toxin-1), was originally associated with superabsorbent tampons
    2. *Strep*
      – From Group A Strep
      – Clindamycin may inhibit *Strep* toxin
  B. Staphylococcal scalded skin syndrome (SSSS)
    – Aka Ritter's disease
    – See primarily in children < 5
    – Can see in adults in context of renal failure (unable to clear toxin) or immunosuppression
    – Can present with erythroderma, scarlatiniform eruption
    – Caused by *Staph* exfoliative toxin A, from *Staph* (group ?, phage 71) against dsg-1
    – Path: granular layer split (unlike apoptotic keratinocytes in TEN, in entire epidermis)
    – *See also Vesiculobullous: Subcorneal blisters and Vascular: Toxic Erythema: Drug Eruptions: Scarlatiniform*

C. Scarlet fever
  – From Group A *Strep*
  – *See also Vascular: Toxic erythema: Scarlatiniform eruptions*
D. Rheumatic fever
  – From *Strep* pharyngitis (not from impetigo, linked to glomerulonephritis)
  – Erythema marginatum (ephemeral figurate erythema) in 11%
  – JONES criteria (J = Joints, O = heart/carditis, N = subcutaneous Nodes, E = Erythema marginatum, S = Syndenham chorea aka St. Vitus's dance)
E. Endocarditis
  – In native valves, often from *Strep viridans* (enterococci) > *Staph*
  – In prosthetics, usually from *Staph epidermidis*; IVDU: *S. aureus*
  Clinical findings:
  – Splinter hemorrhages (but remember, most commonly from trauma)
  – Osler's nodes = tender, erythematous papules/nodules with white centers on finger pads
  – Janeway lesions = painless, small hemorrhagic macules on palms/soles, from embolization of organism
F. *Strep* infection associated with guttate psoriasis

11.1.1.2 Other Gram Positive Bacteria

I. *Corynebacterium* (diphtheroid gram positives)
  Note: "The triad" are the first three
  A. Erythrasma
    – *C. minutissimum*, coral-red fluorescence from coproporphyrin III
    – Path: North/South stranding (vs. East–West of tinea versicolor) in stratum corneum
  B. Pitted keratolysis
    – *Kytococcus sedentarius*, does not fluoresce
  C. Trichomycosis axillaris
    – *C. tenuis* (Mnemonic: tenuously hanging on hair)
    – Superficial infection of axillary and pubic hair, cylindrical sheaths and beading of the axillary hairs
    – Ddx white piedra
  D. *Propionibacterium acnes* (formerly *Corynebacterium*)
  E. Diphtheria
II. *Bacillus anthracis*
  A. Anthrax
    – Black eschar (painless, unlike brown recluse bite), can have sporotrichoid spread
    – Need 3 factors for full virulence: protective, edema, and lethal factors
    – Protective factor + edema factor = edema toxin
    – Protective factor + lethal factor = lethal toxin

    – Edema toxin = impairs neutrophil function, affects water homeostasis, leading to edema

    – Lethal toxin = causes release of TNF-α and IL-1β

    – Tx = ciprofloxacin (for suspected systemic disease, does not affect cutaneous disease, which self-resolves), may use doxycycline for emergency prophylaxis

III. *Clostridium perfringens*

  A. Gas gangrene

  B. Necrotizing fasciitis, polymicrobial type

IV. Others

    – Mnemonic SNAP for treatments of *Nocardia* and *Actinomyces*: sulfa (Bactrim) for *Nocardia*, *Actinomyces* tx with penicillin

  A. *Actinomyces israelii* (Actinomycosis)

    = An anaerobic or microaerophilic gram positive, non-acid-fast organism that can cause suppurative abscesses, granulomas, sinuses

    – Cervicofacial actinomycosis ("lumpy jaw") usually from poor dental hygiene, injury, or procedure

    – Can also involve pulmonary, GI

    – Treatment = penicillin G

  B. *Nocardia* (Nocardiosis)

    = A filamentous, gram-positive, acid-fast organism

    – In immunocompromised can cause systemic disease, in immunocompetent, usually just skin

    – *N. asteroides*—most cases in US

    – *N. brasiliensis*—tropical/subtropical

    – Tx = Bactrim

    1. Actinomycotic mycetoma/Madura foot

      – Mostly caused by *N. brasilensis* and *Actinomadura madurae*

    2. Lymphocutaneous nocardiosis

      – Crusted papule or abscess after trauma

      – Can see sporotrichoid spread of nodules, tender LAD

    3. Superficial cutaneous nocardiosis

    4. Systemic nocardiosis

      – Can see chest wall abscesses, usually fatal

  C. *Erysipelothrix rhusiopathiae* (Erysipeloid)

    – Found in fisherman or people who prepare shellfish, meat, poultry, or fish; usually on hands

    – Tx = PCN

  D. *Listeria*

    Can be associated with extramedullary hematopoiesis (blueberry muffin syndrome), abscesses

11

11.1.2 Gram Negative Bacteria

11.1.2.1 Common Gram Negative Bacteria

I. *Neisseria meningitidis*
  A. Meningococcemia
    – Can cause purpura fulminans
      1. Waterhouse-Friderichsen syndrome
      = DIC, purpura, adrenal hemorrhage causing adrenal insufficiency
II. *Neisseria gonorrhoeae*
    – Aka "the clap"
  A. Disseminated gonorrhea/gonococcemia
    – Can cause tenosynovitis, monoarticular arthritis, pustule over joint, septic vasculitis
    – Cannot find organisms on gram stain, check blood cultures
III. *Pseudomonas aeruginosa*
    – Green pigment from pyocyanin
    – Can colonize wounds, can also cause angioinvasive infection
  A. Ecthyma gangrenosum
    – Macule/ulcer/eschar, an embolic lesion, usually on extremity (from septicemia)
    – Path: necrotic hemorrhagic vasculitis
    – Often in immunosuppressed, HIV, hematologic malignancy
  B. Otitis externa ("Swimmer's ear")
    – Malignant otitis externa usually in diabetics, unresponsive to local tx
  C. Hot tub folliculitis
  D. Botryomycosis
    – Chronic granulomatous infection
IV. *Bartonella*
    – 1st line tx = erythromycin
  A. Cat scratch disease
    – *Bartonella henselae*
    – Sporotrichoid spread
  B. Bacillary angiomatosis
    – *Bartonella henselae* and *quintana*
    – See more in HIV
    – Clinically can resemble Kaposi's
    – Parinaud's—ocular/glandular syndrome; when affects liver, can cause peliosis (more with *henselae*) = hepatic blood-filled cavities
  C. Trench fever
    – *Bartonella quintana*
    – Vector = pediculosis corporis
  D. Bartonellosis (Carrion's disease)
    – *B. bacilliformis* (endemic to Peru), transmitted by *Lutzomyia* (sandfly)

Two biphasic forms:
1. Oroya fever
   = Fever, acute hemolytic anemia
2. Verruga peruana (Peruvian wart)
   = Eruption of angiomatous lesions, chronic
V. *Klebsiella pneumoniae*
   A. Rhinoscleroma
      - *Klebsiella rhinoscleromatis* (subspecies)
      - Granulomatous infection of nose and upper respiratory tract
      - Path: parasitized histiocytes = non-lipidized "foamy" macrophages with small pyknotic nuclei/large vacuolated histiocytes with intracellular bacteria = Mikulicz cells (His GiRl Penelope)
      - Also Russell bodies (large eosinophilic homogeneous immunoglobulin-containing inclusions)
      - Tx = tetracycline (first line)
VI. *Calymmatobacterium (Klebsiella) granulomatis*
   B. Granuloma inguinale (Donovanosis)
      - Chronic indurated red fleshy ulcer/destructive infection, usually painless
      - Also nodular, cicatricial, and hypertrophic types
      - Most common sites = prepuce, glans penis
VII. *Vibrio vulnificus*
   - Usually in older men with chronic liver disease, DM, or immunosuppression
   - From raw seafood ingestion or skin injury exposed to seawater, causes hemorrhagic bullae of the leg/cellulitis
VIII. *Yersinia pestis*—"bubonic plague"
   - Vector = Rat flea, *Xenopsylla cheopis*
   - First line tx = streptomycin
IX. Tularemia
   - *Francisella tularensis*
   - Sporotrichoid spread, can have eschar
   - Most common form = ulceroglandular (punched out indurated ulcer and LAD); worst strain = A1b
   - Can resemble plague
   - Associated with rabbit contact, mostly from deer fly and tick
   - Concern about potential use in bioterrorism
   - Vectors: *Dermacentor andersoni* (American wood tick), *Amblyomma americanum* (Lone Star tick)
   - First line tx = streptomycin > gentamicin
X. *Haemophilus ducreyi* (Chancroid)
   - Purulent, painful, usually multiple ulcers, soft undermined edges
   - Path: "School of fish"
   - Hard to culture, so usually dx of exclusion
   - Tx = one dose of azithromycin or ceftriaxone

XI. Other gram negative bacteria
- A. *Salmonella*
  - – *S. typhi* (typhoid fever)—"rose spots"
- B. *Brucella* (undulant fever)
  - – Can get from raw milk
- C. *Burkholderia mallei* (Glanders)
  - – See only in people with horse contact
  - – Can have sporotrichoid spread
- D. *Burkholderia pseudomallei* (Melioidosis or pseudo-Glanders)
  - – Mostly in SE Asia, Australia
  - – Treatment difficult, broad spectrum abx
- E. *E. Coli (>Pseudomonas>Proteus)*
  - 1. Malakoplakia
    - =Chronic bacterial granulomatous accumulation in immunocompromised hosts
    - – Michaelis-Gutmann bodies = calcified intracytoplasmic phagolysosome
    - – von Hansemann cells = ovoid histiocytes with fine eosinophilic cytoplasmic granules
    - – Non-specific clinical appearance

11.1.2.2 Rickettsial Diseases

Tx: drug of choice = doxycycline; however, chloramphenicol in pregnancy (and no doxy for kids < 8 years old was traditional thought, now this is changing); sulfa drugs can exacerbate

- ▬ Pathologically, affects endothelial cells; it follows that rickettsial diseases may cause vasculitis
- ▬ Can be divided into spotted fever, typhus, scrub typhus, and other groups (see below).

Spotted fever group:
- I. *Rickettsia rickettsii*
  - – Rocky Mountain spotted fever (RMSF)
  - – Purpuric eruption, begins on wrists/ankles, moves centripetally (can involve palms/soles)
    Vectors: Major vector in most of US, not in mountains but in eastern states like NC = *Dermacentor variabilis* (American dog tick); In Rocky Mountains = *Dermacentor andersoni* (American wood tick); also, *Amblyomma americanum* (Lone Star tick)
- II. *Rickettsia akari*
  - – Rickettsialpox
  - – Infected via mite (*Liponyssoides sanguineus*) of *Mus musculus* (house mouse)
  - – On path may see "squiggle cells" = banded lymphocytes (non-specific)

- Tache noir = eschar
- Endemic to New York City (Bronx, Queens)
- Recent report of *R. parkeri* causing rickettsialpox

Typhus group:
III. *Rickettsia prowazekii*
- Epidemic louse-bourne typhus
- Brill-Zinsser disease = milder 2nd episode
- Vector = pediculosis corporis
- Reservoir = flying squirrel
IV. *Rickettsia typhi*
- Murine (endemic) typhus (flea-borne)
- Transmitted by cat and rat fleas

Scrub typhus group:
V. *Rickettsia tsutsugamushi*
- Scrub typhus
- Aka Tsutsugamushi fever
- From chigger (Trombiculid mite)

Other rickettsial diseases:
VI. *Coxiella burnetii*
- Q fever
- Transmitted by inhalation of aerosols
VII. *Ehrlichia chaffeensis*
- Ehrlichiosis
- Major vector = *Amblyomma americanum* (Lone Star tick), but also *Ixodes* (Lyme vectors)
- Organisms grown in small membrane-bound vacuoles in which they form colonies called morulae; can be seen on peripheral blood smears
  A. Human monocytic ehrlichiosis
  B. Anaplasmosis (human granulocytic ehrlichiosis)

11.2 Treponemes and Spirochetes

- The spirochetes, which include treponemes and others, are all gram negative bacteria
- Mnemonic for spirochetes = rat eating a BLT (rat bite fever and *Borrelia*, *Leptospirosis*, *Treponemes*)
  1. Treponemes
     a. *Treponema pallidum* = Syphilis
       - Aka Lues disease (pronounced [Louie's])
       - Path: psoriasiform and lichenoid dermatitis, thin rete ridges, usually increased plasma cells
       - Stain with silver stains (Warthin-Starry, outdated), *T. pallidum* stain (new gold standard)

– RPR = 91% sensitive, 95% specific; FTA-ABS 92% sensitive, 96% specific
– In prozone phenomenon (e.g. with high Ab titer as in HIV), may get false negative, so should request further dilutions
– Screen with RPR/VDRL (sensitive), confirm with FTA-ABS/*T. pallidum* antibody (specific)
– RPR: 1:8 or less = false positive (usually)
– Acute false positive = pregnancy, SLE, mono, leprosy
– Chronic false positive (> 6 months) = Lyme
– Treatment = benzathine penicillin
– Jarisch-Herxheimer reaction = febrile inflammatory reaction to release of endotoxins shortly after receiving therapy
– Successful treatment measured by 4-fold difference in RPR titer (this also determines re-infection if increased × 4)

I. Primary syphilis
= Primary chancre, erosion at site of primary inoculation, classically on coronal sulcus of penis
– 90% on genitals, 10% extra-genital, appears 9–90 days after primary contact, usually 3–4 weeks
– Could use dark field microscopy for definitive dx
– Serology positive 2–4 weeks after chancre
– Non-tender painless, regional non-tender bubo (LN)

II. Secondary syphilis
= Skin eruption with or without lymphadenopathy
– Occurs 6 weeks to 6 months (average 9 weeks) after chancre
– Can go into latent syphilis (only serologically positive)
– Of secondary syphilis, 2/3 develop latent syphilis, 1/3 develop tertiary syphilis
Clinical manifestations of secondary syphilis:
– Papulosquamous eruption that may resemble pityriasis rosea or psoriasis; classically involves palms and soles
– Condyloma lata = papillomatous papules/plaques, look like condyloma, resolve in 2–6 weeks, has the most spirochetes—teeming
– Split papules = fissured papules seen on angles of mouth, base of earlobe, etc.
– Mucous patches, "moth-eaten" alopecia, palm and sole papules and plaques (including "copper penny" spots) with collarette of scale (collarette of Biett), sparse eyebrows (madarosis), large annular syphilid, iritis
– Why not do a dark field on a mouth lesion? Because there are non-pathogenic treponemes naturally in our mouths (will be false-positive)
– Cervical, inguinal, and epitrochlear lymphadenopathy (easiest to palpate on exam, by elbows)

III. Tertiary syphilis
  = Gummas, neurosyphilis, or cardiovascular disease
  – Occurs months to years (4–20 years) after primary infection
  – 1/3 of those infected with syphilis get tertiary
  – Of this 1/3, 15–17% get cutaneous involvement (gummas); these can affect skin, bones, viscera (but not GI or GYN) and can appear as plaques, nodules, ulcers
  – Gummas = "gummy," granulomatous lesions, no organisms found, from delayed hypersensitivity?
  – Can see nasal destruction (saddle nose); ddx TB, syphilis, leprosy, rhinoscleroma, GPA, BCC
  – Arteritis in 10% of tertiary syphilis (aneurysms)
  – Aortic aneurysm (widened mediastinum on CXR)
  – Also, syphilitic glossitis, Charcot joints (enlarged knee with no sensation, osteitis, trauma)
  – Neurosyphilis: tabes dorsalis; tabes = "decay"; this is "decay" of the posterior columns
  – Argyll Robertson pupil = accommodates, but does not react (like a sex worker)
  – Three main forms of neurosyphilis:
  A. Asymptomatic neurosyphilis = only positive serology, would need to check LP
  B. Meningo-vascular = endarteritis leading to focal neurologic signs, stroke
  C. Parenchymatous = actual decay of brain or posterior columns; tabes dorsalis, "general paresis" = demented, optic atrophy
IV. Congenital syphilis
  Note: Hutchinson's triad = interstitial keratitis, Hutchinson incisors (small, notched, widely spaced), sensorineural deafness (CN VIII)
  A. Early signs
    – Parrot's pseudoparalysis, pneumonia alba, snuffles, syphilitic pemphigus, rhagades, Wimberger's sign
  B. Late signs
    – Clutton's joints, 'Mulberry' molars, saber shins, saddle nose
b. *Treponema pertenue* = Yaws (*Framboesia tropica*)
  – Can present with "amber yellow" crust; primary = "Mother yaw"
  – Nasal/palate perforation in tertiary yaws = gangosa
  – Species/name mnemonic = "y'all is pertinent"
c. *Treponema caruleum* = Pinta
  – Endemic to rural Central and South America
  – May cause hypopigmented and hyperpigmented patches
  – Species/name mnemonic—Pinto car
d. *Treponema pallidum endemicum* = Bejel or endemic syphilis
  – Most prevalent in northern Africa and Middle East

11

2. Borrelia
   – Note: *Borrelia* is thought to play a role in the etiology of many primary cutaneous B-cell lymphomas; also associated with pseudolymphomas
   a. *Borrelia burgdorferi*—Lyme disease
      Vector = Ixodes ticks
      I. Lyme disease
         – Causes erythema migrans, ddx Southern tick-associated rash illness (STARI)
         – Nerve defects (Bell's palsy in 10%), Cardiac (AV block in 5%), arthritis (in 60%, preferentially knee)
         – Caused by *Borrelia burgdorferi* (U.S.), *Borrelia afzelii* and *Borrelia garinii* (Europe)
         – Vector = *I. scapularis (aka dammini)* (US east coast), *I. pacificus* (West coast), *I. ricinis* (Europe)
         – Natural hosts = white-footed mouse, white-tailed deer
         – *B. garinii* associated with neurologic symptoms, *B. afzelii* associated more with cutaneous disease
         – Tx = doxycycline; in kids/pregnancy: amoxicillin, alternative—cefuroxime; in disseminated disease, tx with ceftriaxone
      II. Acrodermatitis chronica atrophicans
         – Hastened aging to atrophy of acral skin from chronic borrelial infection; ddx morphea
         – Caused by *Borrelia afzelii*
      III. Pseudolymphoma (Borrelial lymphocytoma)
   b. *Borrelia recurrentis*—relapsing fever
      – Vector = pediculosis corporis
3. *Leptospira interrograns* (leptospirosis)
   – Increased in flooding (e.g. post-Hurricane Katrina outbreak)
4. Rat-bite fever
   = Fever, rash, arthritis; tx with PCN
   – From rat bite or ingestion of rat-contaminated food or drink
   a. *Spirillum minus*—mostly in Asia
      – Sodoku—manifests 2–4 weeks after bite (milder)
   b. *Streptobacillus moniliformis*
      – Haverhill fever—1–3 weeks after bite
5. Alpha-gal syndrome
   – Relatively newly described condition that is a reaction to tick bites from Amblyomma and Ixodes
   – Bites lead to development of an IgE immune response to mammalian oligosaccharides (found in meats) that can cause urticaria, GI distress, angioedema, severe dermatitis or anaphylaxis after eating beef or pork (does not happen with poultry, fish)
   – Epinephrine, systemic steroids for acute episodes and trigger avoidance are only known treatments at this point

11.3 Fungal

11.3.1 Superficial Fungal

a. *Candida*
  – Budding yeast and pseudohyphae on KOH
    I. Cutaneous candidiasis
      – Markedly erythematous or erosive areas, may have fine white pustules, satellite papules/pustules, often in dependent or occluded areas
      – Predisposed by DM, occlusion, systemic abx
      – Ddx pustular psoriasis, AGEP
    II. Oral candidiasis (thrush)
    III. Erosio interdigitalis blastomycetica
      – Mostly caused by *Candida*
      – Finger/toe webspace superficial fungal infection
    IV. Granuloma gluteale infantum
    V. Angular cheilitis
      – Ddx vitamin B deficiency
    VI. Immunodeficiency disorders associated with candidiasis
      A. APECED syndrome
        – Autoimmune PolyEndocrinopathy Candidiasis and Ectodermal Dystrophy
        – Hypoparathyroidism seen in 90%
        – Can be associated with vitiligo
        – From defects in *AIRE* (*a*uto *i*mmune *re*gulator), encodes a transcription factor
      B. IPEX syndrome
        – Immune dysregulation, Polyendocrinopathy, Enteropathy and X-linked
        – Caused by mutations in FOXP3 gene → will lack FOXP3 + regulatory T cells (Treg)
b. Dermatophytes
  – *Trichophyton, Microsporum, Epidermophyton*
  – *T. rubrum* most common
  – Divided based on natural reservoir (humans, animals, soil): anthropophilic, zoophilic, geophilic
  – Septated hyphae on KOH
  – In tinea capitis, think *T. tonsurans* (#1 in US) > *M. canis* (#1 in world)
  – Growth of these fungi on plates and identification no longer clinically relevant as PCR has become prevalent and affordable with fast, high sensitivity results
    I. Tinea capitis
      – "Black dot" tinea capitis—from hair broken off at level of scalp within patches of polygonal shaped alopecia, with finger-like margins

11

- Usually not much inflammation, but some may develop follicular pustules, furuncle-like nodules, or kerion
- Clinically, may also see cervical lymphadenopathy
- Kerion = Tinea capitis presenting as pustular eruption/boggy plaque with alopecia, most common from *M. canis*
- Tx = griseofulvin in kids, griseofulvin/terbinafine/azole in adults

A. Endothrix
  - *T. tonsurans* (does not fluoresce)
B. Ectothrix
  - *Microsporum* and *Trichophyton*
C. Favus
  - *T. schoenleinii*
  - Scutula = yellow cup-like scale

II. Tinea pedis
  - Usually *T. rubrum*; bullous tinea usually *T. mentagrophytes*
  - Patterns: interdigital, moccasin, inflammatory/bullous and ulcerative, and "one hand, two feet syndrome"
  - Important to treat tinea pedis because it is a significant risk factor for cellulits (interdigital > onychomycosis > plantar); may create portal of entry for bacteria
  - Can even be part of cycle that leads to elephantiasis nostra verrucosa cutis (recurrent cellulitis → recurrent lymphangitis → scarred lymphatics → lymphedema and ultimately verrucous changes)
  - Cochrane review did not find any evidence any antifungals better than others for tinea, and though frowned upon by dermatologists, steroids (or combinations with steroids) may marginally improve clinical appearance more than antifungals alone

III. Tinea unguium (dermatophyte onychomycosis)
  - Classic description: "Thickened nail with subungual debris/hyperkeratosis"
  - Tx with terbinafine (1st line); also itraconazole, fluconazole (fluconazole best for older patients with polypharmacy, potential drug interactions and itraconazole best for recalcitrant cases)
  - Vick's VapoRub has been reported to help (has thymol herb/antiseptic); topicals generally considered to have insufficient nail penetration for treatment; some studies have tried lasers with minimal success; efinaconazole is the topical with the best data (still not fantastic)
  - Least likely to be *Microsporum*

A. Distal subungual onychomycosis
  - Most common pattern
B. Superficial white onychomycosis
  - *T. mentagrophytes*
C. Proximal subungual onychomycosis
  - *T. rubrum*

– Considered a marker for HIV (or immunocompromised state); this makes sense since this would be the most difficult location to invade with intact defenses

   D. Scopulariopsis
   – Non-dermatophyte, "beads on a string"
   – Other non-dermatophytes that can cause: *Scytalidium, Fusarium*

IV. Tinea corporis
   – Usually caused by *T. rubrum* (#1), *T. mentagrophytes* (#2)
   – *T. mentagrophytes* has anthropophilic and zoophilic forms
   – *Microsporum canis* (zoophilic) = transmitted from pet
   – Tinea incognito can result if treated with steroids
   – *T. concentricum* causes tinea imbricata (equatorial ring), which consists of polycyclic rings

V. Tinea cruris ("jock itch")

VI. Tinea manuum (on hands)

VII. Tinea incognito
   – Classic appearance of tinea altered by steroid, more difficult to diagnose

VIII. Majocchi granuloma
   – Deep dermatophyte folliculitis/foreign-body granuloma, may be predisposed to by immunosuppression, topical steroids; requires systemic treatment

c. *Malassezia (Pityrosporum)*
   – *Malassezia* is synonymous with *Pityrosporum*; the latter name was given to a new species, but later determined to be the same

   I. Tinea versicolor
      – Caused by overgrowth of normal flora, *Malassezia furfur* (and *globosa*); not contagious
      – Note: *M. furfur*'s = *Pityrosporum ovale/orbiculare*
      – Hyphal and yeast forms seen on KOH, "spaghetti and meatballs"
      – Hypopigmentation caused by release of a dicarboxylic acid (e.g. azelaic acid) from *Malassezia*; these are competitive inhibitors of tyrosinase
      – Treatment with anti-dandruff (antifungal) shampoos, azoles

   II. Pityrosporum folliculitis

   III. Seborrheic dermatitis
      – Implicated as potential etiology
      – Evidence has shown removal of yeasts with antifungals does lead to remission, and relapse associated with reappearance of yeasts

   IV. Neonatal cephalic pustulosis (neonatal acne)
      – Associated with *M. sympodialis*

   V. Confluent and reticulated papillomatosis (CARP)
      – Might be related to *Malassezia*, be a variant of tinea versicolor

d. Superficial phaeohyphomycosis
   – Black hyphae (dematiaceous = pigmented)

11

  I. Tinea nigra
       – Can mimic melanocytic lesion on palms/soles
       – *Hortaea werneckii* (formerly *Exophiala werneckii*)
  II. Black piedra
       Note: piedra = superficial infection of hair shaft, stones along hair shaft
       – Usually on scalp/face
       – *Piedraia hortae*
  e. White piedra
     Note: piedra = superficial infection of hair shaft, stones along hair shaft
     – Non-dematiaceous, usually on face/axillae/pubic areas
     – *Trichosporum beigelii*

11.3.2 Subcutaneous Fungal

  a. Dematiaceous fungi (pigmented)
     – Usually introduced by splinters into the skin
       I. Chromomycosis
            – "Copper pennies" aka Medlar bodies
       II. Phaeohyphomycosis
            – *Exophiala, Phialophora, Alternaria*
            – Another: *Curvularia* ("croissant" appearance)
            – Path: see brown hyphae (in contrast to copper pennies in chromomy-cosis), may see splinter
            – "Phaeomycotic cyst" = pseudocyst of palisated histiocytes
            – Can produce sporotrichoid spread
  b. *Sporothrix schenckii* (sporotrichosis)
     – "Rose gardener's disease," associated with sphagnum moss
     – Dimorphic fungi: yeast in tissues, mycelia outside
     – Path: pseudoepitheliomatous hyperplasia, cigar-shaped organisms ~ 5 μm, asteroid bodies (specific, rarely seen)
     – Treatment: first line = potassium iodide (SSKI) or itraconazole
     – Archetype for sporotrichoid (lymphocutaneous) spread
  c. Mycetoma/Madura foot
     – Three main factors: 1. Tumefaction (tissue swelling), 2. Draining sinuses, 3. Sulfur granules (in exudate)
     – Note: Madura is a region in India
     – Tx = excision and azole antifungals (eumycotic) or Bactrim/streptomycin (actinomycotic)
       I. Actinomycotic mycetoma (not fungal)
            – In Central and South America
            – Caused by filamentous aerobic and anaerobic organisms, e.g. *Nocardia brasiliensis, Actinomadura madurae*
       II. Eumycotic mycetoma (fungal)
            – In Africa
            – Caused by true fungi

III. Botryomycosis (not fungal)
– Caused by bacteria (*Staph, Pseudomonas*)
d. Protothecosis—*Prototheca wickerhamii*
– An algae (not a true fungus, but treated with anti-fungals)
– Clinically causes olecranon bursitis; on path: "soccer balls" (structure called a morula)
e. Lobomycosis—*Lacazia loboi*
– Aka "keloidal blastomycosis"
– Tends to be on head/neck, no systemic symptoms
– Primarily in Central and South America
– Also see in dolphins; ?transmission from dolphins
– Path: "chain-like beads"
– Treatment = surgery
f. Rhinosporidiosis—*Rhinosporidium*
– Path: may resemble coccidioidomycosis, but with much larger spherules
– Has been classified as protist > fungus, most cases from India and Sri Lanka

11.3.3 Deep/Systemic Fungal Infection

Note: CCHP (Cocci, Crypto, Histo, Penicilliosis) can appear cutaneously in HIV patients as masqueraders of Molluscum
- Cocci, Histo can be associated with erythema nodosum and erythema multiforme

11.3.3.1 True Pathogens

= Dimorphic fungi (25 °C mold and 37 °C yeast), Mold = room temperature, Yeast = body temperature (Think: "mold in the cold, yeast in the beast"); sporotrichosis is also dimorphic
I. Histoplasmosis (*Histoplasmosis capsulatum*)
– Aka Ohio valley disease
– Transmitted via bird/bat feces; caves/unoccupied buildings (where birds/bats live) are high-risk
– Can involve lungs > spleen > LNs > bone marrow and liver
– Misnomer—no real capsule, but has halo on path
– Check histo Ag (in urine)
– Can present with molluscum-like papules on the face in HIV patients
– Path: parasitized histiocytes; haloes, cell division by budding (Penicilliosis is by binary fission)
– Tx = itraconazole, amphotericin-B
1. African histoplasmosis
– *Histoplasma capsulatum var. duboisii*
– Larger in size on path compared to American
II. Blastomycosis
– Aka Gilchrist's disease

- In SE United States, in soil, can affect dogs
- Secondary cutaneous dissemination is common (unlike other deep fungae); may be first sign of disease
- Pulm > skin > GU/prostate involvement
- "Broad-based budding," 8–15 μm
- Tx = itraconazole, amphotericin-B

III. Coccidioidomycosis—*Coccidioides immitis*
- Aka San Joaquin valley fever (Southwest)
- Most virulent of fungi, usually pulmonary
- May see erythema nodosum, associated with favorable outcome (stronger immune response?)—first noted in famous case of Stanford medical student Harold Chope contracting Cocci from exposure in a lab by accidental inhalation in 1929
- Has very large endospore-containing spherules measuring 10–80 μm
- Filipinos have high susceptibility (175×)

IV. Paracoccidioidomycosis—*Paracoccidioides brasiliensis*
- Aka South American blastomycosis
- "Path: Mariner's wheel" = large "parent cell" spore with surrounding little buds all around, 60 μm
- Ulcerated lesions usually on face, in nasal/oral mucosa, called "moriform stomatitis"

11.3.3.2 Opportunistic Pathogens

I. Candidiasis (systemic)
- *C. albicans* most common, but *C. tropicalis* often implicated in fungemia in patients with leukemia

II. *Aspergillus*/aspergillosis
- Can be angioinvasive
- Species (with plates): fumigatus (fumes from a point—mostly pointing up from top) and flavus (like a favored lollipop—symmetric around point)
- Hyphae septated, typically at 45° angles

III. Zygomycosis—aka mucormycosis
- Typically in patients with poorly controlled diabetes/DKA
- *Mucor* and *Rhizopus* can be angioinvasive (much like *Pseudomonas*)
- These three can be distinguished by how the sporangium (flower) is positioned compared to the rhizoids (roots)
- Hyphae non-septate, typically at 90° angles (compared to *Aspergillus*)

IV. Cryptococcosis—*Cryptococcus neoformans*
- Can be acquired from pigeons; usually primary pulmonary infection disseminated to skin, rather than primary cutaneous
- Clinical lesions may vary from papulonodules to ulcers and abscesses, and may resemble herpes viral infections or molluscum contagiosum; lesions found mostly on head/neck
- Has gelatinous capsule, surrounded by halo, demonstrated by India ink preparations

– Check cryptococcal Ag (in serum)
  A. Cryptococcus cellulitis
V. *Pneumocystis jiroveci* (PJP, formerly PCP)
  – Treat with Bactrim
VI. Hyalohyphomycosis
  A. Fusarium (Fusariosis)
    – Usually in immunosuppressed; *solani* species may be worst type
    – Presents with erythematous painful papules and nodules
    – Can be angioinvasive
    – Voriconazole may be efficacious
  B. Penicilliosis (*Penicillium marneffei*)
    – Can present with molluscum-like papules on the face in HIV patients
    – Vector = Bamboo rat
    – Path: parasitized histiocytes; cell division by binary fission (Histo is by budding)
    – "Chandelier earrings" on wet mount
    – Mostly in Asia
  C. Paecilomyces
  D. Chrysosporium

11.4 Mycobacteria

11.4.1 Typical Mycobacteria

11.4.1.1 *Mycobacterium tuberculae* (Tuberculosis)

- PPD = purified protein derivative, a test of cell-mediated immunity (Th1) against TB; true positive indicates exposure
- BCG (Bacille Calmette Guerin) = a vaccination against TB that can cause false positive PPD
  I. Exogenous source
    A. Primary inoculation
    B. Tuberculosis verrucosa cutis
      – Aka "Prosector's wart," i.e. from autopsy
      – Represents reaction to inoculation in previously-exposed host
    C. Tuberculosis cutis orificialis (orificial TB)
  II. Direct extension
    A. Scrofuloderma
      – From lymph node direct into skin
  III. Hematogenous source
    A. Lupus vulgaris
      – Primarily from hematogenous spread > lymphatic, other
      – Apple jelly nodules = red-brown papules of gelatinous consistency (granulomatous non-specific)

B. Miliary tuberculosis
IV. Tuberculid eruptions (reactive to underlying TB)
    A. Papulonecrotic tuberculid
    B. Lichen scrofulosorum
        – Firm, typically perifollicular pink or yellow–brown scaly fine papules
    C. Erythema induratum
        – Nodular vasculitis/panniculitis associated with underling TB
        – *See also Dermal: Panniculitis*

11.4.1.2 *Mycobacterium leprae* (Hansen's Disease or Leprosy)

- Chronic infectious disease; has been targeted by the World Health Organization with much progress, but hundreds of thousands of cases still in the world, notably in India and Brazil, and still over a hundred new cases a year in the USA
- Fite stain may show organisms, lepromin skin test (like PPD)
- Notoriously difficult to culture; only possible on mouse footpads
- Only other animal that can get leprosy: armadillo, also maybe in mangabey monkey; most endemic human cases in USA have been associated with armadillo exposure (15% of nine-banded armadillos in Texas and Louisiana are infected, geography is expanding)
- Neurotropism is characteristic, leads to loss of hot/cold first, then light touch
- Organism prefers cooler areas of skin
- *M. leprae* has a unique phenolic glycolipid that binds to Schwann cells
- An estimated 95% self-cure, 5% develop one of three main types
    I. Lepromatous
        – Low cell-mediated immunity, many symmetric lesions, late nerve damage, Th2
        – Leonine facies, madarosis (loss of eyebrows)
        – Many organisms (poor cell-mediated immunity)
        – Path: diffuse dermal infiltrate of histiocytes (Virchow cells), Grenz zone, clusters of organisms = globae, may be neurotropic
        – Bonita leprosy ("Pretty" leprosy) = a form of lepromatous leprosy with infiltrated and shiny skin, in which the disease eliminates wrinkles and improves the patient's complexion
    II. Borderline (BL, BB, BT)
    III. Tuberculoid
        – High cell-mediated immunity, few lesions < 5, anesthetic lesions with no sweating, Th1
        – May have positive lepromin skin test (has cell-mediated immunity)
        – Can see palpable nerve cord (single) in close proximity to lesions → greater auricular, superficial peroneal nerves most common
        – Few organisms
        – Path: epithelioid cell tubercles (like sarcoid); few to no organisms, may be linear (following nerve)

IV. Indeterminate
   = Single hypopigmented patch with slight anesthesia; not well defined
V. Reactions
   – Caused by antimicrobial drugs, pregnancy, infection, mental distress
   A. Type 1 (reversal) reaction
      – Increase in cell-mediated immunity, known as "upgrading" reaction (more tuberculoid/Th1); since cell-mediated immunity is the "correct" immune response to trap the mycobacteria, it makes sense that more Th1 is upgrading or "better" and more Th2 is downgrading or "worse"
      – Type IV delayed-type hypersensitivity reaction
      – Seen in any form of leprosy
      – Can see acute neuritis
      – Tx = prednisone
   B. Type 2 reaction (vasculitis)
      – Formation of immune complexes with excessive humoral immune reaction
      – Seen in patients being treated for lepromatous leprosy
      1. Erythema nodosum leprosum
         – Favors extensor arms/thighs
         – Tx = thalidomide
      2. Lucio phenomenon
         – Reactional thrombosis and necrotizing cutaneous small vessel vasculitis (in Central/South America)
         – Tx = prednisone

11.4.2 Atypical Mycobacteria

- Can follow sporotrichoid spread
- Stain with acid fast stain (Ziehl-Neeson)
   I. *M. marinum*—most common
      – Swimming pool granuloma; has been associated with manicures/spas, cactus-inoculation
      – Sporotrichoid spread
      – Tx with minocycline
   II. *M. kansasii*
      – From cattle/swine
   III. *M. simiae*
   IV. *M. scrofulaceum*
   V. *M. szulgai*
   VI. *M. gordonae*
   VII. *M. avium-intracellulare* (MAI) complex (MAC)
      – Usually in HIV
   VIII. *M. malmoense*
   IX. *M. xenopi*
   X. *M. ulcerans*

11

  A. Buruli ulcer
    – Produces immunosuppressive protein, mycolactone
      = Painless, ddx pyoderma gangrenosum
    – Most patients are children under age 15
    – Note: Buruli is a county in Uganda
a. Fast growers/rapid growers (3–5 days)
  – Know these three! Mnemonic: Fast As a Cheetah!
    I. *M. fortuitum*
  – Associated with pedicures
    II. *M. abscessus*
    III. *M. chelonae*

11.5 Viral

11.5.1 DNA Viruses

Mnemonic: HHAPPPy DNA viruses
  Note: all of these are dsDNA viruses except Parvovirus (ssDNA)
a. Herpes viruses
  – HSV-1,2 and VZV can make umbilicated vesicles and pustules (poxviruses make umbilicated vesicles also)
  – HHV-1,2,3 = alpha herpesviruses (cause herpes)
  – HHV-5,6,7 = beta herpesviruses (CMV, roseola)
  – HHV-4,8 = gamma herpesviruses (oncogenic)
    I. HHV-1 and 2 = HSV-1 and 2 = Herpes simplex virus
      – Classic description = "Grouped vesicles on an erythematous base" (HSV and VZV)
      – Path = multinucleated giant cells, viral changes (margination of chromatin, so can have halo)
      – 3Ms = Margination, Molding, Multinucleation
      A. Orolabial herpes (HSV-1 >> HSV-2)
      B. Herpes gingivostomatitis
      C. Neonatal herpes
      D. Eczema herpeticum
        – Aka Kaposi's varicelliform eruption
        – Disseminated herpetic eruption developing on damaged skin (most commonly in atopic dermatitis, Darier's, ichthyosis, pemphigus, burns, MF)
        – Predisposed by topical tacrolimus/pimecrolimus
      E. Herpetic whitlow/Herpes gladiatorum
      F. Genital herpes (HSV-2 >> HSV-1)

II. HHV-3 = VZV = Varicella-Zoster virus
  A. Varicella (chickenpox)
    – Classic description = "Dew drops on a rose petal"; centripetal spread (head → trunk → extremities)
    – Pneumonia possible in adults
    – Lesions in different stages (unlike smallpox)
    – Congenital varicella → Highest risk 13–20 weeks (first trimester)
    – Neonatal exposure poses serious risk (5 days before to 2 days after delivery)
  B. Herpes zoster (shingles)
    – Can be indistinguishable from herpes simplex on exam (especially if near buttocks/genitals/face), but typically occurs within a dermatome and without a previous history, distinguishing itself
    – Hutchinson's sign = tip of nose, indicating involvement of nasociliary branch of V1 (ophthalmic nerve)
    – Ramsay-Hunt syndrome = involves facial nerve (CN VII) (geniculate ganglion), which innervates anterior 2/3 of the tongue, external ear canal; can cause deafness
  C. Disseminated zoster
    – In immunocompromised
    – Defined as more than 20 vesicles outside primary and immediately adjacent dermatomes
    – Visceral involvement in 10% (lung, liver, brain)
III. HHV-4 = EBV = Epstein-Barr virus
  A. Infectious mononucleosis
  B. Oral hairy leukoplakia
    – Very uncommon, typically on lateral aspect of tongue; may be sign of HIV infection, not pre-malignant
  C. Burkitt lymphoma (in Africa)
  D. Nasopharyngeal carcinoma (in China)
  E. Subcutaneous (panniculitis-like) T-cell lymphoma
  F. Extranodal NK/T-cell lymphoma, nasal type
  G. Gianotti-Crosti syndrome (possible association)
  H. Lipshütz ulcers
    – Ddx aphthous ulcers
    – Large vaginal labial ulcers associated with viral infection
    – *See also Dermal: Inflammatory: Neutrophilic*
IV. HHV-5 = CMV = cytomegalovirus
V. HHV-6 and 7
  – Can be associated with DRESS (HHV-6)
  A. Pityriasis rosea
  B. Roseola
VI. HHV-8
  A. Kaposi's sarcoma
    – *See also Neoplastic: Vascular*

  B. Castleman's disease
  C. Primary effusion lymphoma
b. Pox viruses
   – Like herpes viruses, these can make umbilicated papules
   – These are the largest animal viruses
   I. Molluscum contagiosum (Molluscipox)
      – MCV, molluscum contagiosum virus
      – Classic firm, umbilicated pearly papules
      – The largest virus known to infect humans
      – Can be giant or diffuse with predilection for the face in HIV
      – Intracytoplasmic inclusion bodies, aka Henderson-Patterson bodies (molluscum bodies), "bundles of grapes" on path or crush prep
      – Treatment = cryotherapy, curettage, irritant creams
      – Note: in two large RCTs, imiquimod shown to have no significant effect on molluscum in children
   II. Orf (parapox virus)
      – Aka ecthyma contagiosum
      – Associated with sheep/goat contact
      – Six stages (Mnemonic = PTARPR): papular, targetoid, acute (weeping nodule), regenerative, papillomatosis, regression
   III. Orthopox viruses
      A. Variola (smallpox)
         – Vesicles all in same stage
         – Centrifugal spread (extremities → trunk) vs. chickenpox, which is centripetal (trunk → extremities)
         – Last US case in 1949, last world case in 1977 (Somalia); now completely eradicated and only exists in labs in US (at CDC) and in Russia
      B. Cowpox
         – Used as the first smallpox vaccine by Edward Jenner; word "vaccine" derived from Latin word for cow: "vaccinus"
      C. Vaccinia
      D. Monkeypox (Mpox)
         – Pox virus, initially described in West and Central Africa
         – Presents as fever, followed by rash within 1–3 days, lymphadenopathy
         – Rash generally starts on the face and extremities (including palms and soles of the feet), spreads
         – Macules to papules (umbilicated)/vesicles/pustules then crusting over
         – May affect oral mucosa impacting PO intake
         – During recent outbreak, cases with minimal symptoms, rash starting in groin
         – Has predominantly affected MSM population (95%) in recent outbreak, can spread through any skin-to-skin, not just as STI

- Tx: Smallpox vaccination, isolation (5–14 day incubation); TPOXX (tecovirimat) if severe, antibiotics for superinfection, screen for all STIs

c. Papovavirus (Human papillomaviruses)

HPV-16 and 18 have most oncogenic potential

Gardasil (the quadrivalent HPV vaccine) covers HPV-6, 11, 16, 18

- Clinically, papules with rough, mammillated, hyperkeratotic ("verrucous") surface with black dots (from small thrombosed blood vessels)
- Path: all make coarse hypergranulosis, blue keratinocytes (from viral change), koilocytes (lage vacuolated cells in or immediately below granular layer)
- Compared to a corn, a wart is less likely to retain skin markings (it interrupts them), may hurt on indirect pressure (corn more on direct pressure) and will have black dots (corn will not)
- Mnemonics for HPV types: 3 points in a plane (planar warts), 7 looks like a cleaver (Butcher's warts), 13 is a curse (Heck's)
- *See also Keratotic disease: Hyperkeratotic eruptions*
  I. HPV-1
  A. Verruca plantaris (palmoplantar warts)
  B. Myrmecia (deep palmoplantar warts)
      - Myrmecia means "anthill"
  II. HPV-2, 4
  A. Verruca vulgaris (common warts)
      - Path: + koilocytes, papillomatosis
  III. HPV-3, 10
  A. Verruca plana (flat warts)
      - Path: + koilocytes, no papillomatosis
  IV. HPV-5, 8
  A. Epidermodysplasia verruciformis (EDV)
      - Inherited disease of abnormal susceptibility to HPV infections of specific types
      - Clinical: can look like generalized flat warts, tinea versicolor-like macules, lichenoid papules
      - Path: characteristic cells with grey-blue cytoplasm in epidermis
  V. HPV-6, 11—"Low-risk types"
  A. Condyloma acuminata (genital warts)
      - Can have multiple morphologies: macules, firm or pedunculated papules, "cauliflower" appearance
      - Tx includes cryotherapy, excision/curettage, imiquimod, podophyllin, TCA, green tea extract, 5-FU, topical and IL cidofovir
  B. Verrucous carcinoma
      - *See also Neoplastic: Malignant keratinocyte neoplasms*
      1. Giant condyloma acuminata
         (Buschke-Löwenstein tumor)
         - Large, locally destructive verrucous plaque, usually on penis > other anogenital

11

    2. Oral florid papillomatosis (Ackerman tumor)
- Warts in oral cavity, nasal sinuses
- May be promoted by smoking, radiation

    3. Epithelioma cuniculatum
- Verrucous carcinoma arising from a plantar wart on the foot

C. Recurrent respiratory papillomatosis
- Exophytic laryngeal papillomas that can cause hoarseness, stridor, respiratory distress (may be misdiagnosed as asthma)

VI. HPV-7

A. Butcher's warts

VII. HPV-13, 32

A. Heck's disease (focal epithelial hyperplasia)
- Multiple circumscribed papules on gingival, buccal, or labial mucosa, resembling flat warts or condyloma
- Increased prevalence in American Indians and Inuits (eskimos)

VIII. HPV 16, 18—"High-risk types"
- Mechanism of uncontrolled growth: E6 interferes with p53 braking of replication, while E7 binds to unphosphorylated Rb (tumor suppressor) to allow replication
- *See also Neoplastic: Keratinocyte neoplasms*

A. Bowenoid papulosis

B. Bowen's disease (SCCIS)

C. Squamous cell carcinoma (SCC)

d. Other DNA viruses

I. Hepadnavirus—hepatitis B
- Mnemonic for virus in name = HepaDNAvirus
- Associated with PAN, Gianotti-Crosti syndrome, PCT, vasculitis, urticaria, erythema nodosum, unlikely transfer by bed bugs

II. Parvovirus B19 (ssDNA virus)

A. Erythema infectiosum (Fifth Disease)
- Stage I = "Slapped cheeks," spares nasal bridge, circumoral
- Stage II = lacy, reticulated exanthem on arms
- Can get arthritis, more in adults
- Can affect fetuses in utero (anemia, hydrops fetalis, death); highest risk in first 20 weeks (especially weeks 13–16)
- Can cause aplastic anemia in patients with spherocytosis, sickle cell anemia
- Erythrocyte P antigen-deficient may be protected (cellular receptor for virus)

B. Papular-purpuric gloves and socks syndrome (PPGSS)
= Edema and erythema of palms and soles, with petechiae and purpura
- Burning and pruritus

III. Polyoma viruses

A. Merkel cell carcinoma
- *See also Neoplastic: Other epidermal neoplasms/hyperplasias*

IV. Adenovirus
   A. Viral conjunctivitis (pink eye)
      – Can have Cowdry B bodies (eosinophilic nuclear inclusions in adenovirus and poliovirus)
   V. JC virus
      – Can cause progressive multifocal leukoencephalopathy (PML) in HIV
      – Patients who were on the biologic efalizumab (Raptiva) were at increased risk for PML, pulled from market; has been reported in other biologics

11.5.2 RNA Viruses

a. Arboviruses
   I. West Nile fever
   II. Dengue fever
b. Paramyxovirus
   I. Measles (rubeola)
      – 3Cs = cough, coryza (runny nose), conjunctivitis
      – Koplik's spots on buccal mucosa
      – Morbilliform eruption = exanthem that starts on face/forehead/behind ears and spreads cephalocaudad, clearing in the order it appeared
      – Late manifestation = subacute sclerosing panencephalitis (SSPE) (neurologic)
c. Rhabdovirus
   I. Rabies
      – A neurotropic virus, has intracytoplasmc "Negri bodies," considered pathognomonic
d. Togavirus
   I. Rubella (German measles)
      A. Rubella
         – Associated with Forschheimer spots (petechial enanthem on soft palate, not specific)
      B. Congenital rubella
         – Highest risk in first 16 weeks of pregnancy
         – Cataracts, heart and CNS defects, deafness
         – In blueberry muffin baby ddx
   II. Chikungunya
      – Mosquito-borne disease with recent introduction to the US
e. Picornaviruses
   I. Enteroviruses
      A. Coxsackieviruses
         1. Herpangina
         2. Hand-foot-and-mouth disease
            – Caused by coxsackie A16, enterovirus 71

11

      – Mouth starts first, 2/3 get hand/feet involvement (small perhaps "football-shaped" vesicles), usually more anteriorpharynx, and on lateral hands

f. Retroviruses

  I. HTLV-1
- Associated with adult T-cell lymphoma/leukemia (ATLL)
- Also associated with HTLV-1 associated myelopathy or tropical spastic paresis (HAM/TSP)

  II. HIV

Skin disease associations:
- Candidiasis (thrush)
- Exuberant seborrheic dermatitis
- HPV infection/diffuse verruca vulgaris/condyloma acuminata
- Herpes zoster (and disseminated zoster)
- Molluscum contagiosum (giant, diffuse)
- Kaposi's sarcoma
- HIV-associated eosinophilic folliculitis
- Papular pruritic eruption of HIV
- Lipodystrophy—associated with protease inhibitors (specifically indinavir), NRTIs
- Bacillary angiomatosis
- Exanthem of seroconversion
- Oral hairy leukoplakia (EBV)
- Deep fungal infection (Cryptococcosis, Histoplasmosis)
- Reactive arthritis (psoriasiform)
- Proximal subungual onychomycosis due to *T. rubrum*
- Pruritus
- Stevens-Johnson syndrome (1000× greater incidence); other drug reactions with increased frequency also
- Acquired ichthyosis
- Exacerbations in psoriasis

g. Hepatitis C
- Mostly associated with intravenous drug abuse
- Transmission by needle stick injury most likely with hollow-bore needle and deep puncture

Skin changes associated with hepatitis C:
- Vasculitis (LCV and type II cryoglobulinemia)
- Porphyria cutanea tarda (PCT)
- Lichen planus—stronger association with mucosal/ulcerative LP
- Urticaria
- Cutaneous B-cell lymphoma
- Xerostomia
- Erythema multiforme (possibly)
- Pruritus (in 15% of patients with HCV)
- Necrolytic acral erythema

h. COVID-19 (coronavirus infectious disease 2019)
  – Caused by SARS-CoV-2
  – Associated with many possible cutaneous findings: morbilliform eruptions, pernio-like ("COVID toes" associated with mild disease), urticaria, macular erythema, vesicular papulosquamous, and retiform purpura (exclusively in ill, hospitalized patients).
  – COVID-19 vaccines have been associated with cutaneous findings: delayed large local reactions, local injection site reactions, urticarial eruptions, morbilliform eruptions. Many (43% in one series) recurred with second doses. Other reactions: pernio, cosmetic filler reactions, zoster and herpes simplex flares, pityriasis rosea-like reactions.

11.6 Sexually Transmitted Infections (STIs)

Note: don't forget to consider: psoriasis, lichen planus, fixed drug eruption
1. HIV
  – *See also Infectious Disease: Viral*
2. Gonorrhea
  – *See also Infectious Disease: Gram negative bacteria*
3. Genital herpes
  – *See also Infectious Disease: Viral*
  – Vesicles, erosions, ulcers (painful)
4. Syphilis
  – *See also Infectious Disease: Treponemes and spirochetes*
  – Primary: non-purulent, usually single ulcer, indurated, painless
5. Chancroid—*Haemophilus ducreyi*
  – Purulent, painful, usually multiple ulcers, soft undermined edges
  – Gram stain appears as "school of fish"
  – Tx = azithromycin or ceftriaxone
6. Lymphogranuloma venereum (LGV)
  – *Chlamydia trachomatis* serovars L1–3
  – Transient indurated ulcer, painless
  – Inguinal lymphadenitis (buboes): firm, enlarges, may be painful, and may rupture through skin; along Poupart ligament
  – Tx = doxycycline
7. Granuloma inguinale (Donovanosis)
  – *Calymmatobacterium (Klebsiella) granulomatis*
  – Chronic indurated red fleshy ulcer, usually painless
  – Path: parasitized histiocytes
  – Also nodular, cicatricial, and hypertrophic types
  – Tx = doxycycline

11.7 Congenital Infections: TORCHeS

- These can cause extramedullary hematopoiesis (blueberry muffin baby)
  1. Toxoplasmosis
     – Greatest risk in 3rd trimester, severity worst 1st trimester
  2. Other
     a. HIV
     b. Listeriosis
     c. Parvovirus
- Critical time is 13–16 weeks
     d. Varicella
- Highest risk 13–20 weeks (first trimester)
- Neonatal exposure poses serious risk (5 days before to 2 days after delivery)
  3. Rubella
     – Risk with maternal infection in first 16 weeks, very teratogenic
  4. CMV
  5. Herpes
     – Ascending in utero or at delivery; fetal scalp monitor risk factor
  6. Syphilis

11.8 Parasites

11.8.1 Protozoa

a. Leishmaniasis
   - Aka Baghdad boil, Oriental sore, Delhi boil, etc. etc.
   - Vector = sandfly (*Phlebotomus* in Old World, *Lutzomyia* and *Psychodopygus* in New World), mnemonic = the old phlebotomist
   - Obligate intracellular parasites that exist in two forms: the promastigote (in sandfly) and the amastigote (in histiocytes)
   - In histiocytes—supposedly see inclusions with kinetoplast (at 100×)
   - Sporotrichoid spread
   - Requires NNN (Novy-MacNeal-Nicolle) media for culture growth; can test with Montenegro skin test (like a PPD) (not really used); this has all been replaced by PCR (CDC has free kits)
   - Visceral leishmania mostly old world, mucocutaneous mostly new world, purely cutaneous mostly old world
   - Leishmania recidivans = recurrence at the site of an original ulcer, generally within 2 years and often at the edge of the scar
   - Tx = systemic fluconazole, cryotherapy, topical paromomycin, systemic pentavalent antimony (sodium stibogluconate)

I. New World (Central/South America)
   - Cutaneous leishmaniasis primarily from *L. mexicana*, also *L. panamensis*
   - Mucocutaneous leishmaniasis associated with *L. braziliensis*
   - Chiclero ulcer = most commonly on ear
   - Espundia = mucocutaneous leishmaniasis
II. Old World (Africa/Middle East)
   - Cutaneous leishmaniasis usually due to *L. major* or *L. tropica* > *L. infantum* (in Europe), *L. aethiopica* (in Ethiopia, Kenya)
   - Visceral leishmaniasis (Kala-azar) from *L. donovani*, *L. infantum* (in Europe in setting of HIV), *L. chagasi*; Mnemonic: visceral caused by species with an I (internal) on the outside (first or last letter)
   - Old World Leishmaniasis in US has occurred in vets returning from Iraq
b. Trypanosomiasis
   I. American trypanosomiaisis = Chagas disease (*T. cruzi*)
   - Romana's sign = unilateral periorbital edema
   - Vector = Reduviid bug ("kissing bug")
   - Chagoma = erythema/swelling at site of parasite entrance
   - Can develop CHF, toxic megacolon, achalasia
   - Tx = nifurtimox
   II. African trypanosomiasis = sleeping sickness
   - Winterbottom sign = posterior cervical LAD
c. Toxoplasmosis
   - Path: parasitized histiocytes
d. Amebiasis (*Entamoeba histolytica*)
   - Can cause ulcers or verrucous plaques
e. Acanthamebiasis (*Acanthamoeba castellani*)
   - An opportunistic amoeba in HIV

11.8.2 Helminths (Worms)

a. *Ascaris lumbricoides*
b. Enterobiasis (pinworm)
   - Classic perianal itching
   - Dx with scotch tape test
c. Ancylostomiasis (hookworm)
   - *Necator americanus, Ancylostoma duodenale*
d. Larva currens (*Strongyloides stercoralis*)
   - Generalized or localized urticarial eruption; may be serpiginous
   - *Strongyloides* infection may present severely in the setting of systemic steroids; may see thumbprint purpura
   - Tx = thiabendazole, ivermectin

11

e. Loiasis—*Loa loa*
   - Chrysops fly (mango fly) transmission
   - Can see in eye, episodes of Calabar swellings
f. Dracunculiasis—*Dracunculus medinensis*
   - From ingestion of infected water, water fleas (Cyclops)
   - Tx = gradual extraction of worm (on a stick)
g. Trichinosis—*Trichinella spiralis*
   - From raw/undercooked animal meat (usually pork)
   - Can see periorbital swelling (ddx heliotrope rash)
h. Cutaneous larva migrans
   - Larvae of hookworms that infect domestic dogs and cats (*Ancylostoma caninum* and *A. braziliense*)
   - Ground itch = caused by human hookworms (*A. duodenale, Necator americanus*), can involve internal organs (GI, pulm)
   - Stays superficial (in epidermis), since lacks collagenases to penetrate into dermis
   - Can move 1–2 cm per day
   - If also have pulmonary infiltrates, eosinophilia = Loeffler's syndrome
   - Tx = ivermectin, albendazole or topical thiabendazole
i. Onchocerciasis—*Onchocerca volvulus*
   - Aka "river blindness," second leading cause of infectious blindness
   - Can see "leopard skin" = depigmentation on shins with follicular repigmentation, "hanging groin"
   - Can see "lizard skin" or "elephant skin" = lichenified, hyperpigmented skin
   - Can also have onchocercomas = subcutaneous nodules that contain parasites
   - Transmitted by black fly (*Simulium*)
   - "Skin snip" test for diagnosis
   - Tx = ivermectin (caution DEC, which can cause Mazzotti reaction)
j. Filariasis (*Wuchereria bancrofti*)
   - Two major forms: Bancroftian (due to *Wuchereria bancrofti*) and Malayan (due to *Brugia malayi* and *B. timori*)
   - Vector = mosquitoes (multiple bites)
   - Adults live in blood, microfilaria in lymphatics
   - Can ultimately cause lymphedema/elephantiasis
   - Note: elephantiasis nostra verrucosa = verrucous cobblestone plaques from chronic lymphedema of any cause
   - Tx = diethylcarbamine (DEC), can cause Mazzotti reaction; ivermectin alternative
   - Ddx podoconiosis (non-filarial endemic elephantiasis), *see also Neoplastic: Lymphedema*
k. Schistosomiasis (*S. mansoni, japonicum*, and *haematobium*)
   - Swimmer's itch (cutaneous hypersensitivity reaction) = fresh water; clam digger's itch = salt water; these are self-limiting and do not need treatment
   - Mansoni = lateral spine/oval, Japonicum = no spine, round, Haematobium = terminal spine/oval

- Katayama fever (most common *S. japoncium*) = urticarial eruption, HSM, fever
- Squamous cell carcinoma of bladder—with *S. haematobium*
- Tx = praziquantel
l. Cestodes (tapeworms)
  - Head = scolex
  - When humans infected with larvae, can cause intestinal infection, no dissemination
  - When humans ingest eggs, shell disintegrates in small bowel, releases embryos that penetrate bowel wall, enter circulation, and disseminate widely, developing into larvae; when larvae die, can calcify (as in brain neurocysticercosis)
    I. Cysticercosis—*Taenia solium* (pork tapeworm)
      - Can see subcutaneous nodules, brain cysts
      - Tx = surgical excision of old cysts; praziquantel or albendazole
    II. Echinococcosis—*Echinococcus granulosis* (dog tapeworm)
      - Hyatid cysts in liver and lungs
      - Tx = albendazole
    III. *Diphyllobothrium latum* (fish tapeworm)
      - Can cause B12 deficiency
    IV. Sparganosis (*Spirometra*) (dog/cat tapeworm)
m. Myiasis
  - Pronounced [My ah sis]
  - *Dermatobia hominis* (human botfly), screw-worm, maggots
  - Classically, worm may emerge after lidocaine injection, or with occlusion of air pore by petrolatum
  - Most commonly in tropical areas of the Americas
n. Gnathostomiasis (larva migrans profundus)
  - Associated with eosinophilic panniculitis

11.9 Infestations

11.9.1 Arthropods (Insects)

- Usually have 6 legs
  a. Bed bugs—*Cimex lectularius*
    - "Breakfast, lunch, and dinner" = linear array of bites from an insect that crawls on the skin (mosquitoes bite all over since they fly)
    - May be able to transmit HBV (controversial)
  b. Lice (order Anoplura)
    I. Head lice—pediculosis capitis, aka "Cooties"
      - *Pediculus capitis*
      - Nits = eggs firmly attached to scalp hairs
      - Classically, intense pruritus

11

- Can see erythema, scaliness of scalp, posterior neck
- Tx = permethrin 5%, lindane (risk of CNS toxicity under age 2), and ivermectin (risk of CNS toxicity under 15 kg)

II. Crab lice—pediculosis pubis, aka "Crabs"
- *Pthirus pubis*

III. Body lice—pediculosis corporis
- Aka *Pediculus humanus var. corporis*
- Vector for louse-borne epidemic typhus (*R. prowazekii*), relapsing fever (*Borrelia recurrentis*), and trench fever (*Bartonella quintana*); Mnemonic = BRB, or body louse sitting in a trench, during the war (prowar), drinking (relapsing)
- Body lice eggs in seams of clothing; infestation requires an inability to wash clothes
- Maculae ceruleae = hemosiderin stained purpuric/blue macules from where lice have fed

c. Beetles

I. Blister beetles (order Coleoptera)
- Make cantharidin, a tx for warts

d. Fleas
- Flea bites present as intensely pruritic papulovesicles, usually located on the lower legs (they can only jump, cannot fly)

I. Human flea—*Pulex irritans*
- Shorter, has "lobster claws"

II. Dog flea—*Ctenocephalides canis*
- Has pronodal comb, looks like a "spiked collar"

III. Cat flea—*Ctenocephalides felis*
- Can transmit flea-borne endemic typhus
- Has pronodal comb, looks like a "spiked collar"

IV. Rat flea—*Xenopsylla cheopis*
- Vector for bubonic plague (*Yersinia pestis*)
- Can transmit flea-borne endemic typhus

V. Tungiasis
- Jigger/sand flea, "chigoe flea" = *Tunga penetrans*
- Usually on the feet, in much of the developing world
- Major complications: tetanus, gangrene

e. Flies

I. Sandfly
- *Phlebotomus* in Old World, *Lutzomyia* and *Psychodopygus* in New World
- Vector for leishmaniasis, bartonellosis
- Looks like a hairy mosquito; V-shaped wings

II. Black fly (*Simulium*)

A. Fogo selvagem (endemic pemphigus foliaceus)
- Implicated as a trigger (in Brazil)

  B. Onchocerciasis
   – Vector
 III. Tsetse fly
   – Vector for African trypanosomiasis (sleeping sickness)
 IV. Deer fly/Mango fly (*Chrysops*)
   – Vector for loa loa filariasis, tularemia
  V. Botfly (*Dermatobia hominis*)
   – Can cause myiasis; also caused by screw-worm
   – Can go deep, worms like necrotic tissue
f. Mosquitoes (3500 different species)
 I. Anopheles
  – Transmits malaria
 II. Aedes
  – Transmits yellow and dengue fever, has striped legs (Mnemonic: looks like from the 80s (Ae-des))
g. Reduviid bug (assassin bug)
 I. Chagas disease (American trypanosomiasis)
  – Unilateral eyelid swelling = Romana's sign
h. Lepidopterism—moths/butterflies
 I. Saddleback caterpillar—*Acharia stimulea*
  – "Tram tracks"
i. Fire ants (*Solenopsis invicta*)
 – Toxin = solenopsin
 – Papular/pustular eruption; they latch into skin, pivot around and make extremely painful pustules (they both sting and bite at the same time)

11.9.2 Arachnids

— These all have 8 legs
a. Spiders
 I. Black widow (*Latrodectus mactans*)
  – Red hourglass on back of females
  – Venom—latrotoxin (a neurotoxin)
  – Acute pain and edema at site; can then simulate acute abdomen, cause rhabdomyolysis
 II. Brown recluse spider (*Loxosceles reclusa*)
  – Venom = Sphingomyelinase-D
  – Violin on back
  – Bite can cause black eschar (dermonecrotic reaction)
  – Systemic reactions possible: hemolytic anemia, DIC
 III. Wolf spider
  – Aggressive, hairy like a wolf
  – Venom = histamine

11

    IV. Hobo spider (*Tegeneria agrestis*)
- Looks like wearing a fashionable fluffy hat, rabbit ears with furry balls
- Occurs in northwest US

    V. Jumping spider (*Phiddipus formosa*)
- Venom = hyaluronidase; mnemonic = jumps high

    VI. Tarantula (*Theraphosidae*)
- No venom; but can cause urticaria, ophthalmia nodosa (granulomatous reaction from hairs, can cause blindness)

b. Scorpion (*Centruroides exilicauda*)

c. Mites

    Note: nymphs may have only six legs

    I. Scabies—*Sarcoptes scabiei var. hominis*
- Norwegian (crusted) scabies = teeming with hundreds of mites (in immunocompromised)
- Check mineral oil preparation for mites, feces (scybala), and eggs; Path = look for mites, "curly Q"/pigtail in stratum corneum
- Tx = permethrin 5% (applied twice, a week apart), ivermectin (200 mg/kg, taken twice a week apart), all clothing/linens/towels (fomites) must be washed in hot water or stored in a plastic bag for 7–10 days; permethrin resistance has climbed significantly

    II. Demodex
- Species: *folliculorum* in hair follicles, *brevis* in sebaceous gland
- Usually incidental, can cause folliculitis
- Associated with rosacea

    III. Chiggers (Trombiculid mite)
- Vector for Tsutsugamushi fever/Scrub typhus
- Looks like a raisin with legs

    IV. *Liponyssoides sanguineus* (*Mus musculus* mite)
- Vector for rickettsialpox

    V. Cheyletiella
- "Walking dandruff"
- Compared to scabies, has longer legs
- Non-burrowing mite from cats, dogs, rabbits that can cause a dermatitis from bites

    VI. House dust mite

d. Ticks
- Bites have neutrophilic inflammation
- For tick identification (no longer tested but good to know):
  Ixodes—black legs, black cape, longer mouth part; no festoons, not ornate, no eyes
  Dermacentor—white cape or "bridal veil," short mouth part; festoons, eyes
  Amblyomma—has white spot on back aka "lone star," festooning, ridged pattern on edges; oval-shaped body, eyes, festoons
  Rhipicephalus—tear-drop shape, not ornate

I. *Ixodes scapularis* (deer tick or black-legged tick)
   – *Borrelia burgdorferi* (Lyme disease, East coast)
II. *Ixodes pacificus* (Western black-legged tick)
   – *Borrelia burgdorferi* (Lyme disease, West coast)
   – In Europe, *Ixodes ricinis* is vector for Lyme
III. *Dermacentor andersoni* (American wood tick)
   – RMSF (major vector in Rocky Mountain states)—Colorado tick fever
   – Q fever (*Coxiella burnetii*)
   – Tularemia
IV. *Dermacentor variabilis* (American dog tick)
   – RMSF (major vector of RMSF in US—not in Rocky Mountains, mostly eastern states like NC)
V. *Amblyomma americanum* (Lone Star tick)
   – Tularemia, RMSF, Ehrlichiosis, Q-fever
   A. Southern tick-associated rash illness (STARI)
      – Rash similar to erythema migrans after Lone Star tick bite, with minimal symptoms (fever, headache, joint pains), but none of the complications of Lyme
      – No identified cause, previously speculated to be from *Borrelia lonestari*
   B. Alpha-gal syndrome
      – Aka alpha-gal allergy, or tick bite meat allergy
      – Most associated with Lone Star tick bites, triggers red meat allergies in affected people
      – *See also Infectious Disease: Treponemes and Spirochetes*
VI. *Rhipicephalus* (brown dog tick)
   – RMSF, Boutonneuse fever, and canine ehrlichiosis

11.10 Other Bites and Stings

1. Seabather's eruption
   – From stinging cnidaria larvae of the thimble jellyfish (*Linuche unguiculata*), common in southern waters, or by planula larvae of a sea anemone (*Edwardsiella lineata*) off the coast of Long Island
   – In bathing suit distribution, requires pressure of clothing to cause
2. Swimmer's itch
   – Cutaneous exposure to schistosomiaisis, only in non-covered areas
3. Dog/cat bite—*Pasteurella multocida*
4. Human bite—*Eichenella*
5. Centipedes and millipedes (*Chilopoda, Diplopoda*)
   – Centipedes may inject a neurotoxic venom through venom ducts in the jaws
   – Millipedes do not bite (no jaws), but can cause a chemical dermatitis

Pigmentary Disorders

Contents

12

Abstract

Pigmentary disorders are characterized primarily by an increase or decrease in pigment. In this chapter, the type of pigment change is used to characterize these disorders.

Keyword

Hyperpigmentation · Hypopigmentation · Vitiligo

12.1 Hyperpigmented Conditions

12.1.1 Localized Hyperpigmentation

a. Melanocytic neoplasms
   – *See also Neoplastic: Melanocytic neoplasms*
b. Dermal melanocytosis
   – *See also Neoplastic: Melanocytic neoplasms*
c. Lentigines
   – *See also Neoplastic: Melanocytic neoplasms*
d. Café-au-lait macules
   – *See also Neoplastic: Melanocytic neoplasms*
e. Longitudinal melanonychia
   – Ddx includes racial predisposition, trauma, drugs, pregnancy, Addison disease, Peutz-Jeghers syndrome, Laugier-Hunziker syndrome, SCC, onychomycosis, benign nail matrix nevi, and melanoma
   – Of more concern if involves a single nail, or demonstrates signs concerning for melanoma (e.g. Hutchinson's sign with pigment extending onto the proximal nail fold, 6 mm width or over 40% of nail plate width)

12.1.2 Generalized Hyperpigmentation

a. Post-inflammatory hyperpigmentation (PIH)
   – Aka post-inflammatory pigment alteration (PIPA)
   – Melanin deposits in dermal melanophages secondary to inflammation
b. Erythema dyschromicum perstans (EDP)
   – "Ashy dermatosis" of blue-grey macules; may be post-inflammatory, some consider this a variant of lichen planus

- Path: vacuolar change, perivascular or interface lymphs, and melanin incontinence
- Increased incidence in Latin Americans
- *See also Papulosquamous:Lichenoid*
c. Lichenoid dermatoses
- These tend to leave more post-inflammatory pigment given the infiltrate along the dermal-epidermal junction
- *See also Papulosquamous:Lichenoid*
   I. Lichen planus pigmentosus
- A hyperpigmented form of LP that may may overlap with EDP
d. Pigment deposition
- *See also Dermal:Depositional:Pigment deposition*
   I. Ochronosis
      - Inherited/endogeneous form (alkaptonuria) and exogenous form (typically from long term hydroquinone)
   II. Hemochromatosis (iron deposition)
      - *See also Nutritional Disease*
   III. Argyria (silver deposition)
   IV. Tattoo (pigment deposition)
   V. Drug-induced pigmentary deposition
      A. Minocycline
         - Blue pigment indicates iron on path
         Type 1: blue-black at sites of acne, inflammation; Path = iron in dermis
         Type 2: blue-grey on normal skin; anterior legs; Path = melanin and iron in dermis/subcutis
         Type 3: diffuse muddy brown on sun-exposed areas; Path = increased basal layer melanin, dermal melanophages, no iron
      B. Amiodarone
         - Slate-gray photodistributed pigmentation
      C. Other medications
         - Clofazimine (lipofuscin), diltiazem, imipramine
e. Incontinentia pigmenti
- *See also Vesiculobullous:Intraepidermal blisters*
- Four stages: 1. Vesicular, 2. Verrucous, 3. Hyperpigmentation, 4. Hypopigmentation
f. Addison's disease (adrenal insufficiency)
- Hyperpigmentation, especially of sun-exposed areas, areas of trauma/scars, and creases/areolae/axillae/genitalia
- Cultural note: famous case of President John F. Kennedy, who had hyperpigmented skin likely related to his Addison's disease
g. Necrolytic acral erythema
- Hyperpigmented plaques on dorsal feet/heels, from Hepatitis C

h. Maturational dyschromia
   – Hyperpigmentation of the cheeks > rest of face in darker skin tones, particularly worsening with age and associated with metabolic syndrome
i. Riehl melanosis
   – Hyperpigmentation of the face, sometimes in reticulated fashion due to a pigmented contact dermatitis to cosmetic products

12.2 Hypopigmented Conditions

12.2.1 Localized Hypopigmentation

a. Pityriasis alba
   – *See also Eczematous: Atopic dermatitis*
b. Ash-leaf macules
   = Hypopigmented macules; in tuberous sclerosis
c. Pigmentary demarcation lines
   – Aka Futcher's lines/Voight lines/Ito lines
   – Normal variant; vertically oriented lines of change in skin pigmentation, typically noted in children, especially on the arms, noted more in darker skin

12.2.2 Segmental/Nevoid Hypopigmentation

a. Nevus depigmentosus
   = Blaschkoid hypopigmented (not depigmented) patch
b. Hypomelanosis of Ito
   = More widely distributed variant of nevus depigmentosus
   – Old name = incontinentia pigmenti achromians
c. Nevus anemicus
   – Hypopigmented macule that cannot become erythematous due to localized hypersensitivity to catecholamines (alpha-adrenergic always activated, so blood vessels do not dilate); donor-dominant
   – *See also Vascular: Other*
d. Incontinentia pigmenti
   – *See also Vesiculobullous: Intraepidermal blisters*
   – Four stages: 1. Vesicular, 2. Verrucous, 3. Hyperpigmentation, 4. Hypopigmentation

12.2.3 Generalized Hypopigmentation

a. Postinflammatory hypopigmentation (PIH)
   – Aka post-inflammatory pigment alteration (PIPA)
   – Pigment drop out in dermis post-inflammation

b. Tinea versicolor
   – *See also Papulosquamous: Pityriasisiform and Infectious Disease: Fungal*
c. Idiopathic guttate hypomelanosis
   = Common white spots in elderly, possibly related to UV exposure and aging
d. Hypopigmented mycosis fungoides
   – *See also Neoplastic: Lymphomas*
e. Progressive macular hypomelanosis
   – May be due to *P. acnes*
f. Phenylketonuria (PKU)
   – May have diffuse pigmentary dilution (from resultant tyrosine deficiency)
g. Leprosy
h. Sarcoidosis

12.2.4 Leukodermas (Depigmentation)

Note: poliosis = white forelock

12.2.4.1 Partial/Total Loss of Melanin

I. Oculocutaneous albinism (OCA)
   – From various mutations that cause decreased or absent tyrosinase activity
   – May see nystagmus on exam
   – Risk of melanoma increased in OCA (unlike decreased risk in vitiligo)
   A. Type IA ("tyrosinase negative")
      = Makes no melanin, extreme skin cancer predisposition, white skin/amelanotic nevi
      – Defect in tyrosinase
   B. Type IB and II ("tyrosinase positive")
      = Varied decreases in tyrosinase activity, can have amelanotic or pigmented nevi; one IB form has temperature sensitive tyrosinase
      – Note: Siamese cats all have a similar form of oculocutaneous albinism; their faces, ears, tail, and paws are darker because those areas are colder and so their temperature sensitive tyrosinase can function in those areas and make pigment)
      – Type II has defect in P gene
   C. Type III (Rufous)
      – Defect in TYRP1 gene
   D. Type IV
      – Defect in MATP gene
      – Common in Japan
   E. X-linked ocular albinism (OA1 type)
      – Only in males, only mild skin findings

12.2.4.2 Loss of Melanocytes

I. Vitiligo
  – Depigmentation from loss of melanocytes (unclear autoimmune etiology)
  – Most commonly presents on face, acral sites, genitalia
  – Can be segmental, localized/unilateral, generalized/diffuse
  – "Trichrome" = pattern of unaffected, hypopigmented, depigmented all in sequence
  – "Milk-white" on Wood's lamp
  – Repigmentation happens around hair follicles and then spreads (reason why acral areas so recalcitrant)
  – Can be associated with thyroid disease, pernicious anemia, atopic dermatitis, alopecia areata, APECED
  – Decreased risk of melanoma (3x decrease) (unlike albinism); perhaps etiology from overzealous immune surveillance of melanocytes? Current theory is that the immune response against the melanocytes may be offering protective effect against melanoma.
  – Treatments include TCS, TCI, topical and systemic JAKi (topical ruxolitinib approved) and NBUVB phototherapy/excimer laser, further intentional depigmentation with monobenzyl ether of hydroquinone (e.g. Michael Jackson's treatment for his vitiligo, obviously controversial), as well as surgical grafting (especially for segmental)
II. Vogt-Koyanagi-Harada syndrome
  – Disease that includes vitiligo, poliosis, uveitis, aseptic meningitis, ear problems

12.2.4.3 Defect in Melanosome Biogenesis

I. Hermansky-Pudlak syndrome
  = Defective trafficking of proteins to lysosomes and melanosomes (defect in biogenesis of lysosome-related organelles complex genes (BLOC))
  – Bleeding tendency (defective platelets – do not give ASA), interstitial pulmonary fibrosis, granulomatous colitis
  – Endemic to Puerto Rico
  – 4Ps = Pigmentary dilution, Platelet defect, Pulmonary fibrosis, Puerto Rico
  – No neurologic defect except in HPS2
II. Chédiak-Higashi syndrome
  = Abnormal vesicle trafficking results in giant organelles (uncontrolled fusion from LYST defect)
    – Phenotype = OCA with silvery gray hair, nystagmus, bleeding, immunodeficiency, neurologic problems
    – Giant melanosomes on path, blood smear with giant lysosomes in neutrophils
    – Hair with small regularly spaced clumps of melanin (may appear silvery gray)

12.2.4.4 Defect in Melanosome Transport

- These may present with silvery hair (along with Chédiak-Higashi)
  - I. Griscelli syndrome
    - Pigmentary dilution of skin and silvery gray hair due to pigment clumping within melanocytes
    - GS1 due to defect in gene for myosin-Va (important for transfer of melanosomes from melanocytes to keratinocytes)
    - GS2 due to Rab27A defect; can see hemophagocytic syndrome from uncontrolled T-lymphocyte and macrophage activation leading to death
    - Can have neurologic or immune abnormalities
    - Hair will have large clumps of melanin
  - II. Elejalde syndrome
    - Do not see immune defects

12.2.4.5 Defect in Melanocyte Migration

I. Waardenburg syndromes
  - From AD mutations in various transcription factors important in melanocyte development
  - Characterized by achromia of hair and/or skin, congenital deafness, partial or total heterochromia, synophrys (unibrow), dystopia canthorum (increased distance between medial canthi with unaffected interpupillary distance)

II. Piebaldism
  - From AD mutations in c-KIT or associated c-KIT ligand (steel factor, stem cell factor); these initiate melanoblast migration

12.3 Reticulated Pigmentation

1. Confluent and reticulated papillomatosis of Gougerot and Carteaud (CARP)
   - *See also Keratotic Disease:Papillomatous epidermal eruptions*
2. Macular amyloidosis
   - *See also Dermal:Depositional:Amyloid*
3. Notalgia paresthetica
   - Typically on upper, mid back
   - May have overlap with macular amyloidosis
   - = Focal, intense pruritus over medial scapular borders; see well-defined reticulated hyperpigmented patch
4. Melasma (chloasma)
   - Mostly in women, can occur in pregnancy, "mask of pregnancy" typically on the face, more common in skin of color population
5. Erythema ab igne
   - Reticular pattern from heat injury (e.g. heating pads)
6. Dowling-Degos disease
   - Reticulate pigmentation of flexures, K5 defect

– Path: digitate rete ridges ("antler-like"), horn cysts, basilar pigmentation, ddx seborrheic keratosis
  a. Galli-Galli disease
– Similar to Dowling-Degos, but with acantholysis
7. Prurigo pigmentosa
  – Recurrent pruritic eruption, typically on chest or back, may leave netlike pigmentation
  – Also has been associated with people on keto diets, popularized by people intentionally going into ketosis with their diets, and has been called "keto rash"
  – Commonly in Asians, responds to balanced diet and tetracyclines
8. Reticulate acropigmentation of Kitamura
  – Atrophic reticulate pigmentation on dorsal hands, palmar pits
9. Dyskeratosis congenita
  – Triad: reticulated hyperpigmentation, nail dystrophy (pterygium), and leukoplakia
  – Most common inheritance is XLR > AD, AR
  – *See also Vascular: Regional Erythema: Telangietasia: Genodermatoses with early aging, telangiectasia, sun sensitivity*
10. Naegeli-Franceschetti-Jadassohn syndrome (NFJS)
  – Hyperpigmentation of abdomen, periocular, perioral primarily; dental abnormalities, palmoplantar hyperkeratosis with absent or hypoplastic dermatoglyphics (fingerprints)
  – Defect in keratin 14
11. Dermatopathia pigmentosa reticularis
  – Defect in keratin 14, may be variant of NFJS; also may have absent dermatoglyphics

12.4 Mixed Hyper and Hypopigmentation

1. Follicular repigmentation in vitiligo
2. Scleroderma salt and pepper confetti patches
  – *See also Connective Tissue Disease:*Sclerotic disease
3. Leopard skin in onchocerciasis
4. Pinta
  – *See also Infectious Diseases: Treponemes and spirochetes*

12.5 Treatment Options for Hyperpigmentation

1. Hydroquinone (HQ)-based triple cream (HQ-tretinoin-TCS) qhs x 3-6 months very effective but need to take drug holidays for 3-6 months at a time to prevent ochronosis; may need to push the HQ up to even 12% in recalcitrant cases (pigmentary experts feel that ochronosis risk is highest with inappropriate continuous use > strength of the HQ)

2. Tinted sunscreen (mounting evidence that blocking visible light spectrum in addition to UV is very important in pigmentary disorders)
3. Topical and oral tranexamic acid (TXA)
4. Topical vitamin C, azelaic acid, kojic acid all with evidence (though weak, especially as monotherapy)
5. Polypodium leucotomos supplementation and topical cysteamine available over the counter adjunctive treatments
6. Procedures: microneedling, lasers, chemical peels (expensive and not always effective)

12.6 Treatment Options for Hypopigmentation

- Outside of vitiligo, there is no consistently effective medical therapy for hypopigmentation, but hypopigmentation can improve with tincture of time, sun protection, and minimizing of skin inflammation depending on the etiology

Keratotic Disease

Contents

© The Author(s), under exclusive license to Springer Nature Switzerland AG 2024
J. Lipoff and D. Ruiz Dasilva, *Dermatology Simplified*,
https://doi.org/10.1007/978-3-031-66739-8_13

13

Abstract

Keratotic diseases are clinically characterized by an accumulation of scale or hyperkeratosis. Many inherited disorders of keratin or the cornified envelope may lead to these diseases. Some diseases may be papillomatous without much clinically appreciable scaling.

Keywords

Ichthyosis · Palmoplantar keratoderma · Hyperkeratosis

13.1 Ichthyoses

Note: ichthyosis = "fish-like" scaling, from root "ichthys" meaning fish

13.1.1 Retention of Keratin (Retention Hyperkeratosis)

a. Follicular keratoses
   – Treatment with keratolytics (urea, lactic acid, salicylic acid, glycolic acid), also n-acetylcysteine compounded as topical (10% in 5% urea)
   I. Keratosis pilaris
      = Folliculocentric hyperkeratosis/follicular plugging; most commonly affects upper arms, thighs, buttocks, cheeks
      1. Keratosis pilaris rubra
         = KP with more erythema
      2. Keratosis pilaris atrophicans (ulerythema ophryogenes)
         = KP with atrophy, scarring alopecia
      3. Erythromelanosis follicularis faciei et colli
         = KP with erythema on cheeks/neck
         Note: Graham-Little syndrome
            – Includes LPP, KP, and axillary non-scarring alopecia
   II. Lichen spinulosus
      – Patch of grouped keratotic follicular papules
   III. Phrynoderma
      – "Toad skin," from vitamin A deficiency
b. Ichthyosis vulgaris
   – Most common disorder of cornification, most common ichthyosis
   – Hyperlinear palms, sparing of flexures
   – FLG (filaggrin) defect; decreased profilaggrin
   – Strongly predisposes patients to atopy (atopic dermatitis/allergic rhinitis/asthma)

c. Steroid sulfatase deficiency (X-linked recessive ichthyosis)
   - "Dirty neck," comma-shaped corneal opacities, cryptorchidism
   - Defect in cholesterol metabolism (fatty aldehyde dehydrogenase)
d. Axillary granular parakeratosis
   - Presents as scaly rash classically in axilla, but may be elsewhere
   - Path: unusually thickened stratum corneum with parakeratosis, retention of basophilic keratohyalin granules (?filaggrin defect?)
e. Acquired ichthyosis
   = May be associated with systemic disease: HIV (in 30%), malignancy (most common = Hodgkin's), autoimmune connective tissue disease, sarcoidosis, mycosis fungoides, drugs (nicotinic acid, statins)

13.1.2 Hyperproliferation of Keratin (Proliferative Hyperkeratosis)

a. Epidermolytic ichthyosis
   - Aka bullous congenital ichthyosiform erythroderma (BCIE)
   - On path, aka epidermolytic hyperkeratosis (EHK) = hyperkeratosis with "shot out"/messy granular layer (vacuolization of cells)
   - Clinically, erythroderma initially; later with accentuated skin markings (corrugated appearance)
   - Defect = keratin 1 and 10 mutation, autosomal dominant
   - Can sometimes see EHK in epidermal nevi; risk for phenotypically normal individual with EHK in epidermal nevus having children with epidermolytic ichthyosis (due to mosaicism)
b. Ichthyosis bullosa of Siemens
   - Ddx BCIE, EB simplex; appears as a milder form of BCIE
   - Only mild blistering at birth; can develop trauma-induced blisters, then hyperkeratosis in childhood, especially over joints/flexures, but sparing palms/soles
   - Characteristic feature = superficially denuded areas with collarette-like borders described as 'molting' or 'Mauserung', which develop due to superficial blistering and shedding of the stratum corneum
   - Defect in keratin 2e
c. Lamellar ichthyosis
   - May present at birth with collodion membrane
   - Mutation in transglutaminase-1, AR, defect in protein-lipid envelope crosslinking
d. Non-bullous congenital ichthyosiform erythroderma (NBCIE)
   - Deficiency of loricrin (same as Vohwinkel's with ichthyosis); also can have TGase-1 defect
   - On a spectrum with lamellar ichthyosis
e. Harlequin ichthyosis (Harlequin fetus)
   - Autosomal recessive, ABCA12 deficiency
   - Ectropion, eclabium, death as neonate

13

f. Collodion baby (ichthyosis congenital)
   - Taut, shiny, transparent membrane formed by thickened stratum corneum; resembles a plastic wrap
   - Tautness often leads to ectropion, eclabium
   - Seen in lamellar ichthyosis and non-bullous congenital ichthyosiform erythroderma, self-healing collodion baby, more rarely in some other genodermatoses
   - Babies at risk for hypernatremic dehydration
g. White sponge nevus
   - White plaques of oral mucosa
   - Defects in keratin 4 and 13 (specific to oral keratinocytes)

13.1.3 Genodermatoses with Ichthyosis or Erythrokeratodermia

a. Sjögren–Larsson syndrome
   - Autosomal recessive, fatty aldehyde dehydrogenase deficiency
   - Triad of ichthyosis (like NBCIE), diplegia or quadriplegia (scissor gait), mental retardation
   - On eye exam: perifoveal glistening white dots
   - Mnemonic = "fat Swede dancing with disco ball"
b. Refsum disease
   - From defect in PHYH or PEX7
   - Phytanic acid oxidase deficiency → leads to accumulation of phytanic acid leading to neuropathy and ichthyosis; disease might be stalled by restricting phytanic acid in diet
   - Ichthyosis (can be late-onset), atypical "salt and pepper" retinitis pigmentosa, cerebellar ataxia, chronic polyneuropathy, difficulty hearing
   - Mnemonic = "Deaf ref (black/white like salt and pepper) stumbled over (ataxia) and broke up the PHYH/phytanic acid (fight) then checked his PEX7 (pecs)"
c. KID syndrome (keratitis-ichthyosis-deafness)
   - Autosomal dominant, connexin 26 defect, GJB2 gene (same as Vohwinkel)
   - Symmetric erythematous hyperkeratotic plaques (erythrokeratodermia rather than ichthyosis), usually includes face/cheeks
d. Erythrokeratodermia variabilis (EKV)
   = Disorder of cornification associated with non-inflammatory erythema
   - Clinical hallmark: coexistence of transient erythematous patches and more stable hyperkeratosis
   - The erythema may present in large geographic/figurate patches (more in childhood), while the hyperkeratosis progresses
   - Mostly from defects in connexin 31 and 30.3 (genes GJB3 and GJB4)
e. CHILD syndrome
   - Aka Congenital Hemidysplasia with Ichthyosiform erythroderma and Limb Defects
   - X-linked dominant, NSDHL gene

f. Chanarin-Dorfman syndrome
   – A neutral lipid storage disease
g. Conradi–Hünermann–Happle syndrome (X-linked dominant chondrodysplasia punctata)
   – Defect = emopamil binding protein (EMP); in other types of inheritance, other defects can be found: peroxisomal enzyme defect PEX7 gene (AR), and arylsulfatase E (XR)
   – Erythroderma and linear streaks/whorls of hyperkeratosis; may spontaneously resolve in first year of life, replaced by bands of follicular atrophoderma
   – Follicular atrophoderma → patchy scarring alopecia
   – Skeletal abnormalities (stippled epiphyses)
h. Netherton syndrome
   – Types: ichthyosis linearis circumflexa and congenital ichthyosiform erythroderma (like NBCIE, but no collodion); presents with failure to thrive
   – Ichthyosis linearis circumflexa = "double-edged scale"
   – Autosomal recessive, LEKTI (encoded by SPINK5)
   – Trichorrhexis invaginata (bamboo hairs) most specific, though other hair shaft abnormalities seen
   – Avoid giving topical tacrolimus (Protopic), because of increased systemic absorption
   – Recent case reports of dupilumab and JAKi improving rash and pruritus

13.2 Palmoplantar Keratoderma (PPK)

Transgrediens = does not respect boundaries of palmar/dorsal hands
Non-transgrediens = does respect palmar/dorsal boundaries
When describing, think transgrediens versus non-transgrediens, diffuse versus focal versus punctate

13.2.1 Inherited Palmoplantar Keratodermas

a. Non-transgradiens inherited PPK (respects boundaries, limited to palms)
   I. Unna-Thost syndrome (non-epidermolytic)
      – Autosomal dominant, keratin 1 defect
   II. Vörner type (epidermolytic)
      – Defect in keratins 1 and 9
b. Non-transgrediens inherited focal PPK
   I. Howel-Evans syndrome (tylosis)
      – Focal PPK with esophageal carcinoma in British families, TOC gene (mnemonic TOC/talk from mouth)
   II. Richner-Hanhart syndrome
      = Oculocutaneous tyrosinemia type II

- Defect in tyrosine metabolism
- Painful palmoplantar hyperkeratotic plaques
- Photophobia, dendritic keratitis with corneal ulcerations (pseudoherpetic)
- Will develop retardation if diet not restricted (low phenylalanine and tyrosine diet)
- Mnemonic = Richie's hands and eyes hurt! Hanhart sounds like hands hurt

c. Transgradiens inherited PPK (does not respect boundaries)
  I. Vohwinkel syndrome (keratoderma hereditaria mutilans)
    - Autosomal dominant, connexin 26, GJB2 gene (same as KID)
    - Can have deafness, pseudo-ainhum (constricting bands with auto-amputation of digits), honeycomb palms, starfish keratoses of knuckles
    - Mnemonics = "Rip van Vohwinkel under the stars and a honeycomb," "Twinkle twinkle Vohwinkel"
    - Vohwinkel with ichthyosis = loricrin deficiency (same as NBCIE); no deafness in this form
  II. Mal de Meleda (keratoderma palmoplantaris transgrediens)
    - Autosomal recessive, SLURP-1 defect (transmembrane signal transduction)
    - Diffuse PPK, severe hyperhidrosis, and malodor
  III. Papillon-Lefèvre syndrome
    - Aka palmoplantar keratoderma with periodontitis
    - Autosomal recessive, cathepsin C defect
    - Ddx Haim-Munk
    - May have infections, including hepatic abscesses
  IV. Haim-Munk syndrome
    - Cathepsin C defect, autosomal recessive
    - PPK with severe periodontitis, arachnodactyly, onychogryphosis, and radiographic finger deformity
    - Ddx Papillon-Lefèvre (same defect, same PPK and periodontitis, plus nail/finger changes)
  V. Hidrotic ectodermal dysplasia (Clouston syndrome)
    - Autosomal dominant, GJB6 (connexin 30) defect
    - Affects hair and nails—alopecia, thickened nails, hyperkeratotic palms and soles; teeth, sweating normal
  VI. Bart-Pumphrey syndrome
    = PPK with knuckle pads, leukonychia, deafness
    - Keratoderma may resemble Vohwinkel
    - Defect in GJB2 (connexin 26)

d. Other inherited PPK
  I. Keratosis punctata of the palmar creases (PPPK)
    - Aka keratosis punctata palmaris et plantaris
    - Inherited punctate keratotic papules on palms/soles
    - Ddx pitted keratolysis (*Corynebacterium*)

II. Striate PPK
   – Defect in dsg-1 (also SSSS, bullous impetigo, pemphigus foliaceus)
III. Pachyonychia congenita
   – Thickened and extremely hard "pincer" nails
   1. Type 1 (Jadassohn-Lewandowsky)
      – KRT6a and KRT16
      – Associated with oral leukokeratosis
   2. Type 2 (Jackson-Lawler/Sertoli)
      – KRT6b and KRT17
      – Associated with steatocystoma multiplex, eruptive vellus hair cysts
      – Can have natal teeth
IV. Carvajal disease
   – Desmoplakin defect, autosomal recessive
   – Striate PPK, woolly hair, L ventricular cardiomyopathy
   – Mnemonic (L side of alphabet = C, D, L)
V. Naxos disease
   – Plakoglobin defect, autosomal recessive
   – Diffuse PPK, woolly hair, R ventricular cardiomyopathy
   – Mnemonic (R side of alphabet = N, P, R)
VI. Ichthyosis hystrix
   – *See also Keratotic Disease: Hyperkeratotic/verrucous lesions and eruptions*

13.2.2 Acquired Palmoplantar Keratoderma

a. Pityriasis rubra pilaris
   – *See also Papulosquamous: Psoriasiform*
b. Psoriasis
   – *See also Papulosquamous: Psoriasiform*
c. Darier's disease
   I. Acrodermatitis verruciformis of Hopf
      – AD genodermatosis—looks like planar warts on dorsal hands/feet
d. Bazex syndrome (acrokeratosis paraneoplastica)
   – Don't confuse with other Bazex syndrome (BCC syndrome)
   – Paraneoplastic syndrome associated with carcinoma, usually upper airway "aerodigestive"
   – *See also Neoplastic: Paraneoplastic syndromes*
e. Keratoderma climactericum
   – Associated with menopause
f. Keratolysis exfoliativa (recurrent palmar peeling)

13.3 Papillomatous Epidermal Eruptions

1. Acanthosis nigricans (AN)
   - Velvety thick brown plaques classically on posterior neck and axillae; may also manifest over joints of hands/elbows
   - Associated with obesity, diabetes (insulin resistance)
   - Path: hyperkeratosis, papillomatosis, acanthosis minimal or absent (a misnomer), may have basal layer hyperpigmentation
   - The papillomatous change in AN is similar to that seen in acrochordon; not a coincidence that they may come together
   - If sudden onset, can be paraneoplastic (GI cancers); on palms is called tripe palms
   - Can also be associated with nicotinic acid therapy
   - Tx = topical retinoids, topical vitamin D analogs, topical sirolimus, metformin, isotretinoin/acitretin (many use keratolytics but this is an epidermal hyperplasia not simply hyperkeratosis)
2. Confluent and reticulated papillomatosis (CARP) of Gougerot-Carteaud
   - May look like tinea versicolor, but papular, hyperpigmented, and reticulated
   - Path: hyperkeratosis, papillomatosis, acanthosis minimal or absent, may have basal layer hyperpigmentation
   - CARP and AN are identical on path.
   - Tx = minocycline, doxycycline, or azithromycin; topical sirolimus in case reports
3. Acrochordon
   - Aka skin tag/fibroepithelial polyp (FEP)
   - Ddx intradermal nevus, neurofibroma
   - Can see acrochordon-like lesions in Birt-Hogg-Dubé syndrome (but actually are fibrofolliculomas, trichodiscomas)
4. Dirt-related dermatoses
   - Both of these are easily removed by alcohol wipe
     a. Terra firma-forme dermatosis
        - Reticulate hyperpigmentation despite proper washing
     b. Dermatosis neglecta
        - Dirty dermatosis from neglect (often after nerve injury, surgery)

13.4 Hyperkeratotic/Verrucous Lesions and Eruptions

1. Seborrheic keratoses
   - Path: flat-topped papillomatous epidermis, horned pseudocysts
   Variants:
   a. Dermatosis papulosa nigra (DPN)
      - Common in African-Americans, as in the actor Morgan Freeman
   b. Stucco keratoses

    c. Macular seborrheic keratoses/solar lentigines

    d. Inverted follicular keratosis/irritated seborrheic keratosis
- Slightly enlarged keratinocytes with squamous eddies

    e. Clonal seborrheic keratosis

2. Verruca vulgaris
   - Caused by HPV-2 and 4 most commonly
   - Path: digitated papillomatous epidermis (pointy); spikes with dilated blood vessels, koilocytes, squamous eddies (whorls of eosinophilic keratinocytes)—also seen in SKs
   - Clinically, black dots from thrombosed blood vessels
   - Compared to corn; hurts more on lateral pressure, loses skin markings, has black dots

3. Clavus aka "corn"
   - Thickening due to intermittent pressure/friction forces
   - Compared to wart; hurts more on direct pressure, retains skin markings, no black dots
   - Callus = diffusely hyperkeratotic lesion

4. Actinic keratoses

5. Lichen planus-like keratosis (LPLK)

6. Cutaneous horn
   - Clinical pattern that may be seen in SCC, SCCIS, AK, SK, and verruca
   - Mnemonic SAWS = SK, AK, wart, SCC/SCCIS

7. Angiokeratomas

8. Warty dyskeratoma

9. Epidermal nevi
   - Can sometimes see epidermolytic hyperkeratosis (EHK) in individual epidermal nevi; risk for phenotypically normal individual with EHK in epidermal nevus having children with EHK (due to mosaicism)

   a. Inflammatory linear verrucous epidermal nevus (ILVEN)
   - May have overlap with psoriasis clinically; arises in early adulthood

   b. Nevus sebaceus
   - Hyperkeratotic plaque on scalp of infant
   - May see tumors arise within; #1 trichoblastoma, also BCC and syringocystadenoma papilliferum

   c. Epidermal nevus syndromes
   - I.   Schimmelpenning syndrome
     = Nevus sebaceous (one or more)
   - II. CHILD syndrome
   - III. Phakomatosis pigmentokeratotica
     = Nevus sebaceus plus papular nevus spilus
   - IV. Becker nevus syndrome (pigmented hairy nevus)
   - V. Nevus comedonicus syndrome
     = May have associated ipsilateral cataract
   - VI. Proteus syndrome
     - May have PTEN gene mutation (also seen in Cowden disease, Bannayan syndrome)

13

    d. Ichthyosis hystrix
        – Aka systematized verrucous nevus (a pattern rather than a disease)
10. Incontinentia pigmenti
    – Second stage (verrucous)
    – *See also Vesiculobullous: Intraepidermal blisters*
11. Flegel's disease (hyperkeratosis lenticularis perstans)
    – Multiple yellow-brown flat-topped keratotic papules, ddx stucco keratoses
    – Removal of attached scale can result in bleeding (unlike stucco keratoses)
12. Keratosis lichenoides chronica
    – Violaceous keratotic lichenoid papules, linear/reticulated on limbs/trunk; may have associated facial seborrheic dermatitis-like rash
13. Lichen amyloidosis

13.5 Prurigo and Lichen Simplex

Note: both prurigo nodularis (PN) and lichen simplex chronicus reflect chronic or habitual picking/scratching/rubbing changes to the skin; the itch typically precedes the rash. In the absence of an identified underlying disease, these entities have sometimes been labeled "neurodermatitis." Some dermatologists avoid this term given concern that it implies the patient has a psychiatric condition and is at fault. More recently PN has been associated with atopic dermatitis, and some consider PN a form of atopic dermatitis. Furthermore, the term "neuropathic pruritus" has been encouraged as patients are more familiar with neuropathy as a medical cause of several diseases.

1. Prurigo nodularis
    – Hyperkeratotic nodules with excoriations (sometimes just secondary changes from picking)
    – Similar to lichen simplex chronicus, but nodular
    – In patients with only secondary lesions on exam, consider work-up for underlying cause of generalized pruritus (CBC, BMP for BUN/Cr, LFTs, HIV, TFTs, hepatitis serologies, CXR for lymphoma, SPEP/UPEP, A1c, tryptase, BP180/230 with IIF, age-appropriate cancer screening)
    – May be a form of chronic eczema, *see also Eczematous*
    – Can be superimposed on other primary skin disease
    – Treatments include topical steroids, antihistamines, gabapentin and pregabalin, phototherapy, even thalidomide; dupilumab is the most recently approved medication
    a. Entities that may mimic prurigo nodularis
        I.   SCCs and keratoacanthomas (KAs)
           – *See also Neoplastic: Keratinocyte Neoplasms*
        II. Acquired perforating diseases
           – Some might argue these perforating diseases are simply a different manifestation of prurigo, *see also Keratotic Disease: Perforating Disease*

III. Pemphigoid nodularis
– Bullous pemphigoid presenting with prurigo nodules, *see also Ve-siculobullous: Subepidermal Blisters*
2. Lichen simplex chronicus
– A focal chronic lichenified/eczematous plaque from repeated rubbing/scratching, commonly on bony prominences (malleoli of ankles), posterior neck, anogenital area (labia majora, scrotum)
– Similar to prurigo, but usually more focal or solitary and appears as a plaque
– Path: "Hairy palm sign" = looks like acral skin (thickened), but has hair
– May be a form of chronic eczema, *see also Eczematous*
– Can be superimposed on other primary skin disease
3. Acne mechanica
– Caused by repeated rubbing under occlusion
a. Fiddler's neck
4. Athlete nodules
– From repeated minor trauma
5. Prayer nodules
– From constant praying in same position, typically in Muslim men on knees/forehead
6. Acanthoma fissuratum
– Aka granuloma fissuratum or spectacle-frame acanthoma
– Ulcerated nodule from areas of friction with ill-fitting glasses
– Ddx BCC, SCC, CNH
7. Chondrodermatitis nodularis helicis (CNH)
– Chronic tender ulcerated nodule on helix of ear
– Common in older males, ddx BCC, AK
– Path: hyperkeratosis and acanthosis with central parakeratosis over an erosion with underlying fibrin; may see cartilage

13.6 Perforating Disease

▬ These entities demonstrate transepidermal elimination of connective tissue
▬ Verhoeff-van Gieson stain—stains elastin black, collagen red; though in EPS, elastic fibers high up in dermis may lose ability to stain black
1. Reactive perforating collagenosis
– Path = transepidermal elimination of altered collagen
– May appear in childhood in inherited form or in adults in sporadic form
2. Elastosis perforans serpiginosa (EPS)
– Keratotic papules usually in a serpiginous or annular configuration, most commonly on the lateral neck
– Path = transepidermal elimination of elastic tissue

13

- Mnemonic for associated diseases = CART MOPED: Cutis laxa, Acrogeria, Rothmund-Thomson, Marfan, Osteogenesis imperfecta, PXE/Penicillamine, Ehlers-Danlos, Down's syndrome
- Also, associated eye finding: angioid streaks
- Angioid streaks mnemonic = PEPSI COLA: PXE, Ehlers-Danlos, Paget's disease of bone, Sickle cell, Idiopathic/ITP, Cutis laxa, Osteogenesis imperfecta, Lead poisoning, Acrogyria
- Penicillamine-induced EPS, "lumpy-bumpy" elastic fibers with lateral buds resembling a "bramble-bush" on EM

3. Acquired perforating dermatosis
   - Clinically manifests as nodules with a central hyperkeratotic plug
   a. Kyrle's disease
      - Pronounced [Curly's]
      - Aka hyperkeratosis follicularis et parafollicularis in cutem penetrans
      - Typically occurs in the context of chronic renal failure and diabetes
      - Ddx prurigo
      - Tx: keratolytics, TCS, ILK, cryo, phototherapy, isotretinoin, MTX, HCQ, doxycycline, butorphanol, dupilumab
   b. Acquired elastosis perforans serpiginosa
      - Can be caused by D-penicillamine
   c. Acquired reactive perforating collagenosis
   d. Perforating folliculitis
      - Controversial as an entity

13.7 Porokeratosis

- Recognized on path by *sine qua non* coronoid lamellae = a thin column of parakeratosis; underlying absent/reduced granular layer, dyskeratotic cells
- May be autosomal dominant in Mibelli, DSAP, and PPPD
- SCC reported in traditional variants (a thru d), but not punctate form; highest risk in older patients, linear lesions, longstanding lesions; DSAP has lowest risk
  a. Porokeratosis of Mibelli (classic porokeratosis)
     - In infancy/childhood usually; single plaque with keratotic, well-demarcated border
  b. Disseminated superficial actinic porokeratosis (DSAP)
     - Most common of the porokeratoses
     - Relationship to UV light controversial; almost never on face
  c. Porokeratosis palmaris et plantaris disseminata (PPPD)
  d. Linear porokeratosis
     - May appear along Blaschkoid lines, higher risk of SCC
  e. Punctate porokeratosis
     - Ddx punctate PPK, Darier's, arsenical keratosis

  f. Porokeratosis ptychotropica
- Keratotic or verruclous papules/plaques involving the gluteal folds of the buttocks

  g. Porokeratotic eccrine, ostial, and dermal duct nevus
- New name = porokeratotic adnexal ostial duct nevus

Nutritional Disease

Contents

© The Author(s), under exclusive license to Springer Nature Switzerland AG 2024
J. Lipoff and D. Ruiz Dasilva, *Dermatology Simplified*,
https://doi.org/10.1007/978-3-031-66739-8_14

Abstract

The role of nutrition in medical disease is often underappreciated, but it remains important. In the developed world, nutritional deficiencies are primarily seen in the context of alcohol abuse, post-op, fad diets, psychiatric disease, and bowel disease (e.g. Crohn's and ulcerative colitis).

Keywords

Nutritional disease · Nutritional deficiency · Vitamin deficiency

14.1 General Nutrition Deficiency/Protein-Energy Malnutrition

1. Marasmus
    – Deficiency of protein and calories ("polite term for starvation")
2. Kwashiorkor
    – Deficiency of protein; kids with ascites, big bellies from third spacing of fluid (without albumin, no vessel oncotic pressure)
    – Can produce peeling "enamel paint" on skin
    – Can occur in HIV/AIDS

14.2 Vitamin Deficiencies

Remember: ADEK = fat soluble vitamins, stay in body long-term; all others water soluble, hard to store (except B12 in liver)
- B vitamin deficiencies can be associated with cheilitis
    1. Vitamin A (retinol) deficiency
        – Vitamin A is involved in retinal photoreceptor function, epithelial proliferation, and keratinization
        – Nyctalopia (night blindness) = first manifestation
        – Keratinizing metaplasia affects epithelial surfaces
        – Phrynoderma = "toad skin," keratosis pilaris-like and crateriform papules with plugs
        – Keratomalaciasoftening/ulceration of cornea
        – Bitot spots = grey/white patches on the conjunctivae
    2. Vitamin B1 (thiamine) deficiency = beriberi
        – Coenzyme in many metabolic pathways, associated with Wernicke-Korsakoff
        a. Dry beriberi
            – Symmetric peripheral neuropathy
        b. Wet beriberi
            – Neuropathy and heart failure

3. Vitamin B2 (riboflavin) deficiency
    - Can be caused by acute boric acid ingestion
    - Oral-Ocular-Genital syndrome (cheilitis, photophobia, pruritic genitalia); on scrotum, spares midline
4. Vitamin B3 (niacin) deficiency = pellagra
    - 4Ds = diarrhea, dermatitis, dementia, and DEATH
    - Niacin needed to make NAD, NADP
    - Tryptophan is precursor; its deficiency causes pellagra
    - Hartnup's disease = inability to absorb tryptophan
    - Carcinoid tumordiverts tryptophan to make serotonin
    - Presents as photodistributed eczematous eruption
    - Casal's necklace = photodistributed erosions, hyperpigmentation in V of neck
    - Pellagra-like drug eruption may also occur from INH, 5-FU
5. Vitamin B6 (pyridoxine) deficiency
    - Can occur with INH (which is why B6 is given supplementally)
    - Photodermatitis, glossitis, and cheilitis (like pellagra)
6. Vitamin B7 or H (biotin) deficiency
    - "Fiery red" dermatitis
    - Can see in excessive egg white consumption (contains avidin)
    - Note: biotin sometimes given to improve nail/hair strength (doubt efficacy in patients without a deficiency, has been discouraged due to potential of disrupting certain lab results such as thyroid tests and troponin—the FDA issued a warning in 2019)
7. Vitamin B9 (folate) deficiency
    - Glossitis, cheilitis
8. Vitamin B12 (cyanocobalamin) deficiency
    - Can see atrophic glossitis, angular cheilitis, hair depigmentation, and cutaneous hyperpigmentation
    - Note: angular cheilitis more often seen from drooling, poorly fit dentures, *Candida*
    - French name for angular cheilitis = perleche
9. Vitamin C deficiency (scurvy)
    - Required for the hydroxylation of lysine and proline (lysyl and prolyl hydroxylase) residues on procollagen
    - Perifollicular hemorrhages, corkscrew hairs, gingival hemorrhage
    - 4 Hs: hemorrhage, hyperkeratosis, hypochondriasis, hematologic abnormalities
10. Vitamin D (calcitriol) deficiency
    - Minimal UVB light required for synthesis of pre-D_3, however, vitamin D can be obtained most safely through the diet or supplementation
    - Liver makes 25-D_3; converted by kidney to 1,25-D_3
    - Vitamin D supplementation recommended for babies exclusively fed breast milk
    - Only skin finding: alopecia

a. Rickets in kids

b. Osteomalacia in adults

Note: Calcipotriene (Dovonex) is a 1,25-D_3 analog (has an immunomodulatory effect not well understood)

11. Vitamin K deficiency
    – Required for factors II, VII, IX, X, proteins C and S
    – Easy bruising, bleeding, petechiae
    – Can see in newborns

14.3 Hypervitaminosis/Vitamin Excess

1. Hypervitaminosis A
   – Similar to retinoid side effects (dry, scaly skin; cheilitis)
   – Most serious: retarded bone growth, liver cirrhosis (chronic), pseudotumor cerebri (like with retinoids)
   – Can get from retinoids, overdose of supplements, trivia: risk from eating bear liver
2. Hypervitaminosis D
   – Can cause metastatic calcification
   – *See also Dermal: Depositional: Calcium*
3. Carotenemia
   – Excessive intake leads to yellow-orange pigmentation
   – Spares mucous membranes (unlike jaundice)
   – Does not cause hypervitaminosis A

14.4 Mineral Deficiencies

1. Zinc deficiency
   Signs: alopecia, diarrhea, lethargy, and an acute eczematous and erosive dermatitis favoring acral areas
   – Typical patient = renal failure, alcoholic cirrhosis
   – Check Zn level (RBC Zn level) and alkaline phosphatase
   – Usually appears within 1–2 weeks weaning off breastfeeding, or 4–10 weeks of age if bottle-fed
   – Can lose sense of smell/taste
   – Zinc has been used as treatment for hidradenitis suppurativa (related to zinc deficiency?)
     a. Acrodermatitis enteropathica (inherited zinc deficiency)
        – Mutations in zinc transporter SLC39A4
     Can see similar (or concomitant with zinc deficiency):
     b. Necrolytic migratory erythema (glucagonoma syndrome)
        – *See also Neoplastic: Paraneoplastic syndromes*

    c. Necrolytic acral erythema
       – Hyperpigmented plaques on dorsal feet/heels, from Hepatitis C
2. Copper deficiency
  Note: Copper-dependent enzyme lysyl oxidase is essential for cross-linking of collagen and elastin.
    a. Menkes kinky hair
       – Defect in ATP7A, impaired copper transport, XLR
       – Note: Wilson's disease is defect in ATP7B
       – Classic finding of pili torti (twisted hair), but can also see monilethrix, trichorrhexis nodosa
    b. Copper chelation by penicillamine
       – Can cause PXE, EPS, acquired cutis laxa, pemphigus foliaceus-like drug eruption
       – A treatment for Wilson's disease
3. Iron deficiency
   – Koilonychia, brittle hairs and alopecia, mucous membranes
4. Sulfur deficiency
    a. Trichothiodystrophy
       – Autosomal recessive, sulfur-deficient brittle hair
       – "Tiger-tail banding" on hairs
       – DNA-repair gene mutations
       – Severe neurologic and developmental abnormalities
       – PIBIDS = photosensitivity, ichthyosis, brittle hair, infertility, developmental delay, short stature

14.5 Mineral Excess

1. Copper excess
    a. Wilson's disease
       – Kayser-Fleischer rings in iris, defect in ATP7B
       – Tx = D-penicillamine (can cause reactions, anetoderma)
    b. Green hair (chlortrichosis)
       – Can see in swimmers, from copper concentrating in hair
       – Tx = shampoo with penicillamine
2. Iron excess
    a. Hemochromatosis
       – Aka "bronze diabetes"
       – Causes hyperpigmentation, ichthyotic changes
       – Associated with liver cirrhosis, diabetes, cardiomyopathy
3. Mercury excess
    a. Pink disease
       – Can cause paresthesias in the hands

14

4. Silver excess
   a. Argyria (silver deposition)
      – Blue-gray discoloration
      – From topical application of silver sulfadiazine or from systemic ingestion of silver
      – Path: peri-eccrine deposition of silver salts

14.6 Other Deficiencies/Excesses

Note: tyrosine and phenylalanine necessary to make melanin
1. Essential fatty acid deficiency
   – Only need 2 = linoleic acid (important for skin), α-linoleic acid
2. Phenylketonuria (PKU)
   – Defect in phenylalanine metabolism
   – Characteristic edematous sclerotic disease of the extremities, sparing the hands and feet
   – May have diffuse pigmentary dilution (from resultant tyrosine deficiency)
   – May initially present with early infantile eczema
3. Oculocutaneous tyrosinemia type II (Richner-Hanhart syndrome)
   – Defect in tyrosine metabolism (excess of tyrosine)
   – Painful palmoplantar hyperkeratotic plaques
   – Photophobia, dendritic keratitis with corneal ulcerations (pseudoherpetic)
   – Will develop retardation if diet not restricted (low phenylalanine and tyrosine diet)
   – Mnemonic = Richie's hands and eyes hurt!
   – *See also Keratotic Disease: Palmoplantar keratoderma*
4. Phytanic acid oxidase deficiency (Refsum disease)
   – Leads to accumulation of phytanic acid leading to neuropathy and ichthyosis; disease might be stalled by restricting phytanic acid in diet
   – *See also Keratotic Disease: Ichthyosis: Genodermatoses associated with ichthyosis*
5. Hartnup's disease (tryptophan deficiency leading to pellagra)

14.7 Other Diseases Associated with Malnutrition

1. Noma
   – Aka cancrum oris, necrotizing ulcerative stomatitis/gingivitis
   – A gangrenous condition of the face of young children ages 1–4; thought to be polymicrobial, seen only in developing world with severe nutritional deficiency

Lists and Mnemonics

Lists, Common Differential Diagnoses, and Mnemonics

Contents

© The Author(s), under exclusive license to Springer Nature Switzerland AG 2024
J. Lipoff and D. Ruiz Dasilva, *Dermatology Simplified*,
https://doi.org/10.1007/978-3-031-66739-8_15

Abstract

This chapter contains different groupings and listings of diseases and findings for the purposes of better learning and memorization. Hopefully these differentials, lists, and mnemonics are helpful to you!

Keywords

Lists · Differentials · Acronyms · Mnemonics

15.1 Differentials

15.1.1 Triads and Near-Triads

Triads are useful ways to remember common differential diagnoses for specific presentations. They are not meant to be complete, but rather to assist with quick recall of top possibilities. The mind has trouble recalling more than three or four options, so these help distill certain differentials for better memory.

FLESHY EXOPHYTIC PAPULE

- Acrochordon
- Intradermal nevus
- Neurofibroma

SOLITARY NODULE IN A CHILD

- Spitz nevus
- JXG
- Mastocytoma

SUPERFICIAL PUSTULES

- Candidiasis
- Pustular psoriasis
- AGEP

MOST COMMON KOEBNERIZING DISEASES

- Psoriasis
- Lichen planus
- Lichen nitidus

RETICULATED ERYTHEMA

- Parvovirus (Fifth's disease aka erythema infectiosum)
- Erythema marginatum (rheumatic fever)

15

– Still's disease
Also, erythema ab igne (more brown/violaceous)

SALT AND PEPPER PATCH DDX

Follicular repigmentation in vitiligo
Scleroderma salt and pepper confetti patches
Leopard skin in onchocerciasis

TRACHYONYCHIA (20 nail dystrophy)

Lichen planus
Psoriasis
Alopecia areata

CYSTIC PAPULES ON TEENAGER'S CHEST

Acne
Eruptive vellus hair cysts
Steatocystoma multiplex

FACIAL RASH IN A NEONATE

Seborrheic dermatitis
Atopic dermatitis
Neonatal lupus
Less likely:
Psoriasis
Langerhans cell histiocytosis

HELIOTROPE RASH DDX

Dermatomyositis
Contact dermatitis (think volatiles like nail polish on eyelids)
Trichinosis

CAUSES OF MACROGLOSSIA

Mnemonic = AAA
Amyloidosis
Angioedema
Acromegaly

YELLOW WAXY PERIORBITAL PAPULES

– Syringomas
– NXG
– Amyloidosis
– Xanthelasma

DERMAL PAPULES IN A TATTOO

Allergic reaction to tattoo dye
Sarcoidosis
Keloids/scarring
Atypical mycobacterial infection

MIDLINE FACIAL NODULE IN CHILD

- Dermoid cyst
- Encephalocele
- Nasal glioma
- Also, hemangioma

SOLITARY SCALP PLAQUE IN NEONATE

Aplasia cutis congenita
Nevus sebaceus

MARFANOID CLINICAL APPEARANCE

- Marfan syndrome
- Homocystinuria
- MEN-IIb

TUBEROUS SCLEROSIS APPEARANCE

- Tuberous sclerosis
- MEN-I

MULTIPLE ANGIOFIBROMAS

Tuberous sclerosis
MEN-I
These are only in case reports:
Cowden's disease
Birt-Hogg-Dubé

INTERTRIGINOUS RASH

Intertrigo
Inverse psoriasis
Hailey-Hailey & Darier disease
Pemphigus
Nutritional deficiency
Extramammary paget's disease
Langerhan Cell Histiocytosis

HYPOPIGMENTATION

Vitiligo
Seborrheic dermatitis
Discoid lupus
Chemical leukoderma
Idiopathic guttate hypomelanosis
Leprosy
CTCL

EROSIVE LIP

Erythema multiforme versus SJS
HSV
Lichen planus
Pemphigus vulgaris versus mucous membrane pemphigoid
Fixed drug eruption
Discoid lupus

15.1.2 Important Clinical Differentials

PAINFUL TUMORS

Mnemonic = BLEND AN EGG

- Blue rubber bleb nevus syndrome
- Leiomyoma
- Eccrine spiradenoma
- Neuroma
- Dermatofibroma, Dercum's disease (multiple painful lipomas)
- Angiolipoma
- Neurilemmoma
- Endometrioma
- Glomus tumor
- Granular cell tumor

ERYTHRODERMA

Mnemonic = pretty please don't make beets, dear

- Psoriasis
- Pityriasis rubra pilaris (PRP)
- Dermatitis (Atopic, Contact, Seborrheic, Stasis)
- Mycosis fungoides/CTCL
- Blistering (Pemphigus foliaceous, BP)
- Drug eruption

- Other—lichen planus, Norwegian scabies, GVHD, rarely sarcoid, paraneoplastic
- In infants: don't forget SSSS, ichthyoses

FLESH-COLORED PAPULES ON THE FACE DDX

- Melanocytic nevi
- Syringomas
- Xanthomas/xanthelasma
- Apocrine and eccrine hidrocystomas
- Trichoepitheliomas
- Sebaceous hyperplasia
- Angiofibromas
- Lipoid proteinosis
- Colloid milia
- Favre–Racouchot syndrome = nodular elastosis with cysts and comedones
- Trichilemmomas

Also (less flesh-colored): molluscum, plane warts, DPN

"PURPLE PLUMS"

Can be pink/purple cherry-like to plum-like soft to firm dermal nodules

- Leukemia cutis/lymphoma
- Metastatic cancer
- Kaposi's sarcoma (and bacillary angiomatosis)
- Merkel cell carcinoma
- Angiosarcoma
- Amelanotic melanoma
- Dermatofibrosarcoma protuberans (DFSP)
- Soft tissue sarcoma/Leiomyosarcoma
- Plasmacytoma

BLUEBERRY MUFFIN BABY DDX

Mnemonic = HI Blueberry Muffin

- Hemolysis (spherocytosis, ABO incompatibility)—extramedullary hematopoiesis
- Infection (TORCHeS)—extramedullary hematopoiesis
- Benign (multiple hemangiomas)
- Malignancy (neuroblastoma most common, leukemia)

SPOROTRICHOID SPREAD

Mnemonic = CAT N SPLAT

- Cat scratch disease
- Atypical mycobacteria (esp. *M. marinum*)

- Tuberculosis
- Nocardia
- Sporotrichosis
- Phaeohyphomycosis
- Leishmaniasis
- Anthrax
- Tularemia

Note: most common = sporotrichosis and atypical mycobacteria

RETIFORM PURPURA

- ANCA-associated vasculitides (GPA, MPA, PAN, EGPA)
- Antiphospholipid antibody syndrome
- Calciphylaxis
- Cocaine/levamisole-associated vasculopathy
- Cryoglobulinemia
- Disseminated intravascular coagulopathy (DIC)/Purpura fulminans
- Heparin-induced thrombocytopenia
- Septic vasculitis
- Warfarin skin necrosis
- Cholesterol emboli
- Oxalosis

LEONINE FACIES

- MF/CTCL
- Leprosy (lepromatous)
- Actinic reticuloid
- Scleromyxedema
- Paget's disease of bone
- Amyloidosis
- Acromegaly
- Sarcoidosis
- Leishmaniasis
- Multicentric reticulohistiocytosis

VEGETATING/GRANULATING/ULCERATING PLAQUE DDX

- Tuberculosis (primary inoculation or tuberculosis verrucosa cutis)
- Atypical mycobacterial infection
- Deep fungal infection (chromomycosis, blastomycosis)
- Leishmaniasis
- Mycetoma (Actinomyces/Nocardia)
- Neoplasms (SCC, sarcomas, metastatic)
- Pyoderma gangrenosum
- Gummas (syphilis, TB)
- Halogenoderma (from bromides, iodides)

PALMAR PITTING DDX

- Palmar pits (BCC Nevus syndrome)
- Punctate palmoplantar keratoderma (PPPK)/keratosis punctata palmaris et plantaris
- Punctate porokeratosis
- Punctate keratoses (of palmar creases)
- Arsenical keratoses
- Pitted keratolysis (*Corynebacterium*)
- Keratolysis exfoliativa (more annular collarettes of scale on palms)

CUTANEOUS HORN DDX

Mnemonic = SAWS

- Seborrheic keratosis
- Actinic keratosis
- Wart (Verruca vulgaris)
- Squamous cell carcinoma (including keratoacanthoma and SCCIS)

15.1.3 Differentials by Distribution/Anatomic Location

THE SHINS

- Stasis dermatitis
- Asteatotic eczema/eczema craquele
- Pyoderma gangrenosum
- Leukocytoclastic vasculitis
- Pigmented purpuric dermatosis (Schamberg's)
- Necrobiosis lipoidica
- Pretibial myxedema
- Erythema nodosum
- Diabetic dermopathy (shin spots)
- Lichen amyloidosis
- Hypertrophic lichen planus
- Lipodermatosclerosis
- Disseminated superficial actinic porokeratosis (DSAP)
- Ichthyosiform sarcoid
- Pseudo-Kaposi's sarcoma (acroangiodermatitis)
- Pancreatic panniculitis

ELBOWS AND KNEES

- Psoriasis
- Dermatomyositis
- Dermatitis herpetiformis

15

- Xanthomas
- Rheumatoid nodules
- Papular urticaria

INTERTRIGINOUS AREAS (AXILLAE/INGUINAL FOLDS)

- Intertrigo: candidiasis, irritant dermatitis seborrheic dermatitis, inverse psoriasis, erythrasma, contact dermatitis, inverse pityriasis rosea
- Hidradenitis suppurativa
- Axillary granular parakeratosis
- Pemphigus vegetans
- Hailey-Hailey disease

HANDS AND FEET

- Hand, foot, and mouth disease (Coxsackie)
- Dyshidrotic eczema/hand dermatitis
- Secondary syphilis (classic palms/soles)
- Psoriasis/Palmoplantar pustulosis
- Erythema multiforme
- Tinea manuum and tinea pedis ("one hand, two feet" syndrome)
- Vitiligo
- Warts
- Palmoplantar keratoderma (non-psoriasis types including PRP)
- Acral erythema of chemotherapy (hand-foot syndrome or erythrodysesthesia)
- Raynaud's phenomenon
- Perniosis/Chilblains
- Palmoplantar hyperhidrosis
- Vasculitis/vasculopathy (embolic disease, endocarditis, cryoglobulinemia)
- Papular purpuric gloves and socks syndrome (Parvovirus)

EROSIONS/BLISTERS ON DORSAL HANDS DDX

- Acute contact dermatitis (poison ivy)
- Porphyria cutanea tarda
- Pseudoporphyria
- Epidermolysis bullosa acquisita
- Bullous lupus
- Epidermolysis bullosa simplex

THE EARS

- Keloids
- Ear pit
- Accessory tragus
- Seborrheic otitis
- Discoid lupus

- Otitis externa
- Cocaine/levamisole-associated vasculopathy
- Relapsing polychondritis
- Leprosy
- Lupus vulgaris (tuberculosis)
- Lupus pernio (sarcoidosis)
- Pseudocyst of the auricle
- Chondrodermatitis nodularis helicis
- Angiolymphoid hyperplasia with eosinophilia (ALHE) and Kimura's disease
- Venous lake
- Non-melanoma skin cancers, actinic keratosis, atypical fibroxanthoma

CHRONIC DISEASE OF THE NOSE

- Tuberculosis (lupus vulgaris)
- Leprosy
- Syphilis
- Leishmaniasis
- Rhinoscleroma
- Sarcoidosis
- Granulomatosis with polyangiitis (Wegener's)
- Basal cell carcinoma

THE LIPS

- Angular cheilitis
- Actinic cheilitis
- Cheilitis granulomatosis
- Cheilitis glandularis
- Herpes labialis
- Venous lake
- Labial lentigo
- Pyogenic granuloma
- Angioedema
- Stevens-Johnson syndrome
- Erythema multiforme
- Paraneoplastic pemphigus
- Microcystic adnexal carcinoma
- SCC
- Fordyce spots
- Perioral dermatitis
- Lip licker's dermatitis
- Mucocele
- Condyloma acuminata

WHITE PLAQUE ON ORAL MUCOSA

- Lichen planus
- Thrush
- Leukoplakia (SCCIS)
- Oral hairy leukoplakia (EBV)
- White sponge nevus
- Leukokeratosis associated with pachyonychia congenita (type 1 > 2, not premalignant)
- Leukoplakia associated with dyskeratosis congenita (premalignant)
- Darier's
- Aspirin burn
- HPV: Oral florid papillomatosis, Heck's disease
- Verrucous xanthoma
- Nicotinic stomatitis = fissures/thickened white/red cobblestone papules on hard > soft palate

CAUSES OF GINGIVAL HYPERPLASIA

- Drugs—phenytoin, calcium channel blockers, cyclosporine
- Diseases—AML, sarcoidosis, granulomatosis with polyangiitis (Wegener's), scurvy, pregnancy

THE TONGUE

- Geographic tongue (annulus migrans, benign migratory glossitis)—can see similar in pustular psoriasis
- Fissured tongue (lingua plicata, scrotal tongue); see in Melkersson-Rosenthal syndrome (fissured tongue, Bell's palsy, and lip swelling—non-caseating granulomatous inflammation), Down syndrome
- Black hairy tongue—may be related to poor hygiene, smoking
- Granular cell tumor—tongue is common location

GENITAL LESIONS

- Painful: HSV, Chanchroid
- Painless: LGV, Granuloma Inguinale (Donovanosis), Syphilis (primary chancre, secondary condyloma lata)

RED PLAQUE ON PENIS

- Candidiasis
- Psoriasis
- Lichen planus
- Fixed drug eruption (especially from tetracyclines)
- Irritant balanitis
- Zoon's balanitis

PENILE/SCROTAL PAPULES

- Condyloma acuminata
- Pearly penile papules (angiofibromas)
- Comedones/folliculitis
- Normal hair follicles
- Tyson glands (ectopic sebaceous glands)
- Lichen planus
- Psoriasis
- Non-venereal sclerosing lymphangitis of the penis
- Condyloma lata (secondary syphilis)
- Angiokeratomas
- Acrochordons and nevi
- Idiopathic scrotal calcinosis

NECK FULLNESS DDX

- Goiter
- Madelung disease (benign symmetric lipomatosis)
- Rosai-Dorfman disease (sinus histiocytosis with massive LAD)
- Lymphoma (Hodgkin's and non-Hodgkin's)
- Scrofula

NAIL TUMORS

- Glomus tumor
- Digital myxoid cyst
- Periungual fibromas (Koenen tumors, in tuberous sclerosis)
- Nail matrix nevus
- Onychomatricoma
- SCC
- Melanoma

LONGITUDINAL MELANONYCHIA

- Racial predisposition
- Trauma
- Medication reaction
- Pregnancy
- Addison disease
- Peutz-Jeghers syndrome
- Laugier-Hunziker syndrome
- SCCIS
- Onychomycosis
- Benign nail matrix nevi
- Melanoma

15.1.4 Differentials by Morphology and Configuration

PUSTULES

- Acne
- Superficial folliculitis
- Pustular psoriasis
- Palmoplantar pustulosis
- Acute generalized exanthematous pustulosis (AGEP)/pustular drug eruptions
- Subcorneal pustular dermatosis (Sneddon Wilkinson disease)
- Infantile acropustulosis
- Candidiasis
- Tinea
- Dyshidrotic eczema
- Impetigo
- Varicella/HSV
- Erosive pustular dermatosis of the scalp

ANNULAR LESIONS

1. Vascular

   - Urticarial (< 24 h) = urticaria, erythema marginatum
   - Urticarial, but > 24 h = urticarial vasculitis, erythema multiforme, figurate erythemas (EAC, erythema migrans/Lyme, erythema gyratum repens), exanthematous drug eruptions, urticarial syndromes (Muckle-Wells, FMF), erythrokeratoderma variabilis
   - Purpuric = urticarial vasculitis, purpura annularis telangiectoides (BPP), acute hemorrhagic edema of infancy
   - Serpiginous (larva currens, cutaneous larva migrans)

2. Papulosquamous (Do a KOH!)

   - Psoriasiform = psoriasis, CTCL, even seb derm
   - Pityriasiform = tinea, secondary syphilis, pityriasis rosea
   - Lichenoid = lichen planus

3. Dermal

   - Granulomatous = granuloma annulare, sarcoid, leprosy
   - Lymphocytic = connective tissue disease (SCLE, tumid lupus, Still's disease, Sjögren's), Jessner's
   - Other: Sweet's, Well's syndrome

4. Vesiculobullous

   - Pustular (subcorneal) = pustular psoriasis, Sneddon-Wilkinson, IgA pemphigus
   - Bullous (subepidermal) = urticarial BP, linear IgA
   - Rare = perforating (elastosis perforans serpiginosa)

CATEGORIES OF LINEAR DISEASES

- Blaschkoid/nevoid (mosaicism)
- Dermatomal
- Autoinoculation
- Lymphatic/sporotrichoid
- "Outside jobs" = contact dermatitis, Koebnerized
- Phlebitis

LINEAR ENTITIES

Lichen striatus (in kids)
Blaschkitis (in adults)
Linear lichen planus
Linear Darier's
Linear porokeratosis
Inflammatory linear verrucous epidermal nevus (ILVEN)
Outside jobs: Koebnerized diseases (LP, lichen nitidus, psoriasis), contact dermatitis

LINEAR BULLAE DDX

Epidermolysis bullosa (mechanobullous disease)
Acute contact dermatitis (outside job)

15.1.5 Other Clinical Differentials

CAUSES OF ERUPTIVE KERATOACANTHOMAS

- Grzybowski syndrome
- Ferguson-Smith syndrome
- Muir-Torre syndrome (not really eruptive)
- BRAF inhibitor medications

CAFÉ AU LAIT MACULES

- Coast of California (regular borders): NF
- Coast of Maine (irregular borders): McCune Albright syndrome

CAUSES OF FOLLICULAR ATROPHODERMA

- Keratosis pilaris atrophicans (ulerythema ophryogenes)
- Conradi-Hunermann
- Bazex syndrome (BCCs with follicular atrophoderma)

- Rombo syndrome (BCCs with atrophoderma vermiculatum)

DISCOLORED HAIR

- Green hair = from copper chelation
- Yellow hair = from selenium sulfide

15.1.6 Other Disease Category Differentials

HYPERSENSITIVITY REACTIONS

- Type 1: IgE mediated; e.g. urticaria, anaphylaxis
- Type 2: cytotoxic; antibody-dependent (IgM or IgG); e.g. hemolytic anemia
- Type 3: antigen-antibody immune complex; e.g. serum sickness, vasculitis
- Type 4: delayed-type hypersensitivity; (T-cells) allergic contact dermatitis

BREAST CANCER SKIN MANIFESTATIONS

1. Peau d'orange (can see with any infiltrative disease)
2. Carcinoma erysipeloides (inflammatory breast cancer)
3. Carcinoma en cuirasse (et satellite nodules de Valpeau)
4. Alopecia neoplastica
5. Carcinoma telangiectoides
6. Paget's disease (from direct extension of ductal carcinoma—must involve nipple)

SPIROCHETES

Mnemonic = rat biting into a BLT

- Rat-bite fever (*Spirillium minus*, *Streptobacillus moniliformis*)
- Borrelia
- Leptospirosis
- Treponemes

DIMORPHIC FUNGI

- Sporotrichosis
- Histoplasmosis
- Blastomycosis
- Coccidioidomycosis
- Paracoccidioidomycosis

ANGIOINVASIVE ORGANISMS

- *Mucor*
- *Rhizopus*
- *Pseudomonas* (ecthyma gangrenosum)

- *Aspergillus*
- *Fusarium*

CHILDHOOD VIRAL EXANTHEMS

- First Disease—Rubeola/Measles—*Paramyxovirus*
- Second Disease—Scarlet Fever—*Streptococcus* (not viral)
- Third Disease—Rubella—*Togavirus*
- Fourth Disease—Duke's Disease—not specific
- Fifth Disease—Erythema infectiosum—*Parvovirus B19*
- Sixth Disease—Roseola/Exanthem subitum—*HHV-6/7*

HUMAN HERPES VIRUSES

- HHV-1 = HSV-1, herpes simplex virus-1
- HHV-2 = HSV-2, herpes simplex virus-2
- HHV-3 = VZV, varicella zoster virus
- HHV-4 = EBV, Epstein-Barr virus
- HHV-5 = CMV, cytomegalovirus
- HHV-6 = possibly related to pityriasis rosea and roseola, DRESS
- HHV-7 = possibly related to pityriasis rosea and roseola, DRESS
- HHV-8 = related to Kaposi's sarcoma, Castleman's disease, primary effusion lymphoma

Note:

- Alpha—HHV-1,2,3 (herpes ones)
- Beta = HHV-5,6,7 (CMV, roseola)
- Gamma = HHV-4 and 8 (oncogenic ones)

INSECTS

1. Arthropods (6 legged)

   - Fleas, flies, mosquitoes, bed bugs

2. Arachnids (8 legged): four categories

   - Ticks
   - Spiders
   - Scorpions
   - Mites

ATYPICAL MYCOBACTERIA

- Fast growers (3–5 d) (e.g. *Mycobacterium fortuitum, Mycobacterium abscessus, Mycobacterium chelonae*)

– Mnemonic = "fast as a cheetah"

DISEASES WITH BODY LICE AS A VECTOR

Body lice = *Pediculus humanus var. corporis*
Mnemonic = BRB

- Louse-borne epidemic typhus (*Rickettsia prowazekii*)
- Relapsing fever (*Borrelia recurrentis*)
- Trench fever (*Bartonella quintana*)

TYPES OF CUTANEOUS TB

From external exposure:

- Primary inoculation
- Tuberculosis verrucosa cutis
- Tuberculosis cutis orificialis (orificial TB)

From hematogenous spread:

- Lupus vulgaris
- Miliary tuberculosis

From direct extension:

- Scrofuloderma

Reactive eruptions to TB (tuberculid eruptions):

- Papulonecrotic tuberculid
- Lichen scrofulosorum
- Erythema induratum

CATEGORIES OF DEPOSITIONAL DISEASES

Mnemonic = MACULE[1]

- Mucin
- Amyloid
- Calcium
- Urate
- Lipid
- Exogenous/extra (implanted, pigment, hyaline-like)

---

1   This mnemonic is used with permission from Dr. Donald Rudikoff.

15.2 Associations and Work-Ups

15.2.1 Disease-Specific Associations

HCV SKIN ASSOCIATIONS

(by direct effect and as consequence of associated hepatic damage)

- Cutaneous necrotizing vasculitis (as in type II cryoglobulinemia), usually presents with palpable purpura, can see livedo reticularis, urticaria
- Porphyria cutanea tarda (may have HCV association)
- Lichen planus—stronger association with mucosal/ulcerative LP
- Cutaneous B-cell lymphoma
- Xerostomia
- Erythema multiforme (possibly)
- Pruritus (in 15% of patients with HCV)
- Necrolytic acral erythema

LIVER DISEASE ASSOCIATIONS ON DERM PHYSICAL EXAM

- Prurigo and excoriations (from generalized pruritus)
- Asterixis/tremor
- Palmar erythema
- Spider angiomas
- Caput medusae
- Gynecomastia
- Scleral icterus
- Terry's nails

HIV SKIN ASSOCIATIONS

- Candidiasis (thrush)
- Exuberant seborrheic dermatitis
- HPV infection/diffuse verruca vulgaris/condyloma acuminata
- Herpes zoster (and disseminated zoster)
- Molluscum contagiosum (giant, diffuse)
- Kaposi's sarcoma
- HIV-associated eosinophilic folliculitis
- Papular pruritic eruption of HIV
- Lipodystrophy—associated with protease inhibitors (specifically indinavir), NRTIs
- Bacillary angiomatosis
- Exanthem of seroconversion
- Oral hairy leukoplakia (EBV)
- Deep fungal infection (Cryptococcosis, Histoplasmosis)
- Reactive arthritis (psoriasiform)

- Proximal subungual onychomycosis due to *T. rubrum*
- Pruritus/prurigo
- Stevens-Johnson syndrome (1000x greater incidence); other drug reactions with increased frequency also
- Acquired ichthyosis
- Psoriasis

DERM CONDITIONS ASSOCIATED WITH DIABETES

- Acanthosis nigricans
- Acrochordons
- Diabetic dermopathy ("shin spots")
- Necrobiosis lipoidica (NLD)
- Scleredema
- Granuloma annulare
- Diabetic bullae (bullosis diabeticorum)
- Necrotizing fasciitis
- Erythrasma
- Mucormycosis
- Malignant external otitis

RASH IN PATIENT WITH KNOWN MALIGNANCY DDX

1. Medications (often on many antibiotics, chemo, allopurinol)
2. Metastatic disease
3. Reactive (GVHD, Sweet's)
4. Infectious disease (immunosuppressed and vulnerable)

UMBILICATED PAPULES

Poxviruses

- Molluscum
- Smallpox (*Variola*)
- Cowpox (*Vaccinia*)
- Monkeypox (Mpox)

Herpes viruses

- HSV-1 and 2, herpes simplex
- VZV, varicella and zoster

MOLLUSCUM MASQUERADERS (umbilicated papules) IN HIV PATIENT

Mnemonic = CCHP

- Coccidioidomycosis
- Cryptococcosis
- Histoplasmosis
- Penicilliosis

15.2.2 **Work-Ups**

CLINICAL EXAMINATION OF THE WHITE MACULE

- Check for scale—tinea versicolor
- Check for blanching—nevus anemicus
- Check with Wood's lamp—vitiligo
- Check for anesthesia—leprosy (more in borderline/tuberculoid)

Also remember: PIPA, MF, tuberous sclerosis (ash leaf macules), pityriasis alba, progressive macular hypomelanosis, sarcoidosis

HOW TO WORK UP A PUSTULAR ERUPTION

- Check Tzanck or viral culture/DFA/PCR (to r/o HSV or VZV)
- Check gram stain/bacterial culture (to r/o bacterial impetigo)
- Check KOH (to r/o candidiasis/tinea)
- Check mineral oil (to rule in scabies)
- Check Wright stain (for eosinophils—to rule in erythema toxicum neonatorum or incontinentia pigmenti)
- Check bacterial, fungal, viral PCR and biopsy for H&E if above not definitive

GENERALIZED PRURITUS WORK-UP

Is there a primary skin disease? If not, then search for internal cause of itch.

- Check for dermatographism (urticaria)
- Check for xerosis on exam
- Check mineral oil (rule in scabies)
- Check CBC (for eosinophilia—allergy/neoplasm/parasite, for elevated Hgb—polycythemia vera, other signs of hematologic malignancy)
- Check BMP, A1c: BUN/Cr for renal disease, rule out diabetes
- Check LFTs for liver/cholestatic etiology
- Check HIV, hepatitis B and C serologies
- Check TSH to r/o hyperthyroidism
- Check CXR, r/o Hodgkin's lymphoma
- Check SPEP/UPEP to r/o monoclonal gammopathy
- Check tryptase to r/o mast cell disorder
- Check BP180/230, IIF to r/o pre-bullous BP
- All age-appropriate cancer screening up to date?

SYSTEMIC VASCULITIS WORK-UP

- Assess for systemic involvement: U/A for blood (GU involvement), stool guaiac (GI involvement); CBC and CMP
- Consider etiologies:
  Medication history
  Connective tissue disease (ANA, Rf, C3, C4, Ro, La)
  Infectious disease (HIV, hepatitis serologies, ASLO)
  Other inflammatory (cryoglobulins, p-ANCA, c-ANCA)

15

RETIFORM PURPURA WORK-UP

- Complete systemic vasculitis work-up (as above)
- Check PT, PTT, platelets (r/o DIC)
- Consider ECHO (if septic vasculitis is a consideration) and follow blood cultures
- Has patient been on warfarin (warfarin necrosis) or heparin (heparin-induced thrombocytopenia thrombosis and necrosis)?
- Any cocaine history? Consider urine toxicity for cocaine (cocaine/levamisole-associated vasculopathy)

ERYTHEMA NODOSUM WORK-UP

- CXR—r/o hilar lymphadenopathy (sarcoid)
- PPD—r/o TB
- ASLO—r/o *Strep*
- Consider β-HCG in young women

URTICARIA WORK-UP

- Consider medication and food history, connective tissue disease (ANA, Rf, Ro, La), thyroid disease (TSH), infection (HIV, hepatitis serologies, ASLO)

ALOPECIA WORK-UP

- Clinical exam: Any scalp disease (inflammation)? Any hair shaft abnormalities? Check hair pull test. Dermoscopy very useful but biopsy is most definitive
- Consider CBC, ferritin, vitamin D, zinc, TSH, hormonal evaluation (FSH/LH (depends on stage in menstrual cycle), prolactin, free testosterone (from gonads), DHEAS (from adrenals).

15.3 Acronyms

15.3.1 List of Acronyms

15.3.1.1 Important Acronyms

Dermatologists use *way* too many acronyms, but here is a list of the most common you might not know. Use as needed, but remember that many frown upon their use, especially in clinical notes that may be shared with non-dermatologists. It is easy to get so used to using acronyms and forget what they mean. If you do use an acronym, make sure you know what it stands for!

AFX = atypical fibroxanthoma
AGEP = acute generalized exanthematous pustulosis

AK = actinic keratosis
ALHE = angiolymphoid hyperplasia with eosinophilia
BCC = basal cell carcinoma
BCIE = bullous congenital ichthyosiform erythroderma (EHK)
BP = bullous pemphigoid
BSA= body surface area
BXO = balanitis xerotica obliterans (lichen sclerosis of the penis)
CALM = café-au-lait macule
CARP = confluent and reticulated papillomatosis (of Gougerot and Carteaud)
CCCA = central centrifugal cicatricial alopecia
CTCL = cutaneous T-cell lymphoma
DEJ = dermal-epidermal junction, aka basement membrane zone (BMZ)
DF = dermatofibroma
DFA = direct fluorescent antibody (test for herpes simplex and zoster)
DFSP = dermatofibrosarcoma protuberans
DH = dermatitis herpetiformis
DIF = direct immunofluorescence
DLE = discoid lupus erythematosus
DM = may refer to dermatomyositis or diabetes mellitus
DN = dysplastic (atypical) nevus aka Clark's nevus
DPN = dermatosis papulosa nigra (easy to confuse which word ends in osis!)
DRESS = drug rash with eosinophilia and systemic symptoms (hypersensitivity reaction)
DSAP = disseminated superficial actinic porokeratosis
EAC = erythema annulare centrifugum
EB = epidermolysis bullosa
EBA = epidermolysis bullosa acquisita
EDP = erythema dyschromicum perstans
EDV = epidermodysplasia verruciformis
EED = erythema elevatum diutinumichthyosiform erythroderma)
EHK = epidermolytic hyperkeratosis (pathology term for finding in bullous congenital ichthyosiform erythroderma)
EIC = epidermal inclusion cyst aka follicular/epidermoid/sebaceous cyst
EM = erythema multiforme
EPF = eosinophilic pustular folliculitis
EPP = erythropoietic protoporphyria
EPS = elastosis perforans serpiginosa
FEP = fibroepithelial polyp (skin tag/acrochordon)
GA = granuloma annulare
GVIID = graft versus host disease
HC = hydrocortisone
HS = hidradenitis suppurativa
IDN = intradermal nevus
ILK = intralesional Kenalog (triamcinolone)
ILVEN = inflammatory linear verrucous epidermal nevus
IPL = intense pulsed light

15

IVIg = intravenous immunoglobulin (IgG)
JAKi = JAK inhibitor
JXG = juvenile xanthogranuloma
KA = keratoacanthoma
KP = keratosis pilaris
KS = Kaposi's sarcoma
LCV = leukocytoclastic vasculitis (small-vessel vasculitis dermpath pattern)
LE = lupus erythematosus
LGV = lymphogranuloma venereum
LP = lichen planus
LPLK = lichen planus-like keratosis
LPP = lichen planopilaris
LS and A (LS et A) = lichen sclerosus et atrophicus (technically just lichen sclero-
    sus now)
LSC = lichen simplex chronicus
LyP = lymphomatoid papulosis
MF = mycosis fungoides
MM = malignant melanoma
MMIS = malignant melanoma in situ
NBCIE = non-bullous congenital ichthyosiform erythroderma
Nd:YAG = neodymium-doped yttrium aluminum garnet laser
NF = neurofibroma/neurofibromatosis
NLD = necrobiosis lipoidica diabeticorum (just called necrobiosis lipoidica now
    because not just in diabetics)
NMSC = non-melanoma skin cancer (SCC and BCC)
NXG = necrobiotic xanthogranuloma
PASI = psoriasis area severity index
PCT = porphyria cutanea tarda
PG = may refer to pyogenic granuloma or pyoderma gangrenosum
PIPA/PIH = post-inflammatory pigmentary alteration/postinflammatory hyper-
    pigmentation/hypopigmentation
PLC = pityriasis lichenoides chronica
PLEVA = pityriasis lichenoides et varioliformis acuta
PMLE = polymorphous light eruption
PPK = palmoplantar keratoderma
PR = pityriasis rosea
PRP = pityriasis rubra pilaris
PsA = psoriatic arthritis
PUPPP = pruritic urticarial papules and plaques of pregnancy (aka polymor-
    phous eruption of pregnancy)
PXE = pseudoxanthoma elasticum
SCC = squamous cell carcinoma
SCCIS = SCC in situ
SCLE = subacute cutaneous lupus erythematosus
SJS = Stevens-Johnson syndrome
SK = seborrheic keratosis
TAC = triamcinolone

TCI = topical calcineurin inhibitor
TCS = topical corticosteroid
TBSE = total body skin examination
TEN = toxic epidermal necrolysis
TMEP = telangiectasia macularis eruptiva perstans

15.3.2 Diseases Known Primarily by Acronyms

APECED syndrome

Autoimmune
PolyEndocrinopathy (esp. hypoparathyroidism—90%)
Candidiasis and
Ectodermal Dystrophy

BADAS syndrome

Bowel-
Associated
Dermatosis
Arthritis
Syndrome

CHILD syndrome

Congenital
Hemidysplasia with
Ichthyosiform nevus and
Limb
Defects

CREST syndrome (limited scleroderma)

Calcinosis cutis
Raynaud's phenomenon
Esophageal dysmotility
Sclerodactyly
Telangiectasia

LEOPARD syndrome

Lentigines
EKG abnormalities
Ocular hypertelorism
Pulmonary stenosis
Abnormal genitalia
Retarded growth
Deafness

15

MAGIC (Behçet syndrome/relapsing polychondritis overlap)

Mouth
And
Genital ulcers with
Inflamed
Cartilage

PAPA syndrome

Pyogenic
Arthritis,
Pyoderma gangrenosum, and
Acne

PAPASH syndrome

Pyogenic
Arthritis
Pyoderma gangrenosum,
Acne, and
Suppurative
Hidradenitis

PASH syndrome

Pyoderma gangrenosum,
Acne, and
Suppurative
Hidradenitis

PHACES syndrome

Posterior fossa and other brain malformations
Hemangiomas (mainly facial)
Arterial anomalies typically of the aortic branches
Cardiac defects and coarctation of the aorta
Eye anomalies
Sternal defects and supraumbilical raphe

POEMS syndrome

Polyneuropathy
Organomegaly
Endocrinopathy
Monoclonal gammopathy
Skin changes—remember glomeruloid hemangiomas, hyperpigmentation

SAPHO syndrome

>   Synovitis
>   Acne conglobata
>   Pustulosis (palmoplantar in particular)
>   Hyperostosis
>   Osteitis

TEMPI syndrome

>   Telangiectasias
>   Elevated erythropoietin level and erythropoiesis
>   Monoclonal gammopathy
>   Perinephric-fluid collections
>   Intrapulmonary shunting

15.4 Dermatopathology

15.4.1 Differentials, Lists, and Mnemonics

15.4.1.1 Differentials

EOSINOPHILIC SPONGIOSIS DDX

Mnemonic = HAPPIIE FD

- Herpes gestationis
- Arthropod/allergic contact
- Pemphigus
- Pemphigoid
- Incontinentia pigmenti
- Erythema toxicum neonatorum
- Fungal
- Drug

PAGETOID SPREAD DDX

- Melanoma   → Check S100, Melan-A
- SCC   → Check cytokeratins
- Bowen's disease/SCCIS
- Sebaceous carcinoma
- Paget's disease   → Check CEA, usually preserved
                                basal layer (unlike MM)
- Extramammary Paget's   → Check CK7, CK20

PARASITIZED HISTIOCYTES (ORGANISMS SEEN IN MACROPHAGES) DDX

Mnemonic = His girl Penelope (T!)

- Histoplasmosis
- Granuloma inguinale
- Rhinoscleroma
- Leishmaniasis
- Penicilliosis
- Toxoplasmosis

PAISLEY TIE/TADPOLE/COMMA-SHAPED DDX

Note: aka "sperm in the derm"

- Syringoma
- Microcytic adnexal carcinoma (MAC)
- Morpheaform BCC
- Desmoplastic trichoepithelioma

PSEUDOEPITHELIOMATOUS HYPERPLASIA DDX

- Irregular downward proliferation of epidermis into dermis (mimics SCC)
- Mycobacterial infections
- Deep fungal infections
- Granular cell tumor
- Pyoderma vegetans, pyoderma gangrenosum, borders of ulcers
- Prurigo
- Bromoderma

COMMON "INVISIBLE" ENTITIES ON DERMPATH

- Tinea versicolor
- Dermatophytosis
- Tinea nigra
- TMEP/mastocytosis
- PIPA
- Urticaria
- Amyloid
- Vitiligo
- Ichthyosis vulgaris

INTERFACE DERMATITIS DDX (lichenoid and vacuolar)

1. LP-ish stuff: Lichen planus/nitidus, lichenoid drug, lichen striatus, LPLK
2. EM-ish stuff: EM/TEN, fixed drug, GVHD, paraneoplastic pemphigus, PLEVA
3. Connective tissue disease: lupus, dermatomyositis, poikiloderma
Also: Mycosis fungoides (atypical lichenoid eruption)

DERMAL PALLOR DDX

- PMLE
- Sweet's syndrome
- Porphyria cutanea tarda/pseudoporphyria
- Pernio (on acral skin)
- Lichen sclerosis (hyalinization)

PSORIASIFORM DDX

- Psoriasis
- PRP
- Subacute to chronic spongiotic dermatitis/LSC/prurigo nodularis

ALTERNATING PARAKERATOSIS AND ORTHOKERATOSIS

- Actinic keratosis
- Pityriasis rubra pilaris
- ILVEN

NECROTIC KERATINOCYTES DDX

- Erythema multiforme
- GVHD
- SJS/TEN (if full thickness epidermis)
- PLEVA/PLC
- Fixed drug
- Sunburn (sunburn cells)
- Radiation dermatitis
- Incontinentia pigmenti

PALE EPIDERMIS

- Nutritional deficiency/Necrolytic erythemas
- Normal mucosa
- Necrosis (EM, TEN)

MORPHEA VERSUS RADIATION DERMATITIS VERSUS LICHEN SCLEROSUS

- Pale thickened dermis with square biopsy, loss of periadenexal fat: morphea
- Pale thickened dermis with stellate fibroblasts, loss of adnexae: radiation dermatitis
- Pale thickened dermis with epidermal hyperkeratosis and lymphoid infilatrate: LS&A

15

SALT SPLIT for subepidermal blisters

— Breaks the DE junction at lamina lucida
Epidermal split: bullous pemphigoid, cicatricial pemphigoid
Dermal side/floor: bullous lupus, EB acquisita, cicatricial pemphigoid (anti-epiligrin)

A FEW GROUPS WITH SIMILAR APPEARANCE

— Chondroid syringoma (mixed tumor)
— Proliferating pilar tumor
— Pilomatricoma
— Trichofolliculoma
— Dilated pore of Winer
— Pilar sheath acanthoma
— Folliculosebaceous cystic hamartoma
— Trichostasis spinulosa
— Granular cell tumor
— Xanthoma/xanthelasma

15.4.2 Lists and Notes

PANNICULITIS—septal versus lobular

— Septal = looks like Cheerios in a bowl of milk (i.e. minimal disruption of lobule appearance (the Cheerios))
— Lobular = looks like oil in a bowl of soup (i.e. the lobules are disturbed with large distorted shapes like oil on soup)

SCLEROSIS VERSUS FIBROSIS
(two terms often used inappropriately interchangeably clinically)

Thickened pink collagen with minimal cells = sclerosis (e.g. morphea)
Thickened pink collagen with increased cells = fibrosis (e.g. scleromyxedema)

PINK on PATH

Fibrin
Keratin
Bone
Necrosis

TYPES OF GIANT CELLS

Foreign body
Touton

Osteoclastic
Langhans

TYPES OF GRANULOMAS

Sarcoidal (naked)—sarcoidosis
Tuberculoid—TB, syphilis, leprosy, leishmania
Palisading—NLD, GA, RA
Suppurative—deep fungal
Foreign body—exogeneous/endogenous materials
Miscellaneous—Melkersson-Rosenthal syndrome

PALISADED/PALISADING GRANULOMAS

Mucin—GA
Fibrin—rheumatoid nodule
Degenerated collagen—NLD (horizontal palisading = layer cake)
Urate—gout
Lipids—eruptive xanthomas

15.4.3 Other Factoids

SMALL ROUND BLUE CELL TUMORS OF HEAD/NECK MNEMONIC =
LEMON

Lymphoma
Ewing cell sarcoma
Merkel cell carcinoma
Osteosarcoma
Neuroblastoma

PLEVA HISTOLOGY

Parakeratosis
Lichenoid infiltrate
Extravasated RBCs
V-shaped wedge-shaped infiltrate
Apoptotic keratinocytes

CRYOTHERAPY ARTIFACT PATH = holes/vacuoles in the epidermis

SQUARE BIOPSY
- Morphea
- NLD

FLORET GIANT CELLS

- See in pleomorphic lipomas

THE THREE M'S OF HERPES ON PATH

Molding, margination, multinucleation

NEUTROPHILS IN STRATUM CORNEUM

- Psoriasis, seborrheic dermatitis, tinea, impetigo, candida, subcorneal pustular dermatosis, syphilis

PARAKERATOSIS HELPFUL IN DX

Mounds of parakeratosis + spongiotic dermatitis seen in pityriasis rosea
Shoulder parakeratosis (next to follicular ostia) seen in seborrheic dermatitis
Alternating parakeratosis (sparing adnexal structures) and orthokeratosis seen in actinic keratoses
Checkerboard parakeratosis and orthokeratosis seen in pityriasis rubra pilaris

RBCS IMPORTANT IN DX

Spongiotic dermatitis + RBCs = think pityriasis rosea
Interface dermatitis + RBCs = think PLEVA
RBCs + leukocytoclasis + fibrinoid necrosis = think leukocytoclastic vasculitis

CHOLESTEROL CLEFTS

Cholesterol emboli (clefts in vessels)
NXG (clefts in collagen)
Infantile panniculitis (needle-shaped clefts in fat, with crystals)—subcutaneous fat necrosis of the newborn, sclerema neonatorum, post-steroid panniculitis

MELANIN VERSUS HEMOSIDERIN

Melanin = finer brown clumps
Hemosiderin = thicker more yellowish clumps

SOLAR ELASTOSIS VERSUS MUCIN

Solar elastosis = bluish clumps
Mucin = more wispy bluish strands or spaces in connective tissue

CELLS WITH GRANULAR APPEARANCE

Eosinophils
Mast cells
Granular cell tumor cells
Xanthomatized cells (foamy)

HYALINE-LIKE DEPOSITIONS: LACE

Lipoid proteinosis = diffuse dermal deposits, tend to be vertical, around blood vessels and adnexae
Amyloidosis = papillary dermis pink globs (macular/lichen amyloid), deeper pink globs that may crack (nodular amyloid)

Colloid milium = overlying solar elastosis/atrophy/hyperkeratosis, nodular fissu-
ered masses in papillary dermis

Erythropoetic protoporphyria = deposits in dermis, more around vessels

MUCIN DEPOSITION

Mucin in follicle = follicular mucinosis

Ball of mucin in mucosa = mucocele

Ball of mucin in skin = focal mucinosis

Ball of mucin in acral skin = digital mucous cyst

Mucin in dermis = pretibial or generalized myxedema

Mucin + thickened collagen = scleredema

Mucin + thickened collagen + fibroblasts = scleromyxedema or nephrogenic systemic fibrosis

Mucin + vacuolar + superficial/deep perivascular = lupus/reticular erythematous
mucinosis

Mucin + palisaded granuloma = granuloma annulare

EPIDERMAL PALLOR → VACUOLES → MOTH-EATEN = NECROLYSIS

Zinc deficiency/nutritional deficiency

Necrolytic acral erythema

Necrolytic migratory erythema

15.4.4 Stains and Immunohistochemistry

STAINS VERSUS IMMUNOHISTOCHEMISTRY

Stains are dyes that color different anatomical structures on a slide and may improve visualization of a specific structure

Immunohistochemistry (IHC) involves targeting antigens on cells with antibodies
tagged to an enzyme (catalyzes a reaction which produces color)

IMPORTANT STAINS

Acid fast stain (Aka Ziehl-Neelson) = stains for mycobacteria (leprosy, TB)

Alcian blue = stain mucin

Colloidal iron = stains mucin

Congo red = stains amyloid (apple-green birefringence under polarized light)

Crystal violet = stains amyloid (best for keratin-derived)

Fite stain = acid fast stain, best for leprosy

Fontana-Masson = stains melanin

Giemsa stains = stains mast cells, microorganisms

GMS (Grocott's methenamine silver) stain = stains fungi

Gram stain = stains gram positive bacteria

Hematoxylin/eosin (H&E) = general stain for histopathology

Oil red O = stains fat/lipids (must be frozen section)

PAS (Periodic acid-Schiff) stain = stains fungi

Prussian blue = stains hemosiderin/iron (broken down RBCs, but not intact RBCs)

Sudan black = stains fat/lipids (must be frozen section)

Thioflavin-T = stains amyloid

Toluidine blue = stains mucin, mast cells

Trichrome (Masson's trichrome) = red keratin/muscle, blue/green collagen/bone

Von Kossa = stains calcium black

Verhoeff-van Gieson = stains collagen red, elastin black

Warthin-Starry (a silver stain) = stains spirochetes, treponemes

Wright stain = stains eosinophils

Acid fast stains = Fite stain, Ziehl-Neelson stain

Amyloid stains = Congo red, crystal violet, thioflavin-T

Fat/lipid stains = Oil red O, Sudan black

Fungal stains = PAS, GMS

Mucin stains = Alcian blue, colloidal iron, toluidine blue, mucicarmine

Smooth muscle stain = Masson's trichrome stain

IMPORTANT IMMUNOHISTOCHEMISTRIES

Actin = stains muscle (not specific)

BAX = apoptotic

Bcl-2 = anti-apoptotic

CD1a = Langerhans cells

CD3 = T cell marker (also CD2, CD4, CD5, CD6, CD7, CD8)

CD20 = B cell marker (also CD79a, PAX-5)

CD25 = positive in ATLL (adult T-cell leukemia/lymphoma)

CD30 = positive in ALCL (anaplastic large cell lymphoma), LyP types A and C

CD31 = vascular derivation (expressed in vascular endothelial cells)

CD34 = vascular derivation; negative in DF, positive in DFSP

CD45RO = positive in mycosis fungoides (which is classically CD3 and 4 positive, CD7 and 8 negative)

CD56 = natural killer cells

CD68 = macrophages

CD117 (c-KIT) = stains for mast cells

CD133 = pluripotent stem cell marker

CD207 (langerin) = stains for Langerhans cells

CEA (carcinoembryonic antigen) = may be useful in extramammary Paget's, may stain apocrine and eccrine ducts

Cytokeratins = epithelial derivation

Cytokeratin-7 (CK7) = stains in Paget's disease

Cytokeratin-20 (CK20) = Merkel cells

Desmin = muscle derivation

EMA (epithelial membrane antigen) immunoperoxidase = stains lipids, for confirmation of sebaceous differentiation

Factor XIIIA = positive in DF, negative in DFSP

GLUT-1 = positive in infantile hemangiomas (not in NICH or RICH)

HMB-45 = melanocytic, specific but not sensitive; does not stain desmoplastic MM well

Melan-A/MART-1 = sensitive/specific for melanocytes

Smooth muscle actin (SMA) = muscle derivation

Stromelysin3 = usually positive in DF, negative in DFSP

S100 = stains for neural crest derived cells (neural cells, melanocytes), Langerhan cells

Vimentin = mesenchymal derivation

Epithelial differentiation = cytokeratins

Melanocytic = S100, Melan-A/MART-1, HMB-45

Merkel cells = CK20+, TTF1− (vs. metastatic small cell carcinoma, like lung)

Muscle derivation = smooth muscle actin (SMA) and desmin (see these two with smooth muscle, actin more sensitive, desmin more specific), vimentin (intermediate filaments)

Neural derivation = S100

Vascular = CD34, CD31, Factor VIII

15.5 Lists

15.5.1 Quick Quiz Lists

These lists are not meant to be comprehensive—they are simply for quick quizzing to ensure you know the common answers.

Name an etiology of ERYTHEMA NODOSUM

- Idiopathic
- *Strep*
- Drugs (OCP)
- Other bacterial (*Yersinia*, *Salmonella*)
- Sarcoidosis (Löfgren's syndrome)
- Deep fungal infection (*Cocci*, *Histo*)
- Inflammatory bowel disease
- Tuberculosis

Name a RISK FACTOR for MELANOMA

- Personal history of melanoma
- Family history of melanoma
- Multiple benign nevi
- Atypical/dysplastic nevi and congenital melanocytic nevi
- Fitzpatrick skin type (fair skin, freckling, light hair)
- Ultraviolet light exposure (including tanning)
- Immunosuppression
- Genetic disease (xeroderma pigmentosum, albinism)

Name a gene commonly mutated in melanoma

- BRAF (esp. V600E)
- NRAS
- c-KIT
- CDKN2A
- PTEN

Name a common type of DRUG ERUPTION (not including chemo/radiation reactions)

- Morbilliform drug eruption/exanthematous drug eruption, maculopapular eruption
- Stevens-Johnson syndrome/toxic epidermal necrolysis (SJS/TEN)
- DRESS (Drug reaction with eosinophilia and systemic symptoms)
- Acute generalized exanthematous pustulosis (AGEP)
- Fixed drug eruption
- Drug-induced urticaria/angioedema
- Drug-induced vasculitis
- Drug-induced bullous disease (Linear IgA, BP, pseudoporphyria, pemphigus)
- Erythroderma
- Photo-associated drug eruption
- Drug-induced acne
- Lichenoid drug eruption
- Drug-induced lupus
- Drug-induced interstitial granulomatous dermatitis

Name a potential adverse effect of PREDNISONE

- Osteoporosis
- Increased appetite/Weight gain
- Hyperglycemia
- Hypertension
- Mood changes/psychosis/insomnia
- Peptic ulcers/GI effects
- Acneiform eruptions
- Poor wound healing/striae
- Infection
- CBC changes: neutrophilia/transient lymphopenia
- Adrenal suppression
- Avascular necrosis of femoral head/osteonecrosis
- Cataracts (posterior subcapsular)/glaucoma

Name a potential side effect of ISOTRETINOIN

- Teratogenicity
- Cheilitis/xerosis/epistaxis
- Lipid abnormalities (esp. triglyceridemia)
- Liver abnormalities (esp. transaminitis)

- Pseudotumor cerebri/blurry vision/headaches
- Mood changes/depression/suicidality?
- Inflammatory bowel disease? (not really)
- Premature closure of epiphyses

Name a relative or absolute CONTRAINDICATION to TNF INHIBITORS

- Immunocompromised/HIV
- Infections (e.g. active TB)
- Malignancy
- Congestive heart failure
- Demyelinating disease (e.g. multiple sclerosis)
- Positive ANA or autoimmune disease (relative)

Name a SCLERODERMOID disease (scleroderma-like disease)

- Scleromyxedema
- Scleredema
- Eosinophilic fasciitis (Shulman's syndrome)
- Nephrogenic systemic fibrosis
- Chronic GVHD
- Sclerodermoid changes from porphyria cutanea tarda
- Chronic radiation dermatitis
- Lichen sclerosus
- Acrodermatitis chronica atrophicans
- Atrophoderma of Pasini and Pierini
- Phenylketonuria (PKU)

Name a method for treatment of warts

- Cryotherapy
- Salicylic acids (and other acids, TCA, etc.)
- Topical immunomodulators (imiquimod)
- Podophyllin
- Electrodesiccation/surgical destruction
- Cantharidin/blistering agents
- Injectable immunotherapy (*Candida*, interferon-α)
- Oral cimetidine
- Laser (CO_2 or PDL)
- Occlusion/duct tape
- Topical contact sensitizers (e.g. squaric acid)
- Photodynamic therapy
- Intralesional chemo (Bleomycin, 5-FU)
- Topical green tea catechins (Veragen)
- Topical retinoids
- Topical or intralesional antiviral (cidofovir)

15

Name a type of stitch used in dermatologic surgery

- Simple interrupted (epidermal)
- Buried/deep
- Running epidermal or dermal
- Vertical mattress
- Horizontal mattress
- Subcuticular
- Tip stitch (half-buried horizontal mattress)
- Figure of eight
- Purse string
- Pulley
- Fascial plication

Name a NON-INFLAMMATORY NON-SCARRING ALOPECIA

- Androgenetic alopecia
- Telogen effluvium
- Traction alopecia
- Trichotillomania
- Anagen effluvium
- Loose anagen syndrome
- Temporal triangular alopecia

Name an INHERITED NON-AUTOIMMUNE CONNECTIVE TISSUE DISEASE

- Marfan syndrome
- Ehlers-Danlos syndrome
- Osteogenesis imperfecta
- Pseudoxanthoma elasticum
- Cutis laxa
- Homocystinuria

Name a cause of ESCHARS

- Trauma/burns/chronic wounds
- Brown recluse spider bite
- Ecthyma gangrenosum/Pseudomonas
- Systemic fungal infection
- Rickettsialpox
- Tularemia
- Anthrax
- Plague

Name a well-known NON-LANGERHANS CELL HISTIOCYTOSIS

- Juvenile xanthogranuloma
- Multicentric reticulohistiocytosis
- Necrobiotic xanthogranuloma

- Rosai-Dorfman disease (sinus histiocytosis with massive lymphadenopathy)
- Benign cephalic histiocytosis
- Papular xanthoma

15.5.2 **Often Asked Facts**

COLORS (not including tattoo pigment)

- Red: blood/vessels
- Yellow: jaundice, lipids (sebaceous hyperplasia, xanthomas), elastosis (solar elastosis, PXE), gout, calcinosis cutis, ecchymosis, edema, carotenemia, pus
- Green: pseudomonas
- Blue: blood (venous malformations, venous lakes), minocycline, argyria, erythema dyschromicum perstans, blue nevus/dermal melanocytosis, exogenous ochronosis (from hydroquinone)/endogenous ochronosis, keratin
- Purple: lichenoid, purpura, necrosis, Kaposi's sarcoma (and other purple plums)
- White: vitiligo, lichen sclerosus, morphea, scar
- Black: necrosis, eschar, pigment (melanin), thrombosed vessel, oxidized keratin

TATTOOS: pigment and reactions

- Red: Mercury/cinnabar (red planet)
- Yellow: Cadmium (yellow taxi cad)
- Green: Chromium
- Blue: Cobalt (cobalt blue)
- Purple: Manganese (magenta purple)
- Black: Carbon
- White: Titanium
- Entities in tattoos: sarcoidosis, pigment reaction

IMPORTANT ULTRAVIOLET FREQUENCIES TO KNOW

UVA1: 340–400 nm
UVA2: 320–340 nm
UVB: 280–320 nm
NBUVB: 311 nm
Wood's lamp: 365 nm

INDIRECT IMMUNOFLUORESCENCE SUBSTRATES

- Pemphigus vulgaris = monkey esophagus
- Pemphigus foliaceous = guinea pig esophagus
- Paraneoplastic pemphigus = rat bladder epithelium

DERMATOPHYTES (TINEA)

- *Trichophyton* (corporis mostly rubrum, capitis mostly tonsurans)
- *Microsporum*
- *Epidermophyton*

SIX STAGES OF ORF (ECTHYMA CONTAGIOSUM)

Mnemonic = PTARPR:

Papular, targetoid, acute (weeping nodule), regenerative, papillomatosis, regression

15.5.3 Interesting Factoids

COMMON ETYMOLOGIES IN DERM

Vulgaris = common (like the common or vulgar language)
Pityriasis = scaling
Eczema = "boiling off"
Lupus = "wolf"
Ichthys = "fish"

COMMONLY MISPRONOUNCED

Pityriasis/Tinea amiantacea [am ee ann tay sha]
Sézary syndrome [Sez a ree]
Kaposi's sarcoma [Kap oh sees] and [Kah poe sees] both acceptable
Kyrle's disease [Curly's]
Myiasis [My ah sis]
Letterer-Siwe [See wee]
Porphyrin [pour fir in]
Porphyria [pour fear ee ah]
Buccal [Buck ul, not bue kul]
Cheilitis [Kye lye tis]
Erythema elevatum diutinum [die oo tin um]

COMMONLY MISSPELLED WORDS IN DERMATOLOGY

Pruritus
Guaiac
Jadassohn
Erysipelas
Inoculation
Apocrine and eccrine
Pterygium
Tzanck
Eczema craquele
Condyloma acuminata
Neurilemmoma
Sebaceous gland, nevus sebaceus
Curettage
Acrochordon
Electrodesiccation

Pompholyx
Lichen sclerosus et atrophicus
Lichen amyloidosis

LIST OF DERMATOSES WITH FOOD NAMES OR ASSOCIATED TERMS

Apply jelly—appearance on diascopy of sarcoidosis/granulomatous disease
Banana bodies—pathologic sign of ochronosis (exogenous alkaptonuria)
Beefy red—appearance of clean, healing wound
Blueberry muffin baby—extramedullary hematopoiesis
"Breakfast, lunch, and dinner"—Bedbug (*Cimex lectularius*) bites
Bubble gum—description of collagen in keloids
Café-au-lait macule
Cauliflower—cauliflower ear in wrestlers, also description of condyloma acuminatum
Caviar spots—angiokeratomas on the tongue
Cayenne pepper—benign pigmented purpura
Cheesy exudates—in thrush, like cottage cheese
Cherry—cherry angioma/hemangioma
Corn—clavus
Grapes (in clusters/bunches)—on positive crush prep of molluscum contagiosum
Honey colored crusts—bullous impetigo
Layer cake—pathologic appearance in necrobiosis lipoidica
"Milk white"—vitiligo appearance on Wood's lamp
Mulberry molar—sign of congenital syphilis
Nutmeg grater appearance—pityriasis rubra pilaris
Peach fuzz—hair in anorexia nervosa
Peau d'orange/orange skin—pretibial myxedema and inflammatory breast cancer (or any infiltrative disease)
Plucked chicken skin—pseudoxanthoma elasticum
Port wine stain—nevus flameus
Salmon—color in pityriasis rubra pilaris, Still's disease, "salmon patch" nevus flammeus
Salt and pepper—retinitis in Refsum disease
Sausage digit—in psoriatic arthritis
"Spaghetti and meatballs"—KOH finding for hyphae and spores of tinea versicolor
Strawberry—infantile "strawberry" hemangioma, Strawberry tongue of scarlet fever, Kawasaki disease
Tapioca pudding like vesicles—dyshidrotic eczema
Tripe palms—acanthosis nigricans

15

15.5.4 Nevi, Erythemas, and Other Common Terms

NEVI

Note: These are all called "nevi"; most are not related, not necessarily neoplastic, many are melanocytic

Melanocytic nevi

- Intradermal nevus—melanocytes in dermis (usually exophytic)
- Compound nevus—melanocytes in DE junction and dermis
- Junctional nevus—melanocytes at DE junction (usually macular)
- Spitz nevus—"benign juvenile melanoma"
- Becker's nevus
- Nevus spilus
- Halo nevus
- Balloon cell nevus
- Dysplastic/atypical nevus
- Recurrent nevus
- Congenital melanocytic nevus (small < 1.5 cm, large/giant > 20 cm)
- Blue nevus (dermal melanocytoma)
- Dermal melanocytosis (Mongolian spot—on lumbosacral, Nevus of Ota—by eye, Nevus of Ito—on shoulder)

Blaschkoid nevi

- Epidermal nevus
- Nevus sebaceus (of Jadassohn)
- ILVEN (inflammatory linear verrucous epidermal nevus)

Nevoid/other mosaic malformations

- Nevus anemicus
- Nevus flammeus ("port wine stain") and nevus simplex
- Nevus depigmentosus = Blaschkoid hypopigmented patch
- Nevus araneus (spider angioma/telangiectasia)

Other nevi

- Connective tissue nevus/collagenoma
- White sponge nevus
- Blue rubber blue nevus syndrome
- Porokeratotic eccrine, ostial, and dermal duct nevus

LIST OF "ERYTHEMAS"

Figurate:

Erythema migrans (Lyme disease)
Erythema annulare centrifugum
Erythema marginatum (Rheumatic fever)

Erythema gyratum repens
Eosinophilic annular erythema

Necrolytic:

Necrolytic migratory erythema
Necrolytic acral erythema

Inflammatory:

Erythema elevatum diutinum
Erythema nodosum leprosum

Vascular:

Erythema multiforme
Erythema infectiosum (Fifth disease—Parvovirus)
Toxic erythema
Acral erythema of chemotherapy

Panniculitis:

Erythema nodosum/Erythema contusiforme
Erythema induratum

Other:

Erythema dyschromicum perstans
Erythema ab igne
Erythema toxicum neonatorum
Malar erythema
Flagellate erythema

LIST OF "ECTHYMAS"

Ecthyma gangrenosum = Pseudomonas
Ecthyma contagiosum = Orf
Ecthyma (general) = ulcerative bacterial infection

LIST OF "IMPETIGOS"

Impetigo contagiosum/Impetigo = *Staph* or *Strep*
Impetigo herpetiformis (pustular psoriasis in pregnancy)
Bullous impetigo (*Staph*)

ACRODERMATITIS-ES and ACROKERATOSIS-ES

Acrodermatitis continua of Hallopeau = nail pustular psoriasis
Acrodermatitis enteropathica = inherited zinc deficiency
Acrodermatitis chronica atrophicans = Lyme related aging/atrophy (like morphea)
Acrokeratosis verruciformis of Hopf = seen in Darier's
Acrokeratosis paraneoplastica of Bazex (Bazex syndrome)

15

FASCIITIS-ES

Necrotizing fasciitis
Eosinophilic fasciitis
Nodular fasciitis

15.5.5 Clinical Signs (with Nicknames or Eponymous Names)

Asboe-Hansen sign (pseudo-Nikolsky's sign) = extension of blister with pressure on top

Auspitz sign = in psoriasis, lesions bleed when scale is removed (since capillaries are in dermal papillae close to the surface)

Button-hole sign = in anetoderma

Crowe's sign = axillary/inguinal freckling in neurofibromatosis

Darier's sign = urtication upon palpation of a mastocytoma

Dimple sign = dimpling on palpation of dermatofibroma

Gorlin sign = ability to touch nose with tongue (10% of people can do this; 50% of Ehlers-Danlos)

Gottron's papules = lichenoid papules over MCPs, DIPs, PIPs

Gottron's sign = pink/red/purple atrophic or scaling eruption over knuckles, knees, elbows

Groove sign = vein depressions in indurated skin of eosinophilic fasciitis

Hairy palm sign = in LSC; looks like acral skin on path (thickened), but has hair

Headlight sign = perinasal pallor in atopic dermatitis

Koebner phenomenon ("isomorphic response") = recurrence of dermatosis at site of trauma (often seen in psoriasis and lichen planus); Note: Wolf's isotopic response is occurrence of a dermatosis at the site of a previously resolved unrelated dermatosis

Leser-Trélat sign = Sudden increased size/number of seborrheic keratoses, associated with gastric or colonic adenocarcinoma, breast carcinoma, and lymphoma

Nikolsky's sign = slight rubbing of skin causes denudation; seen in TEN, BP, and pemphigus

Romana's sign = unilateral periorbital edema in Chagas disease

Samitz sign = cuticular changes in dermatomyositis

Shawl sign = erythema and scale ± poikiloderma over shoulders

Teeter totter sign = pressure on one side of pilomatricoma causes elevation on the other side

Tent sign = stretching of overlying skin of a pilomatricoma gives a multifaceted, angulated appearance, likely due to calcification in the lesion

Winterbottom sign = posterior cervical LAD in African trypanosomiasis

Signs of congenital syphilis:

> Early: Parrot's pseudoparalysis, pneumonia alba, snuffles, syphilitic pemphigus, rhagades, Wimberger's sign
> Late: Clutton's joints, 'Mulberry' molars, Saber shins, Saddle nose

15.5.6 Nail and Teeth Findings

NAIL ABNORMALITIES

Remember: Nail matrix → nail plate production; proximal matrix → dorsal nail plate, distal matrix (lunula) → ventral nail plate

Fingernails grow at 3 mm/month (takes 5–6 months to grow out)
Toenails grow at 1 mm/month (8–12 months)

Beau's lines—transverse lines in all nails from acute systemic illness (from inflammation of proximal nail matrix)

Black nails—can be seen with melanoma, but also *Candida* or *Proteus* infection

Clubbing—see loss of the normal < 165° angle (Lovibond angle) b/w nailbed and cuticle

Darier's disease—red and white parallel bands, V-nicking

Digital mucous cyst—impinges upon nail matrix, causes proximal nail dystrophy

Habit tic deformity—median nail ridging

Half-and-half nails (Lindsay's nails)—white proximal nails, brown distal; associated with renal failure (in 10%); (Mnemonic = half/half for 2 kidneys rather than 1 liver)

Koilonychia—spoon-shaped nail, sign of iron deficiency

Leukonychia—white nail

Longitudinal melanonychia—brown linear streak

Median canaliform deformity—"inverted fir tree" (different from habit tic)

Mee's lines—parallel transverse white bands (from arsenic), true leukonychia (in nail plate)

Muehrcke's lines—multiple transverse white bands (in chemo, hypoalbuminemia from nephrotic syndrome), apparent leukonychia (in nail bed)

Nail pitting—from parakeratosis of proximal nail matrix/dorsal nail plate; irregular in psoriasis, grid-like regular appearance in alopecia areata

Onychauxis—nail thickening, subungual hyperkeratosis

Onychogryphosis—ram's horn nails, typically from chronic trauma or neglect

Onychomadesis—proximal detachment of the nail; separation from nail plate, a severe example of Beau's lines

Onychorrhexis—longitudinal ridging and fissuring

Onychoschizia—nail splitting, distal peeling of the nail plate

Paronychia—inflammation of proximal nail folds (can be acute or chronic)

Plummer's nails—onycholysis in thyroid disease

Pterygium—scarring process that involves nail fold overgrowth into nail plate. Dorsal involves proximal nail fold, ventral involves hyponychium (Dorsal in LP, trauma, bullous disease)

Terry's nails—white proximal 2/3 nails, reddish distal; associated with liver cirrhosis (in up to 82%), hypoalbuminemia

15

Thryoid acropachy—clubbing-like appearance of fingers/joints from thyroid disease
Trachyonychia—"twenty nail dystrophy," from lichen planus, alopecia areata, or psoriasis, pachyonychia congenital
Yellow nail syndrome—from lymphatic obstruction in cardiopulmonary disease (bronchiectasis, effusions, COPD, asthma, lymphedema); see loss of cuticle, lunulae

Three most common inflammatory skin diseases with nail changes:

- Alopecia areata—regular "geometric" nail pits, trachyonychia
- Psoriasis—irregular nail pits, onycholysis, oil drops
- Lichen planus—longitudinal ridges/dystrophic changes, dorsal pterygium

Nail-patella syndrome

- Aka hereditary osteo-onychodysplasia (HOOD)
- Defect in LMX-1B (transcription factor that regulates collagen synthesis, dorsal/ventral limb patterning), autosomal dominant, Chr 9
- Clinically, see triangular lunulae (pathognomonic), hypoplastic nails, absent or small patellae, renal dysplasia, hyperpigmentation of papillary margin of iris (Lester iris)
- Check U/A for proteinuria, pelvic XR for iliac horns

TEETH ABNORMALITIES

Pegged teeth—seen in hypohidrotic ectodermal dysplasia (Clouston syndrome), incontinentia pigmenti, congenital syphilis (Hutchinson's incisors)
Natal teeth—seen in pachyonychia congenita
Retention of primary teeth—seen in hyper IgE syndrome (Job's syndrome)—can also see a double row of teeth
Enamel pits—seen in tuberous sclerosis

15.6 Commonly Confused Diseases

15.6.1 Sound-Alikes and Look-Alikes

See ◘ Table 15.1.

▣ Table 15.1	Sound-alike and look-alike terms in dermatology
Acrodermatitis chronica atrophicans	Cutaneous manifestation of chronic Lyme borreliosis (usually *Borrelia afzelii* in Europe; vector *Ixodes ricinus*), specifically atrophic acral morphea-like skin changes
Acrodermatitis continua of Hallopeau	Aka dermatitis repens. Pustular psoriasis of the nail bed, usually just one nail
Acrodermatitis entero-pathica	Inherited form of zinc deficiency, caused by mutations in the zinc transporter SLC39A4. Classically presents with diarrhea, alopecia, and dermatitis
Acrokeratosis paraneo-plastica of Bazex (Bazex syndrome)	A papulosquamous eruption and/or acral keratoderma associated with upper aerodigestive tract malignancy. May precede diagnosis of malignancy
Acrokeratosis verruci-formis of Hopf	Autosomal dominant genodermatosis of flat-topped papules (like flat warts) on the extremities. May be seen with Darier's disease (unclear if represents a separate entity)
Bazex-Dupré-Christol syn-drome (Bazex syndrome)	An X-linked dominant syndrome of multiple basal cell carcino-mas, follicular atrophoderma, hypohidrosis, and hypotrichosis
Acrokeratosis paraneo-plastica of Bazex (Bazex syndrome)	A papulosquamous eruption and/or acral keratoderma associated with upper aerodigestive tract malignancy. May precede diagnosis of malignancy
Buschke-Löwenstein tumor	Giant condyloma acuminata associated with human papilloma-viruses 6 and 11. May develop into a verrucous carcinoma that is locally aggressive, but does not metastasize
Buschke-Ollendorf syndrome	Aka dermatofibrosis lenticularis disseminata, a syndrome of multiple connective tissue nevi (soft yellow-skin colored pap-ules) caused by mutations in LEMD3, which encodes a nuclear envelope protein. Associated with osteopoikilosis—sclerotic opacities typically in carpal bones and phylanges
Scleredema adultorum of Buschke	A disorder of skin induration caused by dermal mucin deposi-tion. Different forms of scleredema are associated with *Strep* infection, monoclonal gammopathy, and diabetes
Cheilitis glandularis	Rare inflammatory painless enlargement of minor salivary glands on the lower lip
Cheilitis granulomatosa	Aka granulomatosis cheilitis. Acute onset swelling of the upper or lower lip. Melkersson-Rosenthal syndrome consists of cheili-tis granulomatosa, facial paralysis (Bell's palsy), and fissured tongue (aka lingua plicata, scrotal tongue)
Dermoid cyst	Cysts formed by retained epithelium along embryonic fusion plane, seen congenitally or in childhood, usually on the fore-head or by the lateral eyes. On pathology, have stratified squa-mous epithelium and adnexal structures in wall

15

◾ **Table 15.1** (Continued)

Desmoid tumor	Deep fibrous infiltrative neoplasm categorized as extra-abdominal or intra-abdominal, associated with Gardner syndrome. Gardner syndrome is an autosomal dominant syndrome of colon polyps, which may also manifest with epidermoid cysts (which may have features of pilomatricoma), osteomas, and congenital hyperpigmentation of retinal pigment epithelium (CHRPE)
Degos disease	Aka malignant atrophic papulosis. A vaso-occlusive/endovasculitic disorder that affects the skin, gastrointestinal tract, and central nervous system. Skin lesions consist of small erythematous papules that heal with atrophic white scars with peripheral ectatic rims
Dowling-Degos disease	Aka reticular pigmented anomaly of the flexures. A disorder of reticulate pigmentation beginning in the groin, axillae, and later involving flexures of then neck, trunk, and extremities. Associated with a defect in keratin 5
Ecthyma	Ulcerative (non-bullous) superficial cutaneous infection usually caused by *Streptococcus pyogenes*
Ecthyma contagiosum	Orf, a poxvirus infection associated with sheep/goat contact. Classically goes through six stages: papular, targetoid, acute (weeping nodule), regenerative, papillomatosis, regression
Ecthyma gangrenosum	Ulcerative superficial cutaneous infection by *Pseudomonas spp.*, typically seen in patients who are immunosuppressed, human immunodeficiency virus positive, or have a hematologic malignancy
Erythema nodosum	Most common panniculitis, which classically presents as tender subcutaneous nodules on the anterior shins. The archetype of a mostly septal panniculitis, associated with infections (tuberculosis, *Strep*, deep fungal), malignancy, sarcoidosis, inflammatory bowel disease, and medications (oral contraceptive pills)
Erythema nodosum leprosum	Type II reversal reaction in the treatment of lepromatous leprosy (a leprosy-specific reaction). May manifest with papules, pustules, vesicles. First line treatment is thalidomide
Fordyce spots	Ectopic sebaceous glands on lips and buccal mucosa
Fox-Fordyce disease	Apocrine miliaria. Pruritic papules primarily in the axillae, caused by obstruction of the apocrine ducts
Angiokeratoma of Fordyce	Angiokeratomas (blue-black hyperkeratotic papules) found on the scrotum, most commonly in elderly males
Goltz syndrome	Aka focal dermal hypoplasia and Goltz-Gorlin syndrome. An X-linked dominant disorder affecting all three embryonic layers. Patients may have perioral and anogenital papillomas, Blaschkoid atrophic telangiectatic lesions, and lobster-claw deformity. Defect in PORCN, which regulates Wnt secretion

Table 15.1 (Continued)

Gorlin-Goltz syndrome	Aka nevoid-BCC syndrome, BCC nevus syndrome, and Gorlin's syndrome. An autosomal dominant disorder of multiple basal cell carcinomas and other congenital abnormalities, including odontogenic keratocysts of the jaw, falx cerebri calcification, palmar pits. Associated with mutations in the PTCH (Patched) gene, which encodes a transmembrane protein that acts in opposition of the hedgehog signaling pathway
Hutchinson's sign (Melanoma)	Clinical sign of extension of pigment onto the nail fold in association with longitudinal melanonychia. Can represent horizontal growth of a subungual melanoma
Hutchinson's sign (Zoster)	Clinical sign of zoster presenting with a nasal tip lesion. This indicates involvement of the nasociliary branch of the ophthalmic nerve (trigeminal nerve) and a risk for developing ophthalmic herpes zoster
Impetigo	The most common bacterial skin infection in children, most commonly caused by *Staphylococcus aureus* (especially phage group II, type 71), and less often by *Strep*. Has both bullous and non-bullous forms. Exfoliative toxin A, associated with bullous impetigo, targets epidermal desmoglein-1
Impetigo contagiosa	Another name for impetigo
Impetigo herpetiformis	Pustular psoriasis in pregnancy. Classically presents in the third trimester and may be treated with systemic corticosteroids
Herpes gestationis	Aka pemphigoid gestationis, a form of bullous pemphigoid in pregnancy or immediately postpartum, presenting with an urticarial or vesiculo-bullous eruption. Direct immunofluorescence classically shows linear C3 at the dermal-epidermal junction. Patients have an increased risk for Graves' disease
Incontinentia pigmenti	Aka Bloch-Sulzberger syndrome, an inherited X-linked genodermatosis most commonly caused by defects in NEMO, the NF-κB essential modulator. Usually lethal in males, characterized by Blashkoid cutaneous lesions in four phases: vesicular, verrucous, hyperpigmented, hypopigmented/atrophic
Urticaria pigmentosa	A form of cutaneous mastocytosis most commonly seen in children and characterized by brown macules or papules. Stroking a lesion typically produces urtication (Darier's sign)
Kimura's disease	Vascular proliferation of nodules and plaques on the head and neck, closely related to angiolymphoid hyperplasia with eosinophilia, though now considered to be a distinct entity
Reticulate acropigmentation of Kitamura	Autosomal dominant disorder of pigmentation presenting with atrophic reticulate pigmentation and angulated pigmented papules on dorsal hands and feet and may have palmar pits. May overlap with Dowling-Degos disease

15

■ **Table 15.1** (Continued)

Lupus miliaris disseminatus faciei	Brown dermal facial papules with histologic finding of caseation necrosis not associated with tuberculosis. May have overlap with granulomatous rosacea
Lupus pernio	A form of sarcoidosis that presents with skin lesions in areas most affected by cold (nose, ears). Has a strong association with chronic pulmonary sarcoidosis
Lupus profundus	Aka lupus panniculitis. A primarily lobular panniculitis associated with systemic lupus erythematosus. Clinically, favors proximal extremities. On histology, classically see hyaline necrosis of the fat lobules
Lupus vulgaris	Chronic form of tuberculosis disseminated by hematogenous spread, or lymphatic or direct extension. Most commonly affects head and neck, such as nose, ears, and cheeks
Milia	Small keratin-filled epidermoid cysts. Can be primary from plugging of pilosebaceous or eccrine sweat ducts, or secondary, from injury to the skin as seen in subepidermal blistering diseases such as porphyria cutanea tarda
Miliaria	Papules resulting from obstruction of eccrine glands (miliaria crystallina, miliaria rubra, miliaria profunda, with increasing depth of obstruction) or apocrine glands (Fox-Fordyce disease)
Parakeratosis	Histologic term for retention of nuclei in stratum corneum keratinocytes
Porokeratosis	A clonal disorder of keratinization (multiple types) characterized by hyperkeratotic papules or plaques with an elevated border. Recognized on histology by *sine qua non* cornoid lamella, a thin column of parakeratosis with underlying absent or reduced granular layer, dyskeratotic cells. Squamous cell carcinoma reported in all types except punctate; linear may have greatest risk
Perniosis/Pernio	Aka Chilblains. Abnormal inflammatory response to cold causing erythematous to violaceous acral macules, papules, and nodules, typically on distal toes and fingers
SLE pernio	Aka Chilblain lupus. The occurrence of pernio lesions in the context of lupus
Lupus pernio	A form of sarcoidosis that presents with skin lesions in areas most affected by cold (nose, ears). Has a strong association with chronic pulmonary sarcoidosis
Phakomatosis	Ectodermal genetic disease affecting the CNS, skin, and retina. For example, neurofibromatosis and tuberous sclerosis
Phakomatosis pigmentokeratotica	Syndrome characterized by nevus sebaceus with papular nevus spilus
Phakomatosis pigmentovascularis	Syndrome characterized by capillary malformations (port wine stain or telangiectasia), vascular (nevus anemicus), and/or melanocytic lesions (nevus spilus, dermal melanocytosis)

◘ Table 15.1 (Continued)

Pyoderma gangrenosum	A neutrophilic dermatosis often associated with inflammatory bowel disease, rheumatoid arthritis, and hematologic malignancy
Pyogenic granuloma	Aka lobular capillary hemangioma, a vascular proliferation associated with trauma, pregnancy, and medications (especially retinoids, HIV protease inhibitors, oral contraceptives, EGFR inhibitors)
Scleredema adultorum of Buschke	A disorder of skin induration caused by dermal mucin deposition. Different forms of scleredema are associated with *Strep* infection, monoclonal gammopathy, and diabetes
Sclerema neonatorum	One of the infantile panniculitides, classically arises in severely ill premature infants in the first week of life. On histology, may see characteristic needle-shaped clefts in lipocytes with minimal inflammation
Scleroderma	Aka progressive systemic sclerosis. One of the classic autoimmune connective tissue diseases, characterized classically by sclerodactyly, hardening of the skin. Greatest mortality is from lung involvement, morbidity from gastrointestinal involvement (esophageal dysmotility)
Scleromyxedema	Aka lichen myxedematosis, papular mucinosis. Disorder of mucin deposition and increased collagen production. Systemic form usually associated with IgG-λ monoclonal gammopathy

Previously published in a different form in *J Drugs Dermatol* (2011). Used with permission

15.6.2 Other Similar Sounding Diseases

THREE EASILY CONFUSED DISEASE NAMES/ENTITIES IN KIDS

Congenital self-healing reticulohistiocytosis (Hashimoto-Pritzker disease, a type of LCH)
Benign cephalic histiocytosis (a non-Langerhans cell histiocytosis)
Benign cephalic pustulosis (neonatal acne)

MORE SIMILAR SOUNDING DISEASES

Dermatopathia pigmentosa reticularis (similar to Naegeli-Franceschetti Jadassohn)
Erythema dyschromicum perstans (ashy dermatosis/possible variant of lichen planus)
Dermatofibrosis lenticularis disseminata (Buschke-Ollendorff syndrome)
Hyperkeratosis lenticularis perstans (Flegel's disease)

15

A FEW EPONYMOUS SYNDROME NAMES THAT CAN BE CONFUSED

Finklestein's disease—acute hemorrhagic edema of infancy, related to HSP? "cockade" appearance

Schnitzler's syndrome—chronic non-pruritic urticaria, FUO, disabling bone pain, monoclonal IgM gammopathy (can progress to Waldenstrom's)

Muckle-Wells syndrome—autosomal dominant, acute febrile episodes with arthritis, urticaria, abd pain. Can have multiorgan amyloid (AA); similar to familial Mediterranean feve

A FEW BACTERIAL INFLAMMATORY DISEASES THAT CAN BE CONFUSED

Malakoplakia

- Chronic bacterial granulomatous accumulation in immunocompromised hosts, from *E. coli* (> *Pseudomonas* > *Proteus*)
- Michaelis-Gutmann bodies, von Hansemann cells

Rhinoscleroma

- Granulomatous infection of nose and upper respiratory tract, from *Klebsiella pneumoniae* (*Klebsiella rhinoscleromatis* (subspecies)), parasitized histiocytes on pathology (Mikulicz cells) and Russell bodies

Granuloma inguinale (Donovanosis)

- Chronic indurated red fleshy ulcerative/destructive infection (usually painless); caused by *Calymmatobacterium (Klebsiella) granulomatis*

15.6.3 Misnomers

MISNOMERS AND TERRIBLY NAMED DISEASES

("Rhode Island is neither a road nor is it an island, discuss")

Acanthoma fissuratum/granuloma fissuratum—A lichen simplex type reaction from chronic rubbing, not neoplastic nor granulomatous

Acanthosis nigricans—A papillomatous eruption, rarely has acanthosis on pathology

Acne keloidalis nuchae—Scarred papules usually on the neck, but not related to acne and scarring is not keloidal on pathology

Adenoma sebaceum—Angiofibromas seen in tuberous sclerosis, not sebaceous-derived, but may have sebaceous distribution on face

Dissecting cellulitis—A disease of follicular occlusion, neither dissecting nor a cellulitis

DRESS syndrome (drug reaction with eosinophilia and systemic symptoms)—A drug reaction syndrome, but may not have eosinophilia in up to 40% of cases

Dyshidrotic eczema—A type of eczema, with etiology not related to eccrine glands

Follicular atrophoderma—Follicular indentations seen in Bazex-Dupré-Christol syndrome and others, does not show any atrophy on pathology

Granuloma faciale—Mixed inflammatory process, not granulomatous and not just on the face

Granuloma gluteale infantum—Inflammatory reaction on the buttocks of infants, not granulomatous

Herpes gestationis—A form of bullous pemphigoid in pregnancy, not related to herpes

Hidradenitis suppurativa—A disease of follicular occlusion, but no primary apocrine inflammation or suppuration (may have secondarily)

Impetigo herpetiformis—A form of pustular psoriasis in pregnancy, not related to any infection (impetigo or herpes)

Keratosis follicularis—Keratotic papules seen in Darier's disease in seborrheic areas, but not follicular

KID (keratitis, ichthyosis, deafness) syndrome—A genodermatosis with skin findings including non-scaly plaques (erythrokeratodermia) rather than ichthyosis, and keratitis not in all patients

Lupus miliaris disseminatus faciei/acne agminate—A granulomatous eruption, previously thought to be a tuberculid reaction, not related lupus or acne, may be related to rosacea

Lupus pernio—A form of sarcoidosis on the nose, not related to lupus or pernio

Mycosis fungoides—A neoplastic disease, etiology not entirely clear, but not fungal

Nevus depigmentosus—A Blashkoid hypopigmentation, no depigmentation

Palisaded encapsulated neuroma—A neuroma, circumscribed but not palisaded or encapsulated on pathology

Pyoderma gangrenosum—A sterile neutrophilic inflammatory disease, with no infection (pyoderma) or necrosis/gangrene

Pyogenic granuloma—A vascular proliferation, neither pyogenic nor granulomatous

Scleredema—Indurated plaques from mucin deposition, but no sclerosis, no edema

Sebaceous cyst—Follicular/epidermoid cyst without sebaceous derivation, but rather from the follicular unit

Tinea versicolor—An eruption caused by a fungus (*Pityrosporum*), but not tinea/dermatophytes

Transient acantholytic dermatosis (Grover's disease)—An acantholytic dyskeratotic disease, with recurrent and often persistent disease rather than transient

15.7 Other Lists

15.7.1 Types of Dermatology Diseases

TYPES OF ECZEMA

Mnemonic = CANDID SCALES[2]

1. Contact dermatitis
2. Atopic dermatitis
3. Nummular dermatitis
4. Dyshidrotic dermatitis/pompholyx
5. Id reaction (autoeczematization) and infectious eczematoid
6. Drug dermatitis
7. Stasis dermatitis
8. Cutaneous T-Cell Lymphoma (Mycosis fungoides)
9. Asteatotic dermatitis (eczema craquele)
10. Lichen simplex chronicus (LSC)
11. Exfoliative dermatitis (erythroderma)
12. Seborrheic dermatitis

By distribution:

Popliteal/antecubital fossae = atopic dermatitis
Pretibial = asteatotic, stasis
Bony prominences (ankles) = LSC
Palmoplantar = dyshidrotic
Generalized = erythroderma

By configuration:

Round = nummular
Pattern = contact
Flare around wound = infectious eczematoid (most common on face; e.g. otitis externa)
No configuration = drug, cancer, psychogenic

TYPES OF POROKERATOSIS

Porokeratosis of Mibelli
Disseminated superficial actinic porokeratosis (DSAP)
Porokeratosis palmaris et plantaris disseminata (PPPD)
Linear porokeratosis
Punctate porokeratosis

---

2   This mnemonic is used with permission by Dr. Steven Cohen.

Porokeratotic eccrine, ostial, and dermal duct nevus
Porokeratosis ptychotropica

- Risk of SCC mostly in linear, any chronic parakeratosis

TYPES OF LICHEN PLANUS

Oral lichen planus
Erosive/ulcerative lichen planus (mucosal)
Lichen planopilaris (LPP)
LP pigmentosus
LP actinicus
LP pemphigoides
Other

- Actinic, annular, atrophic, bullous, hypertrophic (shins), linear (blaschkoid), nail

TYPES OF SARCOIDOSIS

Macular/papular type
Subcutaneous nodular sarcoidosis (includes Darier-Roussy type)
Lupus pernio (on the nose)
Infiltration of scars, tattoos
Angiolupoid sarcoid
Syndromes

- Löfgren's syndrome, Heerfordt's syndrome (uveoparotid fever), Mikulicz syndrome

Other

- Annular, hypopigmented, ulcerative, erythrodermic, ichthyosiform (on shins), alopecia, morpheaform, mucosal

TYPES OF GRANULOMA ANNULARE

Localized GA
Disseminated/Generalized GA
Interstitial GA
Subcutaneous GA
Perforating GA
Arcuate dermal erythema/Patch GA
Actinic granuloma/GA, annular elastolytic giant-cell granuloma

TYPES OF LUPUS (types = clinical presentations, letters list disease entities)

1. Acute
   Types: Malar erythema "butterfly rash," diffuse erythema, bullous
   a. Systemic lupus erythematosus (SLE)
   b. Drug-induced lupus
   c. Bullous SLE

  2. Subacute
     Types: annular (and polycyclic), papulosquamous
     a. Subacute cutaneous lupus (SCLE)
     b. Neonatal lupus erythematosus
  3. Chronic
     Types: discoid, panniculitis, hypertrophic/lichenoid
     Note: Chronic LE is typically associated with scarring (tumid LE is non-scarring)
     a. Discoid lupus (DLE)
     b. Lupus profundus (panniculitis)
  4. Other
     a. Lupus erythematosus tumidus (tumid lupus)
     b. Lichen planus-lupus overlap syndrome
     c. Rowell syndrome (LE with EM)
     d. SLE pernio (Chilblain lupus)

TYPES OF BENIGN PIGMENTED PURPURA (5 CLASSIC ONES)

Schamberg's disease
Lichen Aureus
Doucas-Kapetenakis (Eczematoid Pigmented Purpura)
Gougerot-Blum (Lichenoid Pigmented Purpura)
Majocchi's disease (Purpura Annularis Telangiectoides)
Also: Itchy purpura of Lowenthal
Note: These names are no longer emphasized on exams but occasionally used in texts

15.7.2 Drug Eruption Mnemomics

FIXED DRUG ERUPTION

Mnemonic = Salt Bone PC

  - Sulfa (most common)
  - Acetaminophen/ASA
  - Laxatives
  - Tetracyclines (especially around genitals)
  - Barbiturates
  - OCPs
  - NSAIDs
  - Erythromycin
  - Phenylephrine/pseudoephedrine (can have nonpigmented variant)
  - Carbamazepine

LINEAR IGA DRUGS

Mnemonic = V SAD CLIP

- Vancomycin = the main one
- Sulfa/somatostatin
- Amiodarone
- Diclofenac
- Captopril, gCSF
- Lithium, Lasix
- Interferon-gamma/IL-2
- Penicillin, phenytoin, PUVA, piroxicam

LICHENOID DRUG REACTIONS

Mnemonic = GAP ATAS
Main ones = antihypertensives (BBs, ACEIs, Thiazides), antimalarials, gold, penicillamine

- Gold
- Antimalarials (quinidine)
- Penicillamine/photocolor developer
- Amphetamines
- Thiazides
- ACE inhibitors
- Statins

*Alternative lichenoid mnemonic = HANG PC

- HCTZ
- Antimalarials
- NSAIDs
- Gold
- Penicillamine, PPIs
- Captopril

DRUG-INDUCED PEMPHIGUS

Mnemonic = I CRAP

- Indomethacin
- Captopril (thiols)
- Rifampin
- Ampicillin
- Penicillin/Penicillamine (pemphigus foliaceus-like)
- Note: Sulfhydryl groups of captopril and penicillamine are postulated cross react with the sulfhydryl groups of Dsg-1 and 3

BP-LIKE DRUG ERUPTION

Mnemonic = DAMP Napkin

- Dactinomycin/Diuretics (furosemide/aldosterone antagonists)
- Amoxicillin/Analgesics
- Methotrexate

- Penicillamine
- Neuroleptics

DRUG-INDUCED LUPUS

Mnemonic = HIP SPAM
Note: slow acetylators are more susceptible

- Hydralazine
- Isoniazid/INH
- Procainamide
- Sulfonamides
- Penicillin/penicillamine
- Anticonvulsants (includes phenytoin)
- Minocycline

PELLAGRA-LIKE DRUG ERUPTION

- Isoniazid/INH
- 5-FU

PITYRIASIS ROSEA-LIKE DRUG ERUPTION

- Gold
- ACE inhibitors

SCLE-LIKE DRUG ERUPTION

- HCTZ
- Terbinafine
- Calcium channel blockers
- Griseofulvin
- NSAIDs

EGFR INHIBITORS DRUG REACTIONS

Mnemonic = PPPRIDE

= Papulopustules (acne), Paronychia, Pyogenic granulomas, Regulatory abnormalities of hair growth (alopecia), Itching, Dryness due to EGFR inhibitors

DRUGS THAT CAN INDUCE VARIEGATE PORPHYRIA

Mnemonic = BEGS for Alcohol

- Barbiturates
- Estrogen
- Griseofulvin
- Sulfa drugs
- Alcohol

CHEMOTHERAPY DRUG REACTIONS

- Neutrophilic eccrine hidradenitis
- Sweet's syndrome
- Acral erythema (erythrodysesthesia)
- Radiation recall
- Anagen effluvium
- Hyperpigmentation

IMMUNOTHERAPY DRUG REACTIONS

- "PD1 inhibition causes dermatology"
- Pruritus is the most common cutaneous AE
- Eczematous
- Granulomatous
- Lichenoid
- Psoriasiform
- Vitiligo
- Urticaria
- BP
- SJS/TEN

PSORIASIS EXACERBATION

Mnemonic = SIR BLAM

- Steroid rebound (withdrawal of prednisone)
- Interferon and Ribavirin (HCV treatment)
- Beta blockers
- Lithium
- Anti-Malarials

NON-IMMUNOLOGIC CAUSES OF URTICARIA

Mnemonic = PROMS

- Polymyxin B
- Radiocontrast
- Opioids
- Muscle relaxants
- Salicylates/NSAIDS

G6PD HEMOLYSIS

Mnemonic—DAMN PS

- Dapsone
- Anti-pyretics/analgesics/ASA
- anti-Malarials
- Nitroprusside/Nitroglycerine/Nitrofurantoin
- Procainamide/Phenytoin/Phenobarbital
- Sulfa

15

PENILE ULCERATION

- Foscarnet

15.7.3 Other Lists

HAIR CYCLE: RULE OF 3s

Anagen 3 years
Catagen 3 weeks
Telogen 3 months

SUFFIXES FOR BIOLOGIC MEDICATIONS

-cept = fusion protein creating a receptor
(example = etanercept = Enbrel)
-iximab = a chimeric monoclonal antibody
(example = infliximab = Remicade)
-zumab = a humanized monoclonal antibody (95% human)
(example = risankizumab = Skyrizi)
-umab = a fully human monoclonal antibody
(example = adalimumab = Humira)

X-LINKED RECESSIVE DISORDERS

Mnemonic = "Chad's kinky wife" (is recessive, not that kinky)
Chronic granulomatous disease
Hunter's syndrome
Anhidrotic ectodermal dysplasia
Dyskeratosis congenita
Menke's kinky hair
Wiskott-Aldrich
X-linked Ichthyosis
Fabry's disease
Ehlers-Danlos (types V and IX)

X-LINKED DOMINANT DISORDERS

Mnemonic = "Go in my big hungry child's face" (He can handle it. He's dominant)
Goltz syndrome
Incontinentia pigmenti
MIDAS syndrome
Bazex syndrome
Conradi-Hünermann syndrome
CHILD
PHACES—?if XD, but mostly in females

KERATINS

K1 and 10 = expressed in keratinocytes after basal layer
K1 and 9 = palmoplantar
K4 and 13 = defect in white sponge nevus
K5 and 14 = defect in EB, at basement membrane
K5 (alone) = EB with mottled pigmentation, Dowling-Degos, Galli-Galli diseases
K6 and 16 = increased in psoriasis, atopic dermatitis
K6a and 16 = pachyonychia congenita type 1
K6b and 17 = pachyonychia congenita type 2
K14 (alone) = dermatopathia pigmentosa reticularis and Naegeli-Franceschetti-Jadassohn syndrome
K81 and 86 = defect in monilethrix (aka hair keratins 1 and 6)

INTRACRANIAL CALCIFICATIONS (GENODERMATOSES)

Mnemonic: Picture The Little Brown Stones
Papillon-Lefèvre
Tuberous sclerosis (paraventricular)
Lipoid proteinosis ("sickle-shaped" in temporal lobe)
Basal cell nevus syndrome (falx cerebri)
Sturge Weber syndrome ("tram track")

ETIOLOGIES OF VASCULITIS

Mnemonic = CTD SING

- CTD (SLE, RA)
- Thrombotic (TTP, DIC, septic emboli, HSP, cryo)
- Drugs (including serum sickness)
- Syndromes (Schnitzler's, Muckle-Wells, Finklestein's disease)
- Infection (HCV, HBV, Strep, GC, HIV)
- Neoplasms (Hodgkin's, multiple myeloma, leukemia)
- Granulomatous/Inflammatory (Churg-Strauss, GPA/Wegener's, MPA)

BODY SURFACE AREA RULE OF 9S

Face/Head = 9%
Chest/abdomen = 18%
Back = 18%
Arms = 9%, 9%
Legs = 18%, 18%
Perineum = 1%

DERMATOME REVIEW

Thumb = C6
Nipple = T4

Umbilicus = T10
Top of feet = L5
Bottom of feet = S1

SIGNS OF SUN DAMAGE

- Rhytides—wrinkles
- Furrows
- Elastosis
- Telangiectasias
- Dyschromia/poikiloderma

BURNS

First degree = superficial, limited to epidermis—erythema
Second degree = epidermis and superficial dermis—painful, bullae
Third degree = full thickness epidermis and dermis

ELASTOSIS PERFORANS SERPIGINOSA MNEMONIC

CART MOPED: Cutis laxa, Acrogeria, Rothmund-Thomson, Marfan, Osteogenesis imperfecta, PXE/Penicillamine, Ehlers-Danlos, Down's syndrome

ANGIOID STREAKS MNEMONIC

PEPSI COLA: PXE, Ehlers-Danlos, Paget's disease of bone, Sickle Cell, Idiopathic, Cutis laxa, Osteogenesis imperfecta, Lead poisoning, Acrogyria
Remember: caused by pathologic changes in Bruch's membrane

PIGMENTATION SYNDROMES

- Peutz-Jegher's—morbidity from intussussception
- Laugier-Hunziker = Peutz-Jegher's without GI polyps
- LEOPARD syndrome
- Carney syndrome—NAME (Nevi, Atrial myxoma, Myxoid cutaneous tumors, Ephelides)

JONES CRITERIA for rheumatic fever

- J (joints) = polyarthritis
- O (heart) = carditis
- N (nodules) = subcutaneous nodules
- E = erythema marginatum
- S = Sydenham's chorea

SUBEPIDERMAL NEUTROPHILIC BLISTERING DISEASE

Dermatitis herpetiformis
Linear IgA
Bullous lupus

DERMAL NEUTROPHILIC DERMATOSES

- Sweet syndrome
- Pyoderma gangrenosum
- Dermatitis herpetiformis
- Linear IgA/Chronic bullous dermatosis of childhood
- Behçet syndrome
- Erythema elevatum diutinum
- Cellulitis and other infectious diseases
- Leukocytoclastic vasculitis
- Bullous lupus
- Rheumatoid arthritis neutrophilic dermatosis
- Bowel-bypass syndrome/bowel-associated dermatosis-arthritis syndrome (BADAS)
- Palisaded neutrophilic and granulomatous dermatitis (PNGD)
- Neutrophilic eccrine hidradenitis

LICHEN SCLEROSUS ET ATROPHICUS—VARIETIES

In male genitalia—BXO—balanitis xerotica obliterans
In female genitalia—kraurosis vulvae

SOURCES OF SMOOTH MUSCLE IN THE BODY

Vessel walls
Arrector pili muscles
Dartos muscle (scrotum)
Areolae

DERMATOPHYTE SOURCES

Geophilic = from soil
Anthropophilic = from people
Zoophilic = from animals

SOFT VERSUS HARD NODULES

Soft—fatty, neural
Hard—scar, dermatofibroma, cyst
Rock hard—calcinosis cutis, tophaceous gout

HAMARTOMA VERSUS PHAKOMA

- Hamartoma: benign malformation/hyperplasia of elemental tissue from a given location where that tissue would normally occur.
- Phakoma: a hamartomatous finding in a phakomatosis. This includes retinal hamartomas, lisch nodules, shagreen patches, neurofibromas, etc.
- Phakomatosis: Ectodermal genetic diseases affecting the CNS along with other ectodermal tissues (skin and retina).
- Choristoma: benign neoplasm of "normal" (non-malignant) tissue in an ectopic location.

15

DEFINITION OF PARANEOPLASTIC SYNDROME

Paraneoplastic syndrome = manifestation of neoplasm wherein no neoplastic component is found (reactive to presence of neoplasm)

WOLFF-CHAIKOFF EFFECT

In case of taking potassium iodide (KI)
Excess iodide inhibits binding of iodine in thyroid gland (causes hypothyroid)

TECHNICAL NAME FOR GOOSEBUMPS = Cutis anserina

EPULIS = gingival tumor

High Yield Topics

Medications

Contents

16

Abstract

This section reviews medications commonly used in dermatology, along with side effects and interactions. Generic names are used although most brand names are indicated. Uses of these medications in dermatology are described and many are off-label.

Keywords

Medications · Side effects

16.1 Systemic Immunosuppressants and Anti-inflammatory Agents

Systemic steroids (commonly prednisone)

  Mechanism: Binds to glucocorticoid receptors directly in cell, inhibiting nuclear factor-κB, decreasing inflammation. Also inhibits TNF-α, GM-CSF, and several interleukins

  Immediate side effects: Accelerated release of neutrophils from bone marrow (neutrophilia) and demargination, transient lymphopenia, hyperglycemia, hypertension, mood changes/psychosis/insomnia, acneiform eruptions, weight gain/increased appetite, GI effects/peptic ulcers

  Later side effects: osteoporosis (most significant demineralization in first 6–12 months of therapy), adrenal suppression, avascular necrosis of femoral head/osteonecrosis, cataracts (posterior subcapsular—opposed to anterior cataracts from atopic dermatitis), Cushing syndrome, poor wound healing/striae, risk of infection

  Note: alternate-morning regimens may decrease some effects (hyperglycemia, risk of adrenal suppression), but not cataracts or osteoporosis (effect is from total dose and duration); other methods to decrease SE potential are to administer IM (lower cumulative dose) or to use dexamethasone (no mineralocorticoid effects). Consider PCP/PJP prophylaxis if dose is over 20 mg daily for over 4 weeks

  Interactions: Active TB, systemic fungal infection, depression/psychosis, HTN, DM

Mycophenolate mofetil (CellCept)

  Mechanism: Inhibits inosine monophosphate (IMP) dehydrogenase, blocking guanine (purine) synthesis. Considered more specific inhibition than azathioprine since only affects B and T lymphocyte cell lines (salvage pathway still intact)

  Side effects: GI effects (diarrhea), heme/hepatic toxicity rare

Interactions: With iron, forms complex that decreases absorption Not pregnancy safe

Note: recent study in a large health system showed that lab monitoring abnormalities are quite rare (common practice is baseline labs, repeat in 1m then q3m); takes a few months to "kick in" and can switch to mycophenolic acid if causing GI distress. Rare side effects: hyperglycemia, GI bleeding

Azathioprine (Imuran)

Mechanism: 6-mercaptopurine pro-drug. Inhibits purine synthesis enzymes. Metabolism: metabolized by both thiopurine methyltransferase (TPMT) and xanthine oxidase into non-toxic metabolites, HGPRT into active metabolite, 6-thioguanine (resembles adenosine and guanine). If TPMT deficient or xanthine oxidase blocked (allopurinol), immunosuppression greatly increased.

Side effects: Pancytopenia, increased lympoproliferative malignancies, SCCs, pancreatitis. Can have hypersensitivity reaction (morbilliform eruption) in 1st month, especially when given with MTX or cyclosporine

Interactions: Check TPMT, allopurinol (xanthine oxidase inhibitor), captopril (increase risk leukopenia), or warfarin (decreased effectiveness)

Not pregnancy safe

Note: one of the least favored immunosuppressants in dermatology due to relatively riskier AE profile despite similar efficacy to the other traditional drugs (MMF or MTX)

Review of 6-MP processing (3 pathways)

6-MP

→ (xanthine oxidase) [inhibited by allopurinol]

→ (HGPRT) [mutations cause Lesch-Nyhan syndrome]

→ (thiopurine methyltransferase = TPMT) [this can have variable activity from genetic polymorphism]

Antimalarials:

Hydroxychloroquine (Plaquenil), chloroquine (Aralen), quinacrine

Note: regular eye exam indicated (baseline VF or OCT testing and repeat yearly for HCQ but every 6 months for chloroquine).

Uses: lupus (and most CTD), photodermatoses, porphyria cutanea tarda (PCT)

Mechanism: Not well known (intercalates DNA?); can inhibit IL-2 release, modulates interferon signaling.

Side effects: blue-gray to black discoloration (oral > pretibial > nail > other; yellow with quinacrine), rarely retinopathy, pancytopenia, hemolysis (in severe G6PD deficiency, so rare not routine to check anymore). Only quinacrine has no ocular toxicity (now incredibly difficult to get in the USA). Reversible retinopathy = visual field loss.
Irreversible retinopathy = true retinopathy, greatest for chloroquine.

Interactions: Increased retinal toxicity when hydroxychloroquine and chloroquine together (so these two never combined, only either with quinacrine); smoking may decrease effectiveness of antimalarials in lupus

16

Note: for best safety keep HCQ under 5mg/kg and chloroquine under 2.3mg/kg daily.

Cyclosporine

Uses: psoriasis, atopic dermatitis, TEN, chronic urticaria, DRESS, PG, PRP

Mechanism: Downregulates IL-2 (and thus Th1 T cells)

Specifically, binds to cyclophilin creating a complex that prevents NFATc dephosphorylation (inhibits calcineurin). Normally calcium binds calmodulin, activating calcineurin, which dephosphorylates NFATc (nuclear factor of activated T cells), which would normally upregulate IL-2 gene expression

– In effect, a calcineurin inhibitor like tacrolimus/pimecrolimus

Side effects: Hypertension (check BP), renal failure (check urine), hypertrichosis, gingival hyperplasia, SCCs; hypomagnesemia, hyperkalemia (avoid potassium sparing diuretics)

Interactions: narrow therapeutic window and mostly metabolized by CYP450 3A4

Prior pregnancy category C (categories no longer used but essentially safe to use if necessary and cleared with OB)

– Can use for up to 12 months safely at 2-5 mg/kg/day but meant to be a bridge to maintenance therapy (some experts limit it to 12 weeks).

– Typically taken BID and has most of efficacy by 6 weeks

– Modified (Neoral) is better absorbed than non-modified (Sandimmune)

– Creatinine and blood pressure are most important values to monitor (if necessary use dose reduction and CCB)

Tacrolimus (Prograf systemic, Protopic topical) = calcineurin inhibitor

– Not generally used systemically for dermatologic disease (see other topical medications).

– Mechanism: binds to FK506-binding protein forming inhibitors of phosphatase calcineurin, preventing dephosphorylation of NFAT.

– Pimecrolimus is a topical calcineurin inhibitor in cream vehicle.

– Recent boards fodder for topical—case reports of inducing lentigines and facial flushing upon alcohol consumption.

Dapsone

Uses: neutrophilic dermatoses (EED, linear IgA, DH, bullous LE), leprosy, bullous pemphigoid

Mechanism: Inhibits neutrophil myeloperoxidase, which is required for respiratory burst (a sulfone)

Side effects: hemolysis (in everybody), methemoglobinemia (can be prevented with cimetidine or Vitamin E, tx with methylene blue); long term (rare) = agranulocytosis (occurs in first week to first 3 months presenting with fever, pharyngitis, signs of sepsis), peripheral neuropathy (motor > sensory, e.g. wasting of hands, foot drop), dapsone hypersensitivity syndrome (like DRESS with fever, rash, hepatitis, eosinophilia)

Interactions: G6PD deficiency (always check first)

Prior pregnancy category C

Topical form (Aczone) for acne; methemoglobinemia reported

Colchicine (Colcrys)

    Uses: neutrophilic dermatoses, LCV

    Mechanism: Binds to tubulin and prevents microtubule assembly, blocks neutrophil chemotaxis/adhesion/degranulation (similar to podophyllin, griseofulvin)

    Side effects: GI side effects common (diarrhea)

    Prior pregnancy category C

Thalidomide

    Uses: erythema nodosum leprosum (drug of choice), pruritus, sarcoidosis, lupus

    Mechanism: inhibits TNF-α

    Side effects: symmetric painful paresthesias, teratogenic (phocomelia)

    Monitoring with CBC, CMP every 3 months; CBC, TSH, CMP baseline

    Typical dose 100 mg qhs, can decrease over time to 50 mg every other day

Lenalidomide (Revlimid)

    = Derivative of thalidomide

Rapamycin/Sirolimus (Rapamune)

    Uses: immunosuppression in kidney transplant; now has potential for treating neoplasms given tumor suppressor activity (tuberous sclerosis).

    Note: does decrease risk of SCCs in transplant patients compared to other transplant regimens.

    Mechanism: inhibits mTOR (mammalian target of rapamycin) which is a proto-oncogene in the RAS-PI3K pathway usually inhibited by a tumor suppressor made by hamartin and tuberin (either may be mutated in tuberous sclerosis); despite similar name (sirolimus) to tacrolimus and pimecrolimus, sirolimus/ rapamycin is not a calcineurin inhibitor, but it does similarly suppress IL-2; all three are non-antibiotic macrolides (unlike erythromycin, azithromycin).

    Topical sirolimus can be compounded and used for angiofibromas, CARP, acanthosis nigricans, lymphangioma circumscriptum, angiokeratomas, port wine stains, nevus sebaceous, epidermal nevi

Intravenous immunoglobulin (IVIg)

    Uses: FDA approved for GVHD, dermatomyositis but also used for blistering diseases, SJS/TEN, Kawasaki disease

    Mechanism: provides passive immunity; in TEN, may block Fas–Fas ligand interaction

    Note: Check IgA level (small risk of anaphylaxis if IgA deficient, many hospitals already remove IgA from their blood products); relative contraindications include CHF and renal failure (risk of fluid overload), also history of VTE (pro-thrombotic).

    – Sucrose preparations can induce an osmotic nephrosis → acute renal failure.

    – Prior pregnancy category C

Saturated solution of potassium iodide (SSKI)

    Uses: erythema nodosum, sporotrichosis, Sweet's syndrome (and other neutrophilic dermatoses)

Mechanism: thought to inhibit neutrophil chemotaxis, and by mast cell heparin degranulation

Side effects: Wolff-Chaikoff effect (affects thyroid metabolism, can cause fetal goiter), iododerma, can flare dermatitis herpetiformis (and some neutrophilic dermatoses)

– Difficult to get now, not available at most retail pharmacies

Apremilast (Otezla)

Uses: psoriasis, Behcets disease

Mechanism: a cAMP phosphodiesterase-4 inhibitor (Side effects: nausea/vomiting, weight loss; caution with history of depression

Deucravicitinib (Sotyktu)

Uses: psoriasis

Mechanism: a tyrosine kinase 2 inhibitor (TYK2); non-JAK member of the JAK-STAT pathway; leads to decrease in type I interferon, IL-6, IL-10, IL-12, IL-17 and IL-23

Side effects: Hyperlipidemia, HSV, folliculitis, and acne; no boxed warning typical of JAKi

Janus Kinase Inhibitors (JAKi):

Tofacitinib (pan-JAK), Baricitinib (JAK1/2), Abrocitinib (JAK1), Upadacitinib (JAK1), Ritlecitinib (JAK3/TEC)

Uses: numerous inflammatory skin conditions

Mechanism:Important pro-inflammatory cytokines (IL-4, 13, 5, 31, 22, TSLP, others) activate the JAK-STAT pathway at the cell surface which then leads to immune cell up-regulation and inflammatory disease; by blocking this process the cytokines are unable to trigger this signaling

– The degree to which this is blocked affects the safety profile (tofacitinib is most immune suppressing and carries highest risk of MACE, VTE, malignancy and serious infections)

Side effects: acne, nausea, lymphopenia, lipid elevations are most common

– The selective JAKi are FDA approved to treat AD (abrocitinib, upadacitinib) and alopecia areata (baricitinib, ritlecitinib)

– Ruxolitinib cream (Opzelura) is FDA approved to treat AD and vitiligo

– All of these medications, including the topical, have a "black box" warning similar to the other traditional immunosuppressants used in dermatology

– Not pregnancy safe

16.2 Cytotoxic Medications and Chemotherapy Agents

Methotrexate (MTX)

Uses: derm/rheum diseases, medical abortion, chemotherapy

Mechanism: folic acid analog, irreversible inhibitor of dihydrofolate reductase (DHFR) and required for de novo synthesis of purine nucleotides

Side effects: nausea (relieved by folic or folinic acid), pancytopenia, hepato-toxicity (after years), radiation recall, pulmonary fibrosis, pneumonitis, ter-atogenicity, accelerated rheumatoid nodulosis

Interactions: With sulfa drugs (e.g. TMP/SMX), dapsone, markedly increased pancytopenia (synergistic DHFR inhibition, plus decreased plasma protein binding/renal excretion). NSAIDs/salicylates displace MTX from plasma proteins, lower renal excretion, increasing toxicity. Retinoids, alcohol syn-ergistic for liver disease.

Contraindications: liver disease, alcohol

Liver biopsy was indicated after a cumulative dose of MTX (no longer the case), but serologic testing (e.g. procollagen III peptidase)or imaging (elas-tography) may be an alternative to liver biopsy.

Note: recent studies suggest that adenosine may play a role in MTX resistance.

– Not pregnancy safe—wait at least 3 months after medication stopped to conceive

Leflunomide (Arava)

Uses: rheumatologic diseases

Mechanism: pyrimidine synthesis inhibitor

Hydroxyurea

Uses: psoriasis in HIV patients

Mechanism: inhibits M2 subunit of ribonucleotide reductase

Side effects: Can cause leg ulcers, dermatomyositis (poikiloderma of dorsal hands), megaloblastosis (in 100%), anemia (~25%), radiation recall, hyper-pigmentation

Not pregnancy safe

Cyclophosphamide (Cytoxan)

Uses: granulomatosis with polyangiitis (GPA), MPA, PAN, ocular cicatricial pemphigoid (first line), CTCL, hematologic malignancies

Mechanism: cross-links DNA, derived from nitrogen mustard, alkylating agent

Side effects: hemorrhagic cystitis (can lead to transitional cell carcinoma, pre-vent with mesna)

Not pregnancy safe

5-fluorouracil (5-FU) (topical = Efudex, Carac, others)

Uses: AKs, SCCIS, BCC, keloids, warts

Mechanism: pyrimidine analog, inhibits thymidylate synthetase

Side effects (IV): serpentine supravenous hyperpigmentation

Not pregnancy safe

Note: recent combo with calcipotriene has evidence in treating AKs with shorter duration and similar efficacy (bid × 5–7 days)

Ingenol mebutate (Picato)—off market, but worth knowing about

– Launched with great data for AK treatment in a short topical regimen and gained popularity however it was taken off of the market due to evidence that it may increase the risk of SCC over time

Bleomycin
  Uses: periungual warts (intralesional)
  Mechanism: inhibits DNA synthesis
  Side effects: necrosis, flagellate hyperpigmentation, NEH, radiation recall, Raynaud's
  Not pregnancy safe
CHOP chemotherapy regimen =
  Cyclophosphamide
  Hydroxydaunorubicin (aka doxorubicin or adriamycin)
  Oncovin (vincristine)
  Prednisone
  (Optional: rituximab can be added for R-CHOP)
ATRA (all-*trans*-retinoic acid)
  Uses = acute promyelocytic leukemia
  Side effects: can cause Sweet's syndrome
  Not pregnancy safe

16.2.1 Metastatic Melanoma Systemic Therapies

Dacarbazine, IL-2 = historic standard of care (now rarely used)
  BRAF inhibitors, MEK inhibitors (typically used in combination)

Interferon alfa-2b

Sorafenib (Nexavar)
  Mechanism: first generation nonselective RAF inhibitor; downregulates MAPK signaling, and also targets VEGF and PDGF
  Uses: melanoma, renal cell carcinoma
  – Was disappointing in treatment of melanoma; not efficacious as monotherapy (recognized as a weak BRAF kinase inhibitor)
Vemurafenib, Dabrafenib, Encorafenib
  Mechanism: targeted inhibitor of BRAF with V600E mutation (most common) FDA approved for metastatic melanoma
  Side effects: keratoacanthomas/SCCs (reduced with adding MEKi)
Trametinib, Cobimetinib, Binimetinib
  Mechanism: targeted inhibitor of MEK (part of BRAF pathway)
  FDA approved for metastatic melanoma
  Side effects: keratoacanthomas/SCCs, panniculitis, palmoplantar dysesthesia
Imatinib (Gleevec)
  Mechanism: a receptor tyrosine kinase inhibitor that inhibits BCR-ABL as well as c-KIT (though may be ineffective in c-KIT D816V mutations)
  Uses: c-KIT mutated melanomas (acral, lentigo maligna melanoma, mucosal, other chronic sun exposed); however, few successful treatments reported

Immunotherapy

Ipilimumab (Yervoy)
> Mechanism: a human monoclonal antibody against CTLA-4 (cytotoxic T lymphocyte-associated antigen 4)
> FDA approved for metastatic melanoma in 2011

Pembrolizumab, Nivolumab
> Mechanism: a human monoclonal antibody against PD-1 (programmed cell death receptor); also known as a checkpoint inhibitor.
> FDA approved for stage IIB, IIC and metastatic melanoma; often combined with Ipilimumab (increased efficacy but also increased toxicity).

Relatlimab
> Mechanism: a human monoclonal antibody against LAG-3 (lymphogene activation gene-3, part of the checkpoint inhibitor pathway)
> FDA approved for metastatic melanoma in 2023; often combined with nivolumab
> Side effects: pruritus (most common), inflammatory skin disorders (eczematous, granulomatous, lichenoid, psoriasiform, urticaria, bullous pemphigoid)

Talimogene Laherparepvec (T-VEC)
> Mechanism: injectable viral vector leading to destruction of melanoma cells
> FDA approved for unresectable or metastatic lesions; being studied as a synergistic medication with checkpoint inhibition
> Side effects: pain, ulceration

16.2.2 BCC and SCC Systemic Therapy

Vismodegib, sonedigib
> Mechanism = antagonist of Smoothened receptor in hedgehog pathway
> FDA approved for locally advanced and metastatic BCC
> Side effects: significant GI effects, muscle spasms, dysgeusia, alopecia

Cemilpumab
> Mechanism: a human monoclonal antibody against PD-1 (programmed cell death receptor); also known as a checkpoint inhibitor
> FDA approved for locally advanced and metastatic BCC and SCC
> Side effects: *See Immunotherapy section for melanoma*

16.2.3 Anti-Cutaneous T-Cell Lymphoma Systemic Therapies

– For early stage disease (IA-IIA = topical steroids, phototherapy (PUVA and NBUVB), bexarotene, topical chemotherapy (mechlorethamine and carmustine).
– For advanced MF and Sézary syndrome = total skin electron beam therapy, bexarotene, extracorporeal photopheresis, HDAC (histone deacetylase) inhibitors (vorinostat, romidepsin), interferons, other systemic chemotherapy. The newer therapies of note are mogalizumab and brentuximab vedotin.

16

Mogalizumab

Mechanism: monoclonal antibody against CCR4.

FDA approved in 2018 for advanced CTCL (especially good for blood involvement)

Side effects: inflammatory rash, skin infection.

Brentuximab vedotin

Mechanism: monoclonal antibody against CD-30

FDA approved in 2018 for advanced CTCL (especially good for large cell transformation/LCT)

Side effects: peripheral neuropathy (up to 65% of patients)

16.3 Biologics

Though it can refer to many biological products, the term "biologic" here is generally meant to refer to a medication produced via recombinant DNA technology, such as monoclonal antibodies and fusion proteins that mimic human receptors or cytokines. "Biosimilar" refers to the generic version of a biologic medication.

TNF-α inhibitors

Contraindications for TNF-α inhibitor biologics:

Immunocompromised/HIV, significant active infections (e.g. active TB, HBV), malignancy in past 5 years (lymphoma, solid except NMSC), congestive heart failure, demyelinating disease (multiple sclerosis), positive ANA or autoimmune disease (relative). Many are concerned about possible increased risk of lymphoma in the long term; however evidence thus far has not yet ruled out nor established any causal relationship.

Risks include the above; infection from immunosuppression (including *Legionella* and *Listeria*)

– All below except infliximab are delivered via subcutaneous injection.

Etanercept (Enbrel)

Uses: psoriasis, rheumatoid arthritis

Mechanism: TNF-α inhibitor (blocks soluble form only). A fusion protein ofextracellular domain of TNF-α receptor and Fc domain of human IgG1

Among the biologics, etanercept alone can bind lymphotoxin (TNF-β)

Note: though generally considered less efficacious than other TNF inhibitors, preferred by some given its short half-life and longer experience (first on the market in 1998, first biologic approved by FDA to treat plaque psoriasis in 2004)

Adalimumab (Humira)

Uses: psoriasis, rheumatoid arthritis, Crohn's.

Mechanism: TNF-α inhibitor (blocks soluble form and receptor). A fully human recombinant IgG1 monoclonal antibody against TNF-α.

Infliximab (Remicade)

Mechanism: TNF-α inhibitor (blocks soluble form and receptor). A chimeric (human-mouse) monoclonal antibody against TNF-α
– Drug delivered thru infusion
– May develop anti-drug antibodies

Golimumab (Simponi)

Mechanism: Just like adalimumab (Humira), a TNF-α inhibitor (blocks soluble form and receptor). A fully human recombinant IgG1 monoclonal antibody against TNF-α. Dosed monthly.

Certolizumab (Cimzia)

Mechanism: Just like adalimumab (Humira), a TNF-α inhibitor (blocks soluble form and receptor). It is unique as a pegylated fragment of a humanized monoclonal antibody which stops transplacental migration of drug and is therefore provides no fetal exposure in treated patients

Other biologics

Ustekinumab (Stelara)

Uses: psoriasis
Mechanism: Human antibody against p40 subunit of IL-12 and IL-23 (Th17)
Contraindications for IL-17 inhibitor biologics:
Should not be used in those with known inflammatory bowel disease given potential risk of flare; relative increase in candidal infections (mucosal, cutaneous);
As a class, these agents tend to have more rapid response and best coverage for axial psoriatic arthritis

Ixekizumab (Taltz)

Uses: psoriasis, psoriatic arthritis
Mechanism: Monoclonal antibody against IL-17A

Brodalumab (Siliq)

Uses: psoriasis
Mechanism: Human antibody against IL-17 receptor (blocks all subtypes)
Note: has REMS program for suicidal behavior

Bimekizumab (Bimzelx)

Uses: psoriasis
Mechanism: Human antibody against IL-17A/F
Note: only agent in class that can be dosed every 8 weeks; does have a higher risk of candidiasis than the others in class
Also: FDA mentions potential for suicidal behavior, however no REMS program

Secukinumab (Cosentyx)

Uses: psoriasis
Mechanism: Human antibody against IL-17A
Contraindications for IL-23 inhibitor biologics:
No absolute contraindications
As a class, these agents tend to have fantastic skin improvement but PsA data not as strong as the IL-17s

Tildrakizumab (Ilumya)
  Uses: psoriasis, psoriatic arthritis.
  Mechanism: Antibody against p19 subunit of IL-23 (Th17)
  Note: unique in its administration in the office/infusion center so can go
  through medical benefit instead of prescription (beneficial for medicare)

Guselkumab (Tremfya)
  Uses: psoriasis, psoriatic arthritis
  Mechanism: Antibody against p19 subunit of IL-23 (Th17)

Risankizumab (Skyrizi)
  Uses: psoriasis, psoriatic arthritis, crohn's disease
  Mechanism: Antibody against p19 subunit of IL-23 (Th17)

Rituximab (Rituxan)
  Uses: non-Hodgkin B-cell lymphoma, has also been used in autoimmune bul-
  lous disease, vasculitis, and collagen vascular disease (B-cell mediated disease)
  Mechanism: chimeric monoclonal Ab against CD20 (B cells)
  Contraindications: cardiac arrhythmias, angina, Hepatitis B (may reactivate),
  live vaccines

Anakinra (Kineret)
  Uses: rheumatoid arthritis, Muckle-Wells syndrome, NOMID (neonatal-onset
  multisystem inflammatory disease)
  Mechanism: binds IL-1 receptors (IL-1 antagonist)

Canakinumab
  Uses: rheumatoid arthritis, Muckle-Wells syndrome, NOMID (neonatal-onset
  multisystem inflammatory disease)
  Mechanism: binds IL-1 receptors (IL-1 antagonist)

Tocilizumab
  Uses: rheumatoid arthritis, JIA
  Mechanism: anti IL-6 agent

Mepolizumab
  Uses: eosinophilic disorders
  Mechanism: anti IL-5 agent

Omalizumab
  Uses: chronic urticaria
  Mechanism: anti IgE
  Note: Ligelizumab is a high affinity anti-IgE agent that has been use for recal-
  citrant urticaria cases but is not FDA approved

Dupilumab (Dupixent)
  Uses: atopic dermatitis, prurigo nodularis, chronic pruritus of unknown or-
  igin, bullous pemphigoid, urticaria, and several other pruritic skin disorders
  Mechanism: IL-4 and IL-13 inhibitor
  Side effects: most discussed is conjunctivitis/eye irritation, also erythematous
  eruptions possible

Tralokinumab (Adbry)
  Uses: atopic dermatitis
  Mechanism: IL-13 inhibitor

Note: Has FDA approval for once monthly dosing in well controlled patients; efficacy data not as strong as dupilumab

Nemolizumab

Uses: prurigo nodularis, atopic dermatitis, chronic pruritus of unknown origin

Mechanism: IL-31 inhibitor

Note: Rapid and potent inhibitor of pruritus, uniquely low injection site reaction/pain, monthly dosing from initiation

Off market but still worth knowing about

Alefacept (Amevive).

Mechanism: Fusion protein against LFA-3

Monitoring: must check CD4 weekly to biweekly

Note: The manufacturer stopped producing this medication in 2011; there was not any particular concern or risk for this withdrawal, but the medication was not being prescribed frequently at the time.

Efalizumab (Raptiva)

Uses: psoriasis

Mechanism: Recombinant humanized monoclonal antibody against LFA-1

Monitoring: platelets monthly

Note: Pulled off market in 2009 given cases of progressive multifocal leukoencephalopathy (PML) (occurred at rate of 1 in 500 patients)

16.4 Retinoids

Isotretinoin (Accutane).

Mechanism: binds all RARs, exact mechanism not understood

– Two families of retinoid receptors: RAR (retinoic acid receptors) and RXR (retinoid X receptors), which are ligand-activated transcription factors; direct and indirect effects of RAR/RXR receptors may lead to downregulation of transcription factors, downregulating proliferation/inflammation

– Dimerize to RAR/RXR and RXR/RXR; RAR-γ predominant epidermal receptor; isotretinoin may decrease keratins 6 and 16

Indications: nodulocystic acne, hidradenitis suppurativa, dissecting cellulitis, ichthyoses

Side effects: teratogenicity, dyslipidemia (especially hypertriglyceridemia, liver abnormalities (especially transaminitis), depression/suicidality? (likely minor association if any), inflammatory bowel disease? (likely no association), excessive granulation tissue (PGs), diffuse idiopathic skeletal hyperostosis, premature closure of epiphyses (so recommended preferably after patient has reached adult height)

Interactions: synergistic pseudotumor cerebri with tetracyclines

Contraindications: pregnancy – wait at least 1 month after medication stopped to conceive.

Not pregnancy safe (all sysemic retinoids)

Note: Absorica/Absorica LD are the newest formulations of isotretinoin approved; better absorption in the absence of a fatty meal

Acitretin (Soriatane)

Mechanism: binds all RARs; acitretin is a metabolite of etretinate, which was previously used as a medication

Indications: psoriasis, chemoprevention of NMSC, pityriasis rubra pilaris

Additional concerns: synergistic hepatotoxicity with MTX, re-esterification to etretinate with alcohol → since can be reverse metabolized into etretinate, women must avoid pregnancy for at least three years after being on medication; thus, typically only used in women who cannot get pregnant or have completed any possible child bearing

Bexarotene (Targretin)

Mechanism: a retinoid, binds only RXR-α

Indications: mycosis fungoides

Additional side effects = hypothyroidism (central), leukopenia, agranulocytosis

Topical retinoids

Tretinoin (Retin-A, Altreno, Twyneo) = binds all RARs, Category C (would not give in pregnancy)

Tazarotene (Tazorac, Arazlo, Fabior) = binds RAR-β and RAR-γ (not α), Category X

Adapalene (Differin, Epiduo) = binds RAR-β and RAR-γ (not α), Category C (would not give in pregnancy)

Trifarotene (Aklief) = binds RAR-γ as the newest formulated topical retinoid; meant to be more targeted to the skin and gentle however very similar efficacy and tolerability to other topical retinoids

16.5 Antibiotics

16.5.1 Antifungals

Azole antifungals

Mechanism: inhibition of 14-alpha-demethylase (critical for ergosterol synthesis)

Fluconazole—weak CYP3A4 inhibitor, 2C9

Ketoconazole—strongest CYP450 3A4 inhibitor

Side effects: possible fulminant hepatitis, gynecomastia, impotence

Itraconazole

Prior pregnancy category C

Allylamines:

Mechanism: binds to fungal cell wall sterols (ergosterol) irreversibly, causing formation of aqueous channels, membrane permeability -> cell death

Terbinafine (Lamisil)

Mechanism: Inhibits squalene epoxidase (an allylamine)

Side effects: Reversible taste (dysgeusia)/visual disturbance, subacute cutaneous lupus-like rash; caution in renal/liver disease.
Naftifine (Naftin)
Polyene antifungals:
Mechanism: binds to fungal cell membrane sterols irreversibly, increasing permeability
Note: not effective against dermatophytes
Amphotericin-B
Nystatin
Side effects: Amphotericin "ampho-terrible" may cause nephrotoxicity, though less in lipid-complexed formulations
Griseofulvin
Mechanism: binds to tubulin, interfering with fungal microtubules and mitosis; this mechanism is analogous to podophyllin, colchicine, vincristine (all bind to tubulin)
Interactions: CYP450 3A4 inducer
Ciclopirox
Mechanism: chelates polyvalent cations, inhibiting metal-dependent enzymes in fungus
Other systemic antifungals
Note: these are mostly used for invasive and systemic candidiasis, aspergillosis, etc.
Echinocandins (e.g. caspofungin)
Mechanism: inhibit cell wall synthesis
Triazoles, second generation (voriconazole, posaconazole)
Voriconazole – associated with visual disturbances, phototoxicity, and increased risk of SCCs

16.5.2 Bacteriostatic/Bactericidal Antibiotics: (Divided by Site of Action)

Cell Wall
Beta lactams: 1. Penicillin, 2. Cephalosporins
Vancomycin—may be associated with vancomycin flushing syndrome—previously called 'red man syndrome' (avoid given racist connotations), linear IgA disease
Nucleus
Fluoroquinolones (DNA gyrase aka topoisomerase II)
Metronidazole (DNA strand breakage via cytotoxic metabolites)
Trimethoprim/sulfamethoxazole (TMP/SMX) (Bactrim) (nucleic acid synthesis)
   – Inhibits dihydropteroate synthetase (sulfas compete with PABA) and dihydrofolate reductase (trimethoprim). These two inhibitions synergistically block the pathway that catalyzes formation of folic acid.
   – Sulfas may exacerbate rickettsial disease

16

Rifampin – disrupts RNA synthesis

Ribosome

"Buy AT 30," "CELL at 50"

30S = Aminoglycosides, Tetracyclines

50S = Chloramphenicol, Erythromycin (Macrolides), cLindamycin, and Linezolid

Tetracyclines (doxycycline, minocycline, sarecycline)

– First line tx for acne, rickettsial diseases, Lyme, chlamydia/LGV, granuloma inguinale, *Vibrio vulnificus*, *M. marinum*; second line for syphilis
– Not recommended for under age 8 (tooth discoloration); newer evidence shows it should be fine in short durations but still controversial
– Photosensitizing (especially doxycycline, with photo-onycholysis)
– Most excreted by kidneys, except doxycycline (safe in renal failure)
– Not safe in pregnancy
– Minocycline associated with more side effects
  – Minocycline pigmentation – 3 types
    Type 1: blue-black at sites of acne, inflammation
    Type 2: blue-grey on normal skin; anterior legs
    Type 3: diffuse muddy brown on sun-exposed areas
  – Has been associated with cases of PAN and DRESS, drug-induced lupus, ANCA (+) drug-induced vasculitis

Chloramphenicol

– Second line treatment for rickettsial disease (preferred in pregnancy, despite risk of grey baby syndrome)

Macrolides

– Safe in pregnancy
– Inhibitors of CYP3A4, except azithromycin
– Erythromycin is first line tx for *Bartonella*, also used to tx PLEVA, pertussis, acne, accelerate clearance of pityriasis rosea
– Azithromycin is first line tx for chancroid, also a treatment for CARP

Linezolid

– Risk of thrombocytopenia (more than others)

Note: antibiotic-induced psychosis is known as Hoigné's syndrome or antibiomania.

16.5.3 Anti-viral Medications

Acyclovir/ Valacyclovir (Valtrex)/ Famciclovir (Famvir)

Mechanism: guanosine analog, inhibits DNA polymerase

– Valacyclovir and famciclovir have better bioavailability, fewer doses needed
– Prodrugs that require conversion by viral thymidine kinase phosphorylation; if deficient or mutated, virus may gain resistance
– Risk of TTP/HUS with valacyclovir in immunosuppressed patients

Foscarnet
    Mechanism: a pyrophosphate analog; does not require phosphorylation by viral or cellular kinases
    Side effects: can cause penile ulceration
Cidofovir
    Uses: approved for CMV retinitis; also used for HPV, tumoral HSV
    Mechanism: inhibits viral DNA polymerase
Ganciclovir
    Uses: for CMV
    Mechanism: inhibits viral DNA polymerase
Helicase-primase inhibitors (e.g. pritelivir)—currently in development and not yet approved by FDA

16.5.4 Other Antibiotic Agents

Ivermectin
    Mechanism: blocks glutamate channels. Specifically, binds to glutamate-gated chloride ion channels, which occur in invertebrate nerve and muscle cells. This leads to increased permeability of cell membranes to chloride ions then hyperpolarization of the nerve or muscle cell, and death of parasite
    Side effects: Mazzotti reaction = from release of parasite antigens; less common than with diethylcarbamine (similar to Jarisch-Herxheimer reaction)
    Uses: treatment of scabies, other infections, rosacea (topical form recently brought to market)
Isoniazid
    Mechanism: inhibits synthesis of mycolic acid
    Side effects: can cause drug-induced lupus, pellagra-like reaction, B6 (pyridoxine) deficiency
    Interactions: CYP3A4 inducer
Rifampin
    Mechanism: inhibits bacterial RNA synthesis by binding DNA-dependent RNA polymerase
    Side effects: can cause hepatotoxicity, orange body fluids
    Interactions: most potent CYP3A4 inducer, decreases effectiveness of OCPs
Pentavalent antimony (sodium stibogluconate).
    Uses: leishmaniasis
Clofazamine + dapsone + rifampin = standard leprosy regimen.
Neosporin/triple antibiotic = neomycin + bacitracin + polymyxin

16

16.6 **Other Systemic Medications**

Antihistamines
  H1 antagonists
  First generation (sedating)
  – Includes diphenhydramine (Benadryl) and hydroxyzine (Atarax)
  – Avoid hydroxyzine with ethylenediamene allergy (can cross-react)
  – Doxepin is a potent antihistamine and tricyclic antidepressant Second and third generations (non-sedating)
  – Includes loratadine (Claritin), fexofenadine (Allegra), cetirizine (Zyrtec), levocetirizine (Xyzal)
  H2 antagonists
  – May be useful as adjunct in urticaria (though data may be lacking)
  – Traditionally, oral cimetidine has been a treatment for warts.

Spironolactone (Aldactone)
  Mechanism: aldosterone antagonist, potassium sparing diuretic, and anti-androgen
  Uses: congestive heart failure, hypertension, acne, hyperandrogenism in women (hirsutism, androgenetic alopecia)
  Side effects: urinary frequency, breast tenderness, menstrual irregularities, hyperkalemia (potassium monitoring appears unnecessary during treatment for acne); has not been found to increase risk of breast cancer
  Prior pregnancy category C
Oral contraceptives (OCPs)
  Three combination OCPs with FDA approval for acne:
    Norgestimate/ethinyl estradiol (Ortho Tri-Cyclen)
    Drospirenone/ethinyl estradiol (Yaz)
    Norethindrone acetate/ethinyl estradiol (Estrostep)
  Mechanism: for acne, these OCPs have an anti-androgenic effect
  Contraindications: pregnancy, smokers (over age 35), hypertension, migraine headaches (over age 35), history of thromboembolic disease
  Concerns: increased risk for venous thromboembolism (though less than with pregnancy), can be reduced in effectiveness by rifampin
Vasodilators
  Uses: Raynaud's phenomenon, vascular disease
  Phosphodiesterase inhibitors
    Mechanism of action: inhibit phosphodiesterase, increasing intracellular cAMP
    Pentoxifylline (Trental)
    Sildenafil (Viagra)
  Calcium channel blockers
  Botulinum toxin (has been used for Raynaud's)
D-Penicillamine
  Mechanism: copper chelator

- Interferes with elastin cross-linking (1. By causing low copper bloodlevels that cause reduced lysyl oxidase activity, 2. By directly blocking cross-linking of residues)

Uses: Wilson's disease

Side effects: Can cause PXE, EPS, acquired cutis laxa, pemphigus foliaceus-like drug eruption

Interferon-α

Uses: systemically, for hepatitis; locally, treatment for warts

Side effects: increased eyelashes (trichomegaly), psoriasis exacerbation

Glycopyrrolate (Robinul)

Mechanism: anticholinergic

Uses: hyperhidrosis

Propranolol, Nadolol, carvedilol

Mechanism: beta blocker

Uses: for infantile hemangiomas, rosacea

Risks: hypoglycemia, hypotension, bronchospasm; also "rebound growth," sleep disturbances

Also: topical timolol being used

Gabapentin (Neurontin)

Pregabalin (Lyrica)

These two medications are similar.

Mechanism: binds to alpha-2-delta subunit of voltage-dependent calcium channel in central nervous system; may decrease release of neurotransmitters

Uses: post-herpetic neuralgia, neuropathic pain, pruritus

Side effects: somnolence, vivid dreams/nightmares

SSRIs (paroxetine, sertraline, duloxetine, escitalopram)

Mechanism: selective serotonin reuptake inhibitors

Uses: for anxiety exacerbated skin disease (neuropathic excoriations, skin picking) and cutaneous dysesthesia

Risks: somnolence, GI distress, serotonin syndrome (when combined with other serotonergic drugs)

Mirtazapine

Mechanism: atypical tetracyclic antidepressant

Uses: for anxiety exacerbated skin disease (neuropathic excoriations, skin picking), cutaneous dysesthesia, pruritus

Risks: somnolence, GI distress, weight gain

Tricyclic antidepressants (doxepin, amitriptyline, despiramine)

Mechanism: tricyclic antidepressant

Uses: for anxiety exacerbated skin disease (neuropathic excoriations, skin picking), cutaneous dysesthesia, neuropathic pruritus

Risks: somnolence, GI distress, weight gain, anticholinergic effects, arrhythmia

Antipsychotic (pimozide, risperidone, aripiprazole).

Mechanism: anti-dopaminergic agents

Uses: delusions of parasitosis

Risks: somnolence, GI distress, metabolic syndrome, arrhythmia

346   Chapter 16 · Medications

Naltrexone
    Mechanism: opioid receptor antagonist
    Uses: uremic or cholestatic pruritus, neuropathic pruritus, dysesthesia
    Risks: vivid dreams, nightmares, headache
Difelikefalin
    Mechanism: peripherally restricted opioid receptor kappa agonist
    Uses: uremic pruritus in those on HD
    Risks: somnolence, GI disturbance, paresthesias
Dronabinol
    Mechanism: delta-9-THC canabinoid
    Uses: neuropathic pruritus, dysesthesia
    Risks: euphoria, altered mental status, weight gain
Butorphanol
    Mechanism: partial agonist, antagonist of mu opioid receptor and kappa agonist
    Uses: pruritus of any etiology
    Risks: somnolence, nausea, dizziness
    Note: due to mechanism has lower abuse potential than other opiates

16.7 Other Topical Medications

Notes:
    – Some people use "fingertip units" to estimate amount of steroid that should be prescribed; one fingertip unit = 0.5 g of cream or ointment
    – Ointments are more potent than creams of the same medication and strength
    – Tachyphylaxis = rapid decrease in drug efficacy after repeated doses over a short time
Topical steroids
    Very low potent (Class 7) = hydrocortisone 1%, hydrocortisone 2.5% (Hytone)
    Low potent (Class 6) = hydrocortisone valerate (Westcort), desonide (Desowen)
    Mid potent (Class 4,5) = triamcinolone (Kenalog), mometasone cream (Elocon), betamethasone valerate, fluocinolone acetonide (Synalar, Derma-Smoothe oil)
    High potent (Class 2,3) = fluocinonide (Lidex), betamethasone dipropionate (Diprosone, Diprolene) Superpotent (Class 1) = clobetasol (Temovate, Clobex), diflorasone (Psorcon), flurandrenolide tape (Cordran tape)
    Side effects = cutaneous atrophy, telangiectasias, striae, perioral dermatitis (on face), cataracts and glaucoma (when used around the eyes), possible systemic absorption and HPA axis suppression
Keratolytics
    Includes: ammonium lactate, urea, glycolic acid, salicylic acid, N-acetylcysteine (has been effective in treatment for inherited ichthyoses)
    Mechanism: removes scaling or hyperkeratosis

Azelaic acid (Azelex = 20% cream, Finacea = 15% gel)
  Uses: acne, hyperpigmentation
  Mechanism: competitive inhibition of tyrosinase (like hydroquinone)
Sodium sulfacetamide (Klaron)
  Mechanism: a sulfonamide, just like TMP/SMX
Benzoyl peroxide (BPO)
  Mechanism: active oxygen releaser, oxidizes bacterial proteins by active oxygen
  Side effects: bleaches fabrics
  Note: Epsolay is a new topical BPO for rosacea with modest data and high expense limiting its use
Tacrolimus/pimecrolimus (Protopic, Elidel; topical) = calcineurin inhibitors
  Indications: approved for atopic dermatitis ("steroid sparing")
  Mechanism: bind to FK506-binding protein forming inhibitors of phosphatase calcineurin, preventing dephosphorylation of NFAT
  Side effects: possible allergic contact; black box warning regarding cases of lymphoma (systemically there is risk, no evidence from topicals in long term safety data)
  Contraindications: Netherton syndrome (given increased absorption)
Imiquimod (Aldara, Zyclara)
  Mechanism: stimulates innate immune response (Th1); binds toll-like receptor 7 (TLR7) on APCs; stimulates interferon-α
  Uses: condyloma acuminata, actinic keratoses, BCC
Hydroquinone
  Mechanism: reversible competitive inhibitor of tyrosinases (like azelaic acid)
  Side effects: exogenous ochronosis
Podophyllin (Podocon, Condylox)
  Derived from the mayapple plant (*Podophyllum peltatum*); podophyllin is a crude alcohol extract of the plant's rhizome
  Indications: condyloma acuminata
  Mechanism: binds tubulin and arrests mitosis in metaphase (works similarly to griseofulvin, colchicine)
Sinecatechins (Veregen)
  Indications: condyloma acuminata
  Derived from green tea extract, it is a botanical medication
Eflornithine (Vaniqa)
  Mechanism: inhibits ornithine decarboxylase, which catalyzes the conversion of ornithine into putrescine (which plays a role in hair follicle proliferation)
  Uses: topically used for hirsutism, systemically (Ornidyl) treats African sleeping sickness
  Note: product no longer commercially available but can be compounded
Calcipotriene (Dovonex)
  – 1,25-D_3 analog, has an immunomodulator effect not well understood, used as steroid substitute (like calcineurin inhibitors)
  Side effects: irritant dermatitis

16

Permethrin (Elimite)

   Mechanism: acts on parasite nerve cell membrane to disrupt Na channel current

   Derived from chrysanthemums, a pesticide/scabicide

Ivermectin (Soolantra)

Topical formulation for treatment of rosacea

   – Mechanism: blocks glutamate channels; *see also Antibiotics*

Silver sulfadiazine

   Uses: topical antibiotic for wounds

   Side effects: may actually delay wound healing (per Cochrane review), has been associated with argyria, neutropenia

   Note: one of few topical antimicrobials that is broadly active against gram positives, negatives, anaerobes and fungi

Aluminum chloride

   Uses: hemostatic agent, antiperspirant

   Mechanism of action: aluminum salt precipitates tissue for mechanical obstruction to hemorrhage, or precipitates eccrine ducts for mechanical obstruction to sweating

Monsel's solution (ferric sulfate)

   Uses: hemostatic agent (stronger than aluminum chloride, but has small risk of pigmentation)

Oxymetazoline (Rhofade)

   Uses: rosacea

   Mechanism: alpha adrenergic receptor agonist (primarily alpha-1)

   Side effects: potential for rebound (though much lower than brimonidine)

Brimonidine (Mirvaso)

   Uses: rosacea

   Mechanism: alpha adrenergic receptor agonist (primarily alpha-2)

   Side effects: significant rebound effects have been reported

Ingenol mebutate (Picato)

   Uses: actinic keratosis

   Derived from sap of the plant *Euphorbia peplus*

   Note: no longer available in the USA given concerns of increased development of SCCs

5-fluorouracil (5-FU) (Efudex, Carac)

   Uses: actinic keratosis, SCCIS, superficial BCC, verrucae

Ruxolitinib (Opzelura)

   Uses: atopic dermatitis, vitiligo

   Mechanism: janus kinase inhibitor (primarily JAK1/2)

   Side effects: boxed warning for major adverse cardiovascular events, VTE, serious infection, malignancy and death (taken from oral JAKi), however no risk for these in topical trials

Roflumilast (Zoryve)

   Uses: psoriasis, seborrheic dermatitis, atopic dermatitis

   Mechanism: PDE4 inhibitor (highest affinity compared to apremilast and crisaborole)

Crisoborole (Eucrisa)
   Uses: atopic dermatitis
   Mechanism: PDE4 inhibitor
   Generally seems to be less effective and more expensive, but a non-steroidal option'
Tapinarof (Vtama)
   Uses: psoriasis, atopic dermatitis
   Mechanism: aryl hydrocarbon receptor agonist (only drug of its class)
   Side effects: folliculitis
Clascoterone (Winlevi)
   Uses: acne
   Mechanism: androgen receptor inhibitor
   Note: perhaps conceived as a topical spironolactone that is safe to use in males, may have increased risk for adrenal suppression
Tirbanibulin (Klisyri)
   Uses: actinic keratosis
   Mechanism: microtubule inhibitor (works on the SRC tyrosine kinase pathway)
   Note: gentler than other field therapies but difficult coverage due to expense (also not as effective compared to other field therapies, especially 5-FU)

16.7.1 Combination Products for Acne

Note: these may be much more expensive without added benefit compared to separately prescribed ingredients. Ultimately only worth a consideration if you have significant concerns for compliance

Acanya = 2.5% benzoyl peroxide + 1% clindamycin
Benzaclin = 5% benzoyl peroxide + 1% clindamycin
Benzamycin = 5% benzoyl peroxide + 3% erythromycin
Duac = 5% benzoyl peroxide + 1.2% clindamycin
Epiduo = 2.5% benzoyl peroxide + 0.1% adapalene
Onexton = 3.75% benzoyl peroxide + 1% clindamycin
Veltin = 1.2% clindamycin + 0.025% tretinoin
Ziana = 1% clindamycin + 0.025% tretinoin
Epiduo Forte = 2.5% benzoyl peroxide + 0.3% adapalene
Twyneo = 3% benzoyl peroxide + 0.1% tretinoin

16.8 Drug Metabolism and Interactions

– Epoxide hydrolase deficiency – ? association with DRESS
– Slow N-acetylation associated with drug-induced lupus (INH, hydralazine, procainamide)
– G6PD deficiency:

16

Defect = single base substitution (asparagine to aspartic acid) involved in metabolism of several drugs: antimalarials (hydroxychloroquine, primaquine, chloroquine), dapsone, sulfa drugs, aspirin
– May also lead to hemolysis with fava beans (favism), infection
– Thiopurine methyltransferase (TPMT) deficiency – phase 2 reaction, must check before azathioprine; when deficient, metabolism produces different metabolites leading to greater immunosuppression

Cytochrome P450 3A4 Inducers
– Note: Takes weeks to cause induction.
Aromatic anticonvulsants:
    Phenobarbital
    Phenytoin
    Carbamazepine
Anti-tuberculous therapy:
    Isoniazid
    Rifampin (most potent inducer—caution with OCPs)
Griseofulvin
Dexamethasone
St. John's wort

Cytochrome P450 3A4 Inhibitors
– Note: these can inhibit immediately
Azole antifungals
    Ketoconazole (most potent inhibitor)
    Itraconazole
    Fluconazole (weak inhibitor)
Macrolides (but not azithromycin!)
    Erythromycin
    Clarithromycin
Cimetidine
    Grapefruit juice
    HIV protease inhibitors
    Ca channel blockers
    SSRIs

Procedures, Cosmetics, and Surgery

Contents

© The Author(s), under exclusive license to Springer Nature Switzerland AG 2024
J. Lipoff and D. Ruiz Dasilva, *Dermatology Simplified*,
https://doi.org/10.1007/978-3-031-66739-8_17

Abstract

This section reviews the most high yield facts regarding procedures in dermatology, including cosmetics and surgery.

Keywords

Cosmetics · Skin surgery · Lasers · Neurotoxins · Procedural dermatology

17.1 Procedures and Cosmetics

17.1.1 Neurotoxins

Botox (onabotulinumtoxin A):
- Mechanism: binds SNAP-25 (BTX-1) or other SNARE complex protein (such as synaptobrevin (VAMP) by BTX-2). The SNARE complex is responsible for allowing neurotransmitter (acetylcholine) vesicle fusion at neuromuscular junction (postsynaptic cholinergic)
- Duration: takes 24–72 h to start effect, full effect by 2 weeks, lasts 3–5 months
- Use: for dynamic rhytides, primary axillary hyperhidrosis; originally for strabismus, blepharospasm, cervical dystonia, also approved for migraine headaches
- Muscles of the brow:
    - Depressors (4): procerus, orbicularis oculi, depressor supercilli, corrugator supercilli
    - Elevator: frontalis
- Associated effects: ptosis (if affect levator palpebrae superioris, so inject at least 1 cm above superior orbital rim, avoid lateral aspect above brow), lip drop (if affect zygomaticus major/minor—be careful when injecting lateral/inferior orbicularis oculi)
- Other neurotoxins:
    - Dysport (abobotulinumtoxin A) = ~2.5–3:1 conversion ratio with Botox
    - Xeomin (incobotulinumtoxin A) = 1:1 conversion ratio with Botox
    - Juveau (prabotulinumtoxin A-xvfs) = 1:1 conversion ratio with Botox
    - Daxxify (daxibotulinumtoxin A-lanm) − 2:1 conversion ratio with Botox
    - Note: Daxxify is newest approved toxin and only one with average duration of 6–9 months

17

17.1.2 Fillers

Semi-permanent fillers:
  Bovine collagen (Zyderm)—historic, no longer used
  Hyaluronic acid (Restylane, Juvéderm, Teosyal, Revanesse)
    – Derived from bacterial fermentation of *Streptococci*
  Poly-L-lactic acid (Sculptra) (longer-lasting)
    – Works by stimulating collagen production (collagen neosynthesis)
    – This filler has been specifically used for HIV lipodystrophy
  Calcium hydroxyapatite microspheres (Radiesse) (longer-lasting)
Permanent fillers:
  Polymethylmethacrylate beads suspended in bovine collagen (Artefill, rebranded as Bellafill)
Risks: nodules/granulomatous reactions
Danger areas:
  Glabella, nose
    Risk of glabellar, nasal necrosis
    Risk of embolization to ophthalmic artery and blindness due to retrograde movement of material
  Nasolabial folds
    Risk of vascular occlusion of angular artery

17.1.3 Peels

Alpha hydroxy acids=trichloroacetic acid (TCA), glycolic acid; can penetrate into dermis depending on concentration and anatomic location
  Glycolic acid peels must be washed off with water or neutralized with sodium bicarbonate; TCA frosts and does not neutralize, and rinsing is only for patient comfort
Note: TCA medium depth peels (25–40%) are good for AKs and actinic damage
Beta hydroxy acids=salicylic acid (the only one); can enter sebaceous unit, only penetrates stratum corneum; good for acne
Jessner solution=salicylic acid, lactic acid, resorcinol in ethanol
Phenol=a deeper peel, but given risk of arrhythmias from systemic absorption, traditionally needs EKG monitoring (almost nobody uses phenol because of this risk); also has risk of acute kidney injury

17.1.4 Lasers

Basic principles
  – LASER=Light Amplification by Stimulated Emission of Radiation
  – Lasers are monochromatic, high intensity, coherent (in phase), and collimated (in parallel)

- Three main chromophores: water, hemoglobin, and melanin
- These chromophores all absorb best at different wavelengths. The principle is to choose a laser wavelength which will be absorbed by your target chromophore and not be absorbed by the chromophores you wish to leave unaffected (principle of selective photothermolysis)
- The higher the laser wavelength, the deeper it penetrates into the skin (however, once above 1300 nm, water absorption in stratum corneum limits penetration)
- If you are targeting a specific color pigment as a chromophore, the best laser should have a different color from the target. The color of an object reflects the wavelengths of light it does not absorb, and thus how it appears that color to our eyes. The ideal laser color may be the opposite end of the color wheel
- Thermal relaxation time = time required for chromophore to cool to 50% of heated temperature; dependent on square of diameter of chromophore
- Pulse duration = must equal or be less than thermal relaxation time; if too long, heat will diffuse and damage normal tissue
- In order to eliminate pigment, one should use a q-switched or pico laser, which uses a very short pulse duration (nanoseconds/picoseconds as opposed to milliseconds) and effectively targets the melanosome
- In hair removal, melanin is the target chromophore; thus it follows that the ideal patient for hair removal is a light skinned person with dark hair. In dark-skinned patients, it could be hard to remove hair without causing hypopigmentation of the skin as well. That said, a deep penetrating laser (higher wavelength) should target dermal > epidermal pigment. E.g. could use a Nd:Yag laser in type IV–VI skin for hair removal. Also, a long pulsed laser is recommended, as a longer pulse duration is needed for heat to go from the hair follicle to the stem cells in the bulge (most of these lasers have a protective cooling mechanism to limit damage to the epidermis)
- In laser skin resurfacing, high wavelength lasers are used for their higher coefficient of absorption for water
- Fractional laser resurfacing = produces microcolumns of damage with normal surrounding skin, allows for faster healing
- To increase depth of laser penetration, in general: increase wavelength, spot size (less photo scatter), and pulse duration

Terms:

Fluence = energy per unit area for a single pulse = J/cm^2 (fluence = irradiance × time)

Irradiance = power per unit area for a single pulse (power density) = W/cm^2

Energy is proportional to frequency; frequency and wavelength are inversely proportional

Know the UV spectrum:

Below 400 nm = ultraviolet light

400–700 nm = visible light

Above 700 nm = infrared light

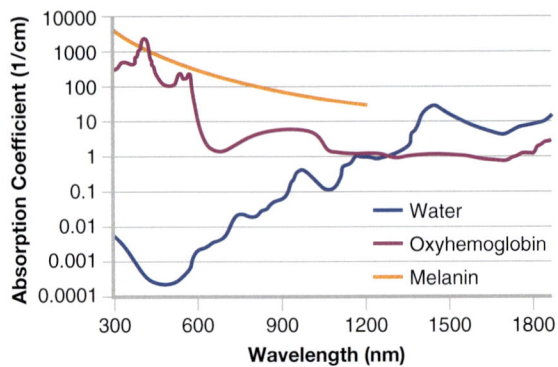

■ **Fig. 17.1**   Laser absorption spectra for hemoglobin, melanin, and water

Know the absorption spectra of hemoglobin, melanin, and water (■ Fig. 17.1):
  Hemoglobin (oxyhemoglobin): absorbs best at 500–600 nm (peaks at 540 (alpha peak) and 580 (beta peak))
  Melanin: absorbs at 300–1000 nm, though generally target 600–800 nm when specifically targeting pigment to avoid hemoglobin absorption
  Water: absorbs best above 1000 nm
Toxicities/complications:
  Ocular toxicity:
    Cornea absorbs like water (damage with Er:YAG and CO_2)
    Retina (rod and cones) absorbs like melanin (damage with lasers in melanin spectra)
Tattoo removal complication:
  Can see paradoxical darkening of tattoos containing beige, red, white or light brown color; thought to be from reduction of ferric oxide to ferrous oxide, leading to immediate gray-black color
Purpura:
  Short pulse durations effectively target in PDL, but may lead to purpura, which can be reduced with greater pulse durations (though purpuric settings known to be most effective)
Know the commonly used lasers:
  Excimer: 193, 308, 355 nm (in UV range, can cause cataracts)
  Argon: 488, 514 nm (green)—risk of scarring
  KTP: 532 nm (green)—good for vascular lesions
  Pulsed dye laser (PDL): 585–600 nm (yellow)=good for vascular lesions
  Ruby: 694 nm (red)
  Alexandrite: 755 nm—good for hair removal up to fitz IV
  Diode: 800, 810 nm—good for hair removal up to fitz V
  Nd:YAG: 1064, 1320 nm (frequency-doubled Nd:YAG=532 nm)—safest for hair removal in Fitzpatrick type VI
  Er:YAG: 2940 nm—resurfacing
  CO_2: 10,600 nm—resurfacing

Intense Pulsed Light (IPL): 500–1200 nm (not a laser; can use filters to narrow wavelength range)—works for variety of conditions but significant caution in Fitzpatrick types IV–VI

Note:

UVB = 280–320 nm, UVA-2 = 320–340 nm, UVA-1 = 340–400 nm

Soret band = 400–410 nm (blue); Oxygen (ozone) absorbs UVC 100–200 nm

Shortest UV wavelength = infrared

Longest UV wavelength = radiowaves

17.1.5 Phototherapy

UVB phototherapy (NBUVB = 311 nm)

= light therapy without any photosensitizers

Mechanism = reduces DNA synthesis, induces expression of tumor suppressor p53, various cytokine release; this would explain how it works in psoriasis; in CTCL, may work by impairing Langerhans cell function

Indications = psoriasis, CTCL, vitiligo; also atopic dermatitis, GVHD, PLEVA/PLC, pruritus

MED (minimal erythema dose) = lowest dose that causes minimally perceptible erythema; this peaks at 24 h, so doses may be increased with each treatment

Efficacy = UVB inferior to PUVA, but NBUVB may be nearly as effective

UVA-1 phototherapy (UVA-1 = 340–400 nm)

Indications = sclerotic diseases (morphea, eosinophilic fasciitis, chronic GVHD, lichen sclerosus) thought to have greater penetration, less carcinogenic risk than PUVA (not widely available in USA)

Mechanism = Unclear, but may upregulate matrix metalloproteinases (collagenase) and decrease production of collagen

PUVA/Psoralen (UVA = 320–400 nm)

Background: Psoralens = naturally occurring linear furocoumarins found in a number of plants. In PUVA (Psoralen + UVA), typically use 8-methoxypsoralen (8-MOP), which is orally ingested or applied topically; 5-MOP is less efficacious, but has fewer side effects

Mechanism: In the absence of UV, psoralen intercalates with DNA. With absorption of UVA photons, this leads to cross-links with the pyrimidine bases and the production of reactive oxygen species. It is thought that this interaction with DNA inhibits replication and causes cell cycle arrest. Some effects even in absence of DNA crosslinks

Side effects = nausea/vomiting (from 8-MOP), erythema (peaks 72–96 h after exposure), pigmentation, pruritus, cataracts (eye protection mandatory), long-term risk of photocarcinogenesis (though perhaps not as much as once feared)

17.1.6 Photodynamic Therapy

Photosensitizer + photoactivating light + target cell + tissue oxygen
  PDT works by producing cytotoxic oxygen radicals and may cause oxidative damage that leads to cell death
Light source: must have wavelength > 400 nm (to limit UV light penetration, avoiding photocarcinogenesis), but < 800 nm
  Absorption spectrum of protoporphyrin IX has blue (417 nm) and red (630 nm) peaks
Indications: actinic keratoses, superficial BCCs; also acne, photoaging, MF, CTCL
  Topical ALA + red light approved for tx of BCC, AKs, SCC; topical ALA + blue light approved for tx of AKs
Photosensitizers:
  5-ALA (5-aminolevulinic acid) and methyl-esterified ALA (mALA)
Mechanism:
  In a way, causing a transient iatrogenic erythropoietic protoporphyria
  5-ALA (pro-drug) → protoporphyrin-IX (wait an hour after application to apply light; conversion can be checked with Wood's lamp). On exposure to light, singlet oxygen species may be produced. The 5-ALA is preferentially absorbed by cells with high turnover; stops at protoporphyrin-IX since lack next enzyme in cascade
  Note: this is markedly painful and so "painless PDT" has been used where there is no incubation and the light is turned on directly after applying ALA with studies showing similar efficacy to traditional PDT

17.1.7 Radiofrequency Microneedling

Indications: facial rejuvenation, rhytides, skin tightening, acne scarring
  - Device that places small needles at a programmed depth to cause a controlled injury leading to neocollagenesis but also deposits radiofrequency energy that leads to further collagen, elastin and skin tightening, some fat burning as well depending on depth and energy
  - Safe for all skin types given energy is deposited under the epidermis so no damage to the DEJ where melanocytes are
  - Low risk for significant complications but erythema, bruising, pain is common

17.1.8 Sclerotherapy

Indications: telangiectasias and reticular veins
Agents:
  Detergents (sodium tetradecyl sulfate = Sotradecol)
    – Disrupt vein membrane

Osmotic agents (hypertonic solution)
– Damage cells by shifting water balance
Chemical irritants (glycerin)
– Damage cell wall by direct destruction
Greatest risk of arterial clot = injection into popliteal fossa

17.1.9 Dermabrasion

- Microdermabrasion and mechanical dermabrasion are techniques for resurfacing skin defects; most commonly used for treatment of acne scarring
- Recommendations are to wait 6–8 weeks post-surgery, 6–12 months post-isotretinoin (may be more than necessary)
- Risk of scarring greatest over bony prominences (e.g. mandible)
  Note: no longer common practice as lasers and radiofrequency microneedling have been more effective and safe

17.1.10 Hair Transplantation (Follicular Unit Transplantation)

= Techniques of restorative surgery to relocate hair follicular units
- Should not be done on patients who are too young or have too diffuse hair loss
- Requires aesthetic sense for hairline design, anticipation of future hair loss
- Donor strip may be harvested using triple-bladed scalpel, typically done from posterior scalp
  Note: there has been significant innovation in this space with machines and new tools to harvest hair follicles

17.1.11 Liposuction

= A technique for removal of fat; not a treatment for obesity
- Uses tumescent anesthesia with lidocaine; allows large volumes of fat to be removed with minimal blood loss
- Contraindications include bleeding disorders
  Note: this was invented by dermatologists, not plastic surgeons

17.1.12 Platelet Rich Plasma (PRP)

A technique for using a patient's own PRP to stimulate growth of hair (has been used to a lesser extent in skin rejuvenation as well, and for various other purposes in different specialties)

17

- First a patient's blood is drawn, placed in a particular centrifuge device to isolate the PRP, then aspirated into syringes and injected across areas of alopecia subdermally
- Treatment regimens vary, however a typical schedule is one treatment monthly × 3 followed by a maintenance treatment every 6–12 months
- Note: PRP can be quite expensive for patients, and also may best utilized as part of comprehensive alopecia treatment plan (not monotherapy); further, while a systematic review showed results that seemed promising, one analysis noted that "even among patients who improve, the potential benefits of PRP may not be clinically significant" with changes that were not meaningful

17.2 Surgery

17.2.1 Anatomy of the Face: Nerves, Arteries, Veins

Motor innervation of muscles of facial expression = facial nerve (◘ Fig. 17.2)
Branches of the facial nerve = TZBMC (Mnemonic = To Zanzibar by Motor Car), Temporal, Zygomatic, Buccal, Marginal mandibular, Cervical

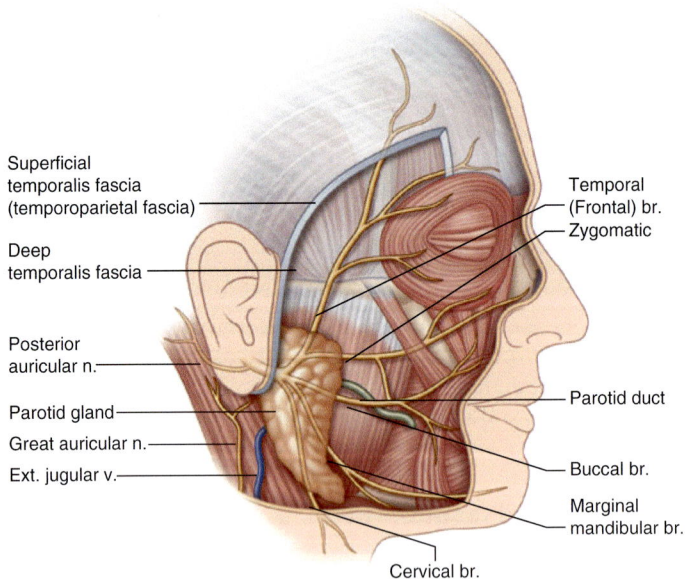

◘ **Fig. 17.2**   The facial nerve and its branches. Reproduced with permission from *Cosmetic Surgery: Art and Techniques* (2013), Shiffman, M. A., Di Giuseppe, A. (Eds.), Chap. 2, Springer

Sensory innervation of the muscles of facial expression = trigeminal nerve
(V1, V2, V3): V1 = supraorbital, V2 = infraorbital, above lips, V3 = mental,
below lips, includes auriculotemporal nerve

Superficial muscle aponeurotic system (SMAS)
= fibromuscular layer that connects and organizes muscles of face into co-
ordinated movement. Need to undermine above SMAS to avoid injury to
motor nerves

Scalp layers = SCALP (Skin, subCutaneous tissue, Aponeurosis/galea aponeu-
rotica, Loose connective tissue, Periosteum)
– Undermine in subgaleal space (avoid all vessels except emissary veins)

Ear anatomy/innervation
Superior helix, tragus = auriculotemporal nerve (of V3)
Middle helix = lesser occipital nerve
Lobule, antitragus, and most of posterior pinna = greater auricular nerve
External auditory meatus = auricular branch of vagus nerve

Nasal anatomy/innervation/supply
Nasal dorsum/root = V1 innervation (Hutchinson's sign in nasociliary
branch of V1), dorsal nasal artery (ophthalmic artery)
Nasal tip = VI innervation (anterior ethmoidal)
Lateral side walls/alae = V2 innervation, angular artery (facial artery)

Arterial supply of the face (☐ Fig. 17.3)
Internal carotid artery = supplies brain, forehead, nasal septum
Ophthalmic artery
Supraorbital artery (lateral forehead)
Supratrochlear artery (median forehead)

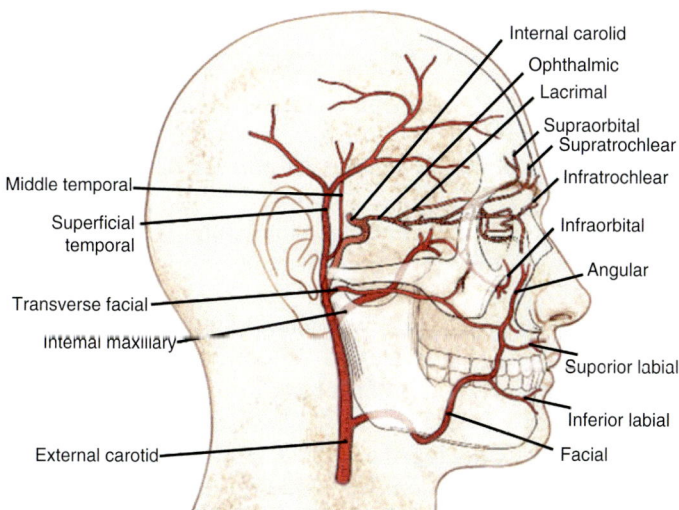

☐ **Fig. 17.3** Arterial supply to the face. Reproduced with permission from *Cosmetic Surgery: Art and Techniques* (2013), Shiffman, M. A., Di Giuseppe, A. (Eds.), Chap. 2, Springer

Anterior ethmoid artery (nasal septum)
Dorsal nasal artery (dorsum of nose)
External carotid artery = supplies face (except forehead, nasal septum)
  Facial artery
    Inferior and superior labial arteries
    Angular artery (nasal alae)
    Superficial temporal artery (temple, terminal branch of ECA)
  Anastamoses between internal and external carotid arteries =
    – Dorsal nasal artery (ophthalmic) (ICA) to angular artery (facial) (ECA)
Facial nerve innervation of facial muscles:
  Temporal nerve = frontalis, upper orbicularis oculi, corrugator supercili, procerus (Botox muscles)
    Defect = ptosis, brow drop
  Zygomatic nerve = lower orbicularis oculi, procerus, nasalis, levator anguli oris (LAO), zygomaticus major
    Defect = Ectropion, loss of nostril flare, poor eyelid seal
  Buccal = buccinator, nasalis (transverse), orbicularis oris, levator labii superioris (LLS), levator anguli oris (LAO), zygomaticus major and minor, risorius
    Defect = Mouth seal poor (drooling), facial droop, muffled speech
  Marginal mandibular = orbicularis oris, depressor anguli oris (DAO), depressor labii inferioris (DLI), mentalis, platysma
    Defect = cannot evert lower lip, crooked smile
  Cervical nerve = platysma
    Defect = unable to grimace
Anatomy of the face (muscles) (▣ Fig. 17.4):
  Muscles of the brow:
    Depressors (4): procerus, orbicularis oculi, depressor supercilli, corrugator supercilli
    Elevator: frontalis
    Opens eyelid = levator palpebrae superioris (CN III)
  Muscles of the mouth:
    Zygomaticus major and minor=lift corners of the mouth, upper lip
      Mentalis
      – Raises and protrudes lower lip, raises chin
      – Assists with drinking, expresses doubt
    Buccinator
      – Assists with mastication, shortens cheek vertically and horizontally (presses cheek against teeth)
      – Allows for whistling (trumpet muscle)
    Orbicularis oris
      – Presses lips tightly together
      – Closes, protrudes, purses lips; pouting, kissing

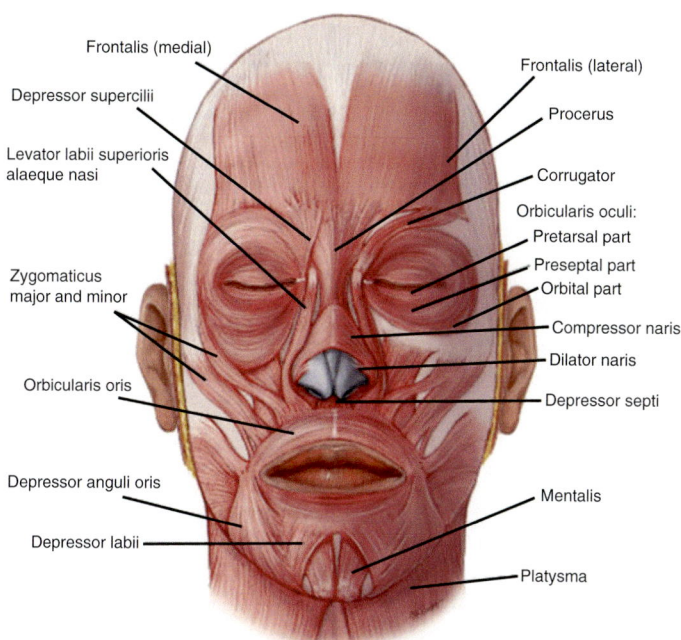

Frontalis (medial)
Frontalis (lateral)
Depressor supercilii
Procerus
Levator labii superioris alaeque nasi
Corrugator
Orbicularis oculi:
Pretarsal part
Preseptal part
Zygomaticus major and minor
Orbital part
Compressor naris
Dilator naris
Orbicularis oris
Depressor septi
Depressor anguli oris
Mentalis
Depressor labii
Platysma

◻ Fig. 17.4 Muscle anatomy of the face. Reproduced with permission from *Cosmetic Surgery: Art and Techniques* (2013), Shiffman, M. A., Di Giuseppe, A. (Eds.), Chap. 2, Springer

Risorius
 – Widens mouth when person is smiling widely
Platysma
 – Draws lower lip and angles of mouth inferolaterally
Other facial muscles:
Masseter
 – One of the muscles contributing to mastication (along with temporalis, medial and lateral pterygoid; may be treated with Botox for TMJ)
Nasalis
 – Compresses nasal cartilage
Depressor anguli oris (DAO)
 – Depresses angle of mouth
Levator anguli oris (LAO)
 – Elevates angle of mouth
Depressor labii inferioris (DLI)
 – Depresses lower lip
Levator labii superioris (LLS)
 – Raises upper lip
Levator labii superioris alaque nasi
 – Dilates the nostrils and elevates the upper lip, allows one to snarl

Three danger zones in head and neck:
1. Temporal nerve injury (protected only by thin superficial temporal fascia)
2. Marginal mandibular nerve injury
   – Could occur during liposuction of neck or kybella injection
3. Spinal accessory nerve injury
   Erb's point (at posterior margin of SCM muscle, where cervical plexus emerges)
   Posterior triangle: formed by posterior aspect of SCM muscle, trapezius, and middle 1/3 of the clavicle
   Risk of injuring: the spinal accessory nerve, greater auricular nerve, lesser occipital nerve (and transverse cervical nerves) pass within 2 cm
   – Face lifts risk injury to greater auricular nerve most commonly

Sensory innervation of hand
   Remember: anatomic position is palms facing forward, 1st finger (thumb) is lateral
   Medial hand/1.5 fingers (5th finger and medial 4th finger) = ulnar nerve
   Palm and remaining 3.5 fingers on lateral hand = median nerve
   Lateral dorsal hand = mostly radial nerve (fingertips are median nerve)
   Medial dorsal hand = mostly ulnar nerve

Sensory innervation of the foot
   Dorsal foot (except 1st webspace) = superficial peroneal nerve
   1st webspace = deep peroneal nerve
   Plantar foot (except 1st webspace) = posterior tibial nerve
   Medial foot (including instep, medial malleolus) = saphenous nerve
   Lateral foot (including lateral malleolus) = sural nerve

Foot blocks:
   Saphenous and superficial peroneal block = injected on dorsal foot between medial and lateral malleoli
   Deep peroneal block = inject lateral to extensor hallucis longus down to the bone (or simply locally infiltrate 1st webspace, which may be easier)
   Posterior tibial block = palpate posterior tibial artery (by medial malleolus); nerve is lateral to artery, so inject in between medial malleolus and Achilles tendon
   Sural nerve block = inject in between lateral malleolus and Achilles tendon

Local anesthetics
   Mechanism = reversibly inhibit nerve conduction via interfering with Na^+ influx
   Smaller fibers (A-delta, C fibers) blocked first, causing pain/temperature to be affected before vibration/pressure
   Low pH impairs action (as in acidic environments like infected tissues)
   Two types: amides and esters
      Mnemonic = Amides are your amigos! (They rarely cause allergic reactions, and lidocaine is one of our friends/amigos!)
      Amides have at least 2 Is in their names, Esters only have 1 I (except dibucaine)

Amides (lidocaine, bupivacaine = longest acting)
- Metabolized by liver (cytochrome P450), excreted by kidneys
- Use esters in patients with liver failure
- Allergy to amide is allergy to Paraben preservative
- Lidocaine is pregnancy safe; bupivacaine, mepivacaine can cause fetal bradycardia, so are to be avoided
- Lidocaine max dose = 4.5 mg/kg (without epinephrine), 7 mg/kg (with epinephrine); standard concentration 1% = 10 mg/mL
- Tumescent lidocaine maximum dose 35–55 mg/kg

Lidocaine toxicity
  Mild: circumoral parasthesia, drowsiness, nausea/vomiting
  - Tx: Hold lidocaine, observe
  Moderate: nystagmus, twitching, seizures
  - Tx: Diazepam for seizure prophylaxis/treatment, maintain airway
  Severe: Tx: apnea, coma
  - Respiratory support
  Note: tachycardia + high BP can be from epinephrine, tachycardia + low BP can be from anaphylaxis

EMLA = lidocaine + prilocaine topically; careful in infants since risk of methemoglobinemia with prilocaine; presents with cyanosis, treat with methylene blue

Esters (procaine, tetracaine, benzocaine)
  Metabolized by pseudocholinesterases, excreted by the kidneys
  = can cross react with PABA, sulfa drugs (allergies more common)

Epinephrine = enhances efficacy by keeping lidocaine localized; added since most anesthetics are vasodilating; vasoconstriction requires 7–15 min
  Toxicity = increased BP, tachycardia (rare)
  Contraindications = pheochromocytoma, uncontrolled HTN, pregnancy (relative contraindication and most use plain lidocaine for biopsies in pregnant women)

Lidocaine anesthesia enhanced by benzoyl alcohol preservative, which has anesthetic properties itself

Sodium bicarbonate = reduces pain on infiltration, increases pH (alkalinizes), faster onset of anesthesia, shortens duration of action of epinephrine and shelf life

17.2.2 Antiseptics

- Note: broadest coverage = alcohol > iodine > chlorhexidine
  Isopropyl alcohol
    = Fastest onset, broadest antiseptic coverage, but minimal sustained activity once evaporated (so often combined)
    = Flammable, so allow to dry before electrocautery or laser

17

Chlorhexidine (Hibiclens)
- Broad coverage (gram positive and negative bacteria, viruses, mycobacteria, excellent sustained activity)
- Risk of ototoxicity and ocular toxicity if gets into globe or ear canal

Hexochlorophene (pHisoHex)
- Teratogen, possible neurotoxicity in infants

Povidone-iodine
- Potential systemic toxicity in neonates
- Must dry to be bacteriostatic, has broad coverage
- May cause a contact dermatitis
- Inactivated by contact with blood or sputum

Hydrogen peroxide
- Used for cleansing, removal of debris

17.2.3 Sterilization

Steam autoclave
- Most popular, may dull sharp instruments

Cold sterilization (glutaraldehyde)

Gas sterilization (ethylene oxide or formaldehyde)
- Best for moisturize sensitive instruments

17.2.4 Pre-surgery Medication

Prophylactic antibiotics
- Antibiotics do reduce the incidence of surgical site infections, however, surgical site infections are uncommon and antibiotics carry other risks, so antibiotics are usually not necessary
- If deemed necessary, dose antibiotics 1–2 h prior to first incision, so that adequate concentrations are present in tissue; however some only give post-op so lack of standardization in practice can be frustrating
- Can use 2 g of cephalexin or amoxicillin versus 1 DS TMP-SMX (if PCN allergi can also use 600 mg of clindamycin or 500 mg of azithromycin); for those who give post-op typically use cephalexin, doxycycline, or cefadroxil however drug choice and dosing varies widely with no consensus in this setting
- Rarely needed; current recommendations are to consider if in:
  1. Infected wound
  2. High risk patient in high risk area
  3. High risk of surgical site infection

     High risk patient = prosthetic valve, mitral valve prolapse with mitral regurgitation, history of subacute bacterial endocarditis, prosthetic joint, etc.

High risk areas = oral/nasal, lower extremities (especially leg), groin, lip/ear wedge excisions, flaps on nose, feet, axilla, grafts, extensive inflammatory skin disease
  - In ear surgery cover for *Pseudomonas* with fluoroquinolones (important especially if you breach cartilage)

Aspirin and Clopidogrel (Plavix)
  - May discontinue 10–14 days preoperatively if used for primary prevention; however, generally do not recommend stopping if prescribed by a doctor/needed for active prevention of clot (e.g. atrial fibrillation); most surgical derm literature supports not interrupting anticoagulation as we can always control intra-op bleeding but potential stroke, clotting can be catastrophic

NSAIDs
  - Variable, but can discontinue 3–4 days before

Warfarin (Coumadin) or other direct acting anticoagulants
  - Do not discontinue (see above) unless it is warfarin and it is supratherapeutic and directed by the prescribing physician

Herbals/supplements
  - Arnica, garlic, ginseng, Vitamin E, and others may affect wound healing and bruising and increase risk of hematoma

17.2.5 Wound Healing

Three overlapping stages:
  - Inflammatory (days to weeks)
  - Proliferative (days to months)
  - Remodeling (days to months)

First cells to appear: platelets (secrete PDGF)

Most important regulatory cells in inflammation: macrophages, which are critical to repair and mediate actions via cytokines

Important in proliferative phase, contraction: fibroblast, attracted by macrophages

Wound strength
  At 2 weeks = 5%
  At 3 weeks = 20%
  At 1 month = 40%
  Final healing (unlimited time) = 80%

Wound debridement
  - May be required for removal of necrotic tissue for proper wound healing
  - May convert a chronic wound into a more acute wound more likely to heal
    Types:
      - Mechanical (by wet to dry dressings)
      - Surgical (by curette under local anesthesia)
      - Enzymatic (e.g. collagenase ointment (Santyl))
      - Other (includes use of medical maggots)

17

17.2.6 Wound Dressings

Functions of dressings: cover wound, absorb wound drainage, compression, provide moist environment

Types:

Absorptive dressings

Note: absorb drainage well, may not preserve moisture
- Gauze (usually not put directly on wounds since adherent and causes pain and mechanical debridement when removed)
- Hydrophilic non-adherent fabrics
- Foams
- Alginates (derived from seaweed)

Occlusive dressings

Note: preserve moisture well, may absorb drainage poorly
- Hydrophobic non-adherent fabrics (e.g. Vaseline gauze, Telfa, Xeroform)
- Hydrogel
- Hydrocolloid (e.g. Duoderm)
- Films (e.g. Tegaderm)
- Foams
- Alginates
- Collagen dressings

Biologic/biosynthetic dressings
- Grafts (*see also Grafts*)
- Skin substitutes
  - Often expensive, second line
  - E.g. Apligraf, made from bovine collagen and keratinocytes and fibroblasts from human neonatal foreskin

17.2.7 Mohs Surgery

- Developed by Frederic Mohs
- Aka microscopically controlled surgery, a tissue sparing procedure
- Performed in stages (many bevel their layers at 45° angle), tissue mapped and stained, frozen sections examined to evaluate deep and peripheral margins
- Unlike standard excisions, Mohs has the ability to examine 100% of the surgical margins

17.2.8 Indications for Mohs Surgery

- Head/neck, hands, feet, genital tumor
- >2 cm in size any location
- Recurrent or high risk for recurrence
- Irregular borders/poorly defined margins

- Perineural invasion
- Ease of closure, to avoid need for graft
- Site of previous irradiation
- Aggressive tumors: e.g. DFSP, Merkel cell carcinoma, AFX
- Immunosuppression
  Note: Mohs for MMIS and superficially invasive melanoma is gaining traction as evidence mounts for its efficacy at several centers in the USA

17.2.9 Reconstruction

You must remember:
1. Skin tension lines—try to orient/hide scar in tension lines
2. Cosmetic units—more distracting/possible functional impairment if you cross cosmetic units

Closure options = primary closure, secondary intention healing, flap, graft

17.2.10 Healing by Secondary Intention

- Ideal on concave surface such as temple, medial canthus, alar crease, ear (concha, not helical rim)
- Bad in areas that are free margins; a free margin is a margin that has unopposed tension vectors such as lips, eyebrows, eyelids, helices, nasal alae (no skin on opposite/other side), lacks ability to counteract tension forces

17.2.11 Flaps

Advancement flaps
  = Simple advancement, bilateral advancement, V to Y (aka island pedicle flap (IPF)), A to T flap
  = Mobilizes tissue by undermining and advancing skin in a single direction of pedicle (wound axis)
Rotation flaps
  = Simple rotation, O to Z flap (bilateral rotation)
  = Mobilizes tissue around a pivot point (can be seen as advancing in two different directions), may have back cut to counter tension
  – O to Z good for scalp since convex/curved surface and tissue not that mobile
Transposition flaps
  = Rhombic/rhomboid flap, bilobed, Z-plasty
  = Mobilizes a rectangle of skin on a pivot point to cover immediately adjacent defect, passing over intact skin
  – Close secondary defect first, then primary defect

Interpolation flaps (subtype of transposition flaps)
  = Paramedian forehead flap, Abbe lip flap
  = Two-stage transposition flap in which the base of the flap is not immediately adjacent to the recipient site
  – Paramedian forehead = from forehead down to nose, utilizing supratrochlear artery
  – Typically divided at 3 weeks (called a take down)
Scar revision
  Z-plasty = reorients scar, lengthens scar
  M-plasty = shortens wound to stay in cosmetic unit/avoid free margin
Point of maximum tension = will be at key suture, usually that closes primary defect (except in rhomboid/transposition, where secondary defect closed first)

17.2.12 Grafts

- Full-thickness skin graft (FTSG)
  Advantages: best potential for good cosmetic match
  Disadvantages: donor-site morbidity, more metabolically demanding than split thickness grafts, which may increase risk of failure
- Split-thickness skin graft (STSG)
  Advantages: thinner, requires less metabolic support so survives better
  Disadvantages: may contract/produce poorer cosmetic result (hypopigmentation), no adnexal structures; may not resist contraction near free margins, no sweating
- Composite graft
  = A modified full-thickness skin graft of skin plus cartilage, fat, or perichondrium
  – Commonly used to repair alar rim defects; donor site = ear
  – Four stages: blanches at first, pink by 6 h, dusky blue by 24 h (from venous congestion), pink by day 7 again indicating graft survival
- Healing process:
  (1) Plasma imbibition (first 48 h): may appear cyanotic and edematous (normal); the graft is surviving by absorbing wound exudate and passively diffusing nutrients
  (2) Inosculation (days 2–3): vessels and fibrin mesh established
  (3) Neovascularization (days 4–7): blood flow evident by days 5–7

17.2.13 Sutures

Needle characteristics
  Three parts of a needle = Tip/point, Body (grasp the needle 1/2–2/3 from the tip), Shank (attaches to suture, weakest part due to hollow nature)

- Typically made of stainless steel, typically curved 3/8 circle ones used in dermatologic surgery
- Should only be handled by instruments to prevent injury
- Cutting: standard is reverse cutting with the cutting edge of the outside of the needle arc (which decreases chance of suture tearing through tissue) versus conventional cutting with the cutting edge on the inside of the arc

Suture characteristics

Capillarity
= ability of suture to absorb/transfer fluid

Elasticity
= ability of suture to regain original length after being stretched

Plasticity
= ability of suture to retain new length/form/tensile strength after being stretched

Memory
= suture's tendency to regain former shape after bending (how stiff it is); determined by elasticity, plasticity, and tensile strength of a suture

Pliability
= how easily a suture can be bent, opposes memory

Tissue reactivity
= degree of foreign body inflammatory response when placed in a wound (natural > synthetic); natural (gut, silk), multifilament, absorbable usually cause more

Tensile strength
= force required to snap a suture

Absorbable versus non-absorbable
- Absorbable defined as losing majority of tensile strength within 60 days

Multifilament/braided = may increase risk of infection

Note: elasticity and plasticity are opposing properties, and both contribute to suture memory; memory and pliability are opposing properties

Common non-absorbables

Nylon (Ethilon)
- Monofilament, high tensile strength, low tissue reactivity

Polypropylene (Prolene)
- Monofilament synthetic, does not degrade in tissue (long term support), stiff/has high memory, requiring extra knots, but also quite plastic, lowest reactivity

Silk
- Multifilament, soft, used in mucosal, intertriginous areas, most inflammatory suture

Polyester
- Multifilament, highest tensile strength (except metal sutures, steel used in thoracic surgery)

Polybutester
- Monofilament, high tensile strength (less than polyester)

Common absorbables
  Note: absorbable suture defined as most of tensile strength lost within 60 days of placement
  Gut (Catgut, fast gut)
    – Natural, high tissue reactivity, tensile strength half life < 1 week
  Polyglactin 910 (Vicryl)
    – Braided multifilament synthetic
    – 50% absorbed by 3 weeks, gone by 56–70 days
    – Most prone to spitting sutures
  Polyglycolic acid (Dexon)
  Polydioxanone (PDS)
    – Very slow absorption (90–180 days)
  Polytrimethylene carbonate (Maxon)
    – Monofilament synthetic (similar to PDS)
  Poliglecaprone 25 (Monocryl)
    – Monofilament synthetic, increased pliability, knot strength
    – Highest initial tensile strength
Suturing techniques
  Simple interrupted
    – Basic, for approximating wound edges
  Buried suture (deep)
    – Closes dead space, apposes wound edges
  Vertical mattress
    = Best suture for additional edge eversion (far-far, near-near)
    – Suture line perpendicular to wound edge
  Horizontal mattress
    = Helpful for hemostasis of nonspecific wound edge oozing
    – Suture line parallel to wound edge
  Tip stitch (half-buried horizontal mattress)
    = Primarily to position corners and tips of flaps; provides increased blood flow to tips
  Running sutures
    = Faster; can be modified (locked) to create more pressure on wound edges for greater hemostasis
  Pulley stitch
    = Multiple passes through tissue to close wound under tension
  Subcuticular stitch
    – Running parallel to surface in high dermis, avoids epidermal punctures, eliminating railroad tracks
  Figure of eight suture
    = Ties off a bleeding vessel
  Purse string
    = Buried horizontally oriented stitches placed continuously along circumference of wound to at least partially close a wound

Basting/Tacking/Pexing suture
  = May be placed to anchor the central portion of a graft (5–0 or 6–0 gut sutures) or flap to a fixed surface (e.g. periosteum)
Retention suture
  – A suture placed deep (fascial plication) or superficial (grabbing large amount of epidermis through full thickness) with the goal of taking tension off of the wound edges and allowing approximation
  – There are also devices that can be placed over wound to function as a retention suture (more commonly used in general surgery)
Skin closure tapes (Steri-Strips)
  = Typically applied with tincture of benzoin or mastisol
  – Should be applied non-overlapping, perpendicular to wound
Tissue adhesives (Dermabond)
  = Cyanoacrylate
  – Can be used in place of epidermal sutures, especially in low tension areas
Suture removal: pull tail of suture over and away from wound (avoiding tension that would pull wound apart) and cut suture. Remove suture pulling across wound or up

17.2.14 Safety/Needlesticks

- Needlesticks and sharps injuries are very common; important to report all injuries
- Risk of exposure to HIV, hepatitis B and C
- Risk of exposure to HIV through percutaneous injury ~ 0.3–5% (similar risk to exposure from unprotected sexual intercourse)
- Greater risk with hollow-bore needle, deep injury, exposure to patient with high viral load or advanced disease
- Post-exposure prophylaxis for HIV should be started within 24–36 h of exposure; there are no recommendations for exposure to HBV or HCV, though most health care workers required to have immunization against HBV

17.2.15 Other Surgical Rules

Ellipse = should be in a 3–4:1 length to width ratio with 30° apical angles
Rule of halves = purpose is to prevent dog ears
Railroad tracks from sutures = may be prevented by early removal of sutures, use of bolsters, or tissue adhesives
Trap door deformity = from insufficient undermining of periphery; transposition flaps most susceptible
Step-off deformity = occurs when wound is closed by suture placed at different levels on different edges of wound
Step-off deformity correction: can be corrected by either removing original suture, or by placing a compensatory stitch that is deeper on low wound edge and superficial on high wound edge

17

17.2.16 Margins

Note: this depends on individual case
- Surgical excision of SCCs:
  Low risk (in situ) $= 3$–4 mm margin
  High risk (invasive) $= 5$ mm margin or Mohs surgery
- Surgical excision of BCCs:
  < 2 cm $= 3$–4 mm margin
  ≥ 2 cm $= 5$ mm margin or Mohs surgery
- Surgical excision of DN and MM by depth:
  Dysplastic nevi $= 2$–3 mm margin
  MMIS $= 0.5$ cm (some say 0.9 cm esp. head/neck)
  MM < 1 mm $= 1$ cm
  MM < 1–4 mm $= 1$–2 cm
  MM > 4 mm $= 2$ cm

Sentinel lymph node biopsy (in melanoma):
- Dye is injected into lesion site; drainage of dye indicates which are the sentinel lymph nodes that should be sampled
- Controversial because it improves staging and prognostic accuracy, but has not been shown to provide any survival benefit to patients
- Generally offered to patients with MM of depth > 1 mm, or for less deep lesions if has aggressive features (mitoses > 1, ulceration)

Note: the goal is to consider the procedure if likelihood of positivity is 5–10% and to recommend it if over 10% but this is not a simple calculation and genetic testing (GEP) is being validated to help with this

17.2.17 Cryosurgery/Cryotherapy

Objective $=$ selective necrosis of tissue by reduction of skin temperature
Liquid nitrogen (-196 °C boiling point)
- Rapid freeze–thaw cycles produce maximum destruction
- For malignant lesions, -50 to -60 °C recommended (would need a thermocouple in order to determine exact temperature); benign need at least -25 °C (cryonecrosis); it takes -50 °C to destroy a keratinocyte; melanocytes are more fragile and can be destroyed at -5 °C
- Caution in pigmented skin (hypopigmentation), corners of mouth, vermillion borders, eyebrows, inner canthi, auditory canal, nasal ala, free margins

17.2.18 **Electrosurgery**

These are superficial, high voltage, low amperage (weak)
Electrodesiccation
Electrofulguration (the same, but no electrode contact with skin)
At low setting, these may be tolerated in patients with pacemakers, but any current can cause a problem potentially (particularly if working near the pacer)
These are deep, low voltage, high amperage (strong); both have second electrode (biterminal)
Electrocoagulation
Electrosection (tissue cutting)
These cannot be tolerated in patients with pacemakers (controversial, probably okay in modern pacemakers but avoided out of caution)
Electrocautery
- Low voltage, high amperage current to heat a surgical tip to cause tissue desiccation, coagulation, or necrosis by direct heat transference to tissue (no current passes through patient, so not actually electrosurgery)
- Excellent for pinpoint hemostasis
- Compatible with patients who may not tolerate current flow (implantable cardiac pacemaker or defibrillator)

17.2.19 **Superficial Radiation Therapy (SRT)**

- Used to treat non-melanoma skin cancer, and has been available for decades but over the last few years has had a resurgence of interest by clinicians, device companies, and patients
- There is an emerging body of evidence that this can be useful, safe and effective for select patients/cases however the lack of margin control, expense, number of treatments needed and paucity of high quality long term data limits its use currently
- Radiation also may be a useful modality in treatment of keloids

Basic Science

Contents

Note to trainees studying for exams: basic science minutia has been removed from board exams, but we do include this information for completeness' sake and because a strong understanding does help build the foundation for the practicing clinician.

© The Author(s), under exclusive license to Springer Nature Switzerland AG 2024
J. Lipoff and D. Ruiz Dasilva, *Dermatology Simplified*,
https://doi.org/10.1007/978-3-031-66739-8_18

Abstract

This section reviews high yield facts behind the most important areas of basic science relevant to dermatology.

Keywords

Basic science · Genes

18.1 Keratinocyte Adhesion

Occluding
- Tight junctions (zonula occludens)
  Transmembrane proteins: claudins and occludins (cytoskeletal component: actin)
  Intracellular proteins: e.g. ZO-1, ZO-2, ZO-3 (zonula occludins)

Anchoring
- Desmosomes (macula adherens): "slow, strong"
  Desmosomal plaque (■ Fig. 18.1) = Intermediate filament → desmoplakin → plakoglobin → desmosomal cadherins (transmembrane proteins) = desmocollin, desmoglein (desmosomes connected by homo- and hetero-dimers of cadherins)
  Intermediate filaments = keratin in epithelia/skin (desmin in muscle, vimentin in fibroblasts and endothelial cells)
  Cadherins = calcium-dependent adhesion transmembrane proteins, includes both desmocollin and desmoglein
  Dsg1 = more in upper layers of epidermis, less in mucosae; Ab causes pemphigus foliaceus, also *Staph* exfoliative toxin A (*Staph* group 2, phage 71) against Dsg1 causes SSSS and bullous impetigo. Genetic defect in striate PPK. Homozygous mutant may cause severe dermatitis, allergies (to food), and metabolic wasting (SAM syndrome)
  Dsg2 = mostly in heart and simple epithelia (e.g. gut), small amount in skin and increased expression in SCC
  Dsg3 = more in lower layers of epidermis, but all throughout mucous membranes (Ab causes pemphigus vulgaris)
  Dsg4 = mostly in hair follicles, mutated in AR monilethrix
  Desmocollin-1 = Ab causes IgA pemphigus (subcorneal pustular dermatosis)
  Desmocollin-2 = mutation can cause R-sided cardiomyopathy along with mild PPK and woolly hair
  Desmocollin-3 = mutation associated with hypotrichosis and vesicles

18

Desmosome

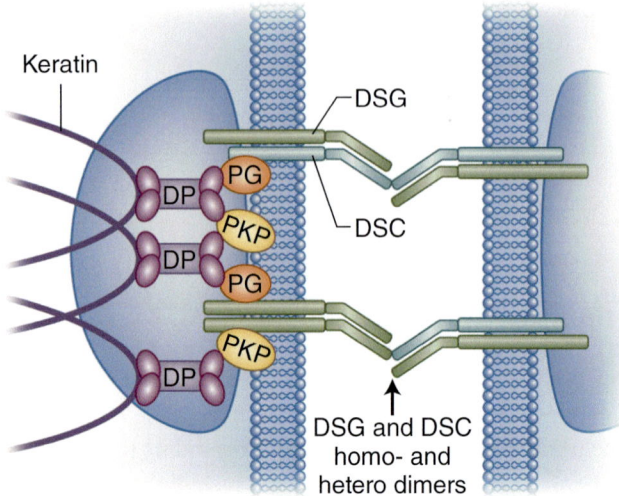

Keratin

DSG

DSC

DSG and DSC
homo- and
hetero dimers

DP=desmoplakin; PG=plakoglobin; PKP=plakophilins;
DSG=desmoglein; DSC=desmocollin

▣ Fig. 18.1 Components and structure of the desmosome

Desmoplakin = defect causes Carvajal syndrome (Woolly hair, L-sided cardiomyopathy, epidermolytic PPK) also linked to striate PPK and lethal
acantholytic epidermolysis bullosa

Plakoglobin = defect causes Naxos syndrome (Woolly hair, R-sided cardiomyopathy, PPK); can also cause lethal congenital EB

Plakophilin-1 = defect causes ectodermal dysplasia-skin fragility (McGrath)
syndrome

— Adherens junctions (zonula adherens): "quick, weak"

E-cadherin attached to actin via α- and β-catenin

E-cadherin = defect in gastric cancer, E-cadherin also expressed by
Langerhans cells to allow homing to epidermis

β-catenin = mutated in pilomatricomas; inactivation of APC in Gardner's
causes β-catenin accumulation and pilomatricoma-like changes in
associated EICs

Communicating

— Gap junctions (nexus)

Six connexins form connexon

Two connexons (two hemichannels) form gap junction

Connexins preferentially expressed in inner ear/cornea, epidermis and follicular unit (affects hearing, hair/skin)

Connexin 26 = defect causes Vohwinkel's syndrome (with deafness), KID (keratitis, ichthyosis, deafness) syndrome, PPK with deafness, Bart-Pumphrey syndrome

Connexin 30 = defect causes hidrotic ectodermal dysplasia (Clouston's syndrome)

Connexin 30.3, 31 = defect causes erythrokeratodermia variabilis

18.2 Basement Membrane

The structure of the basement membrane zone (BMZ) contains many components (◻ Fig. 18.2).

Note: the hemidesmosome (at the BMZ) and the desmosome (keratinocyte to keratinocyte adhesion) share similarities, but are different. The BMZ can be divided into 4 zones:

Zone 1—plasma membrane and hemidesmosome (keratin 5 and 14) = basal keratinocyte, plectin/BPAG1

Zone 2—lamina lucida (cleavage plane of salt-split skin) = BPAG2, α6β4 integrin (anchoring *filaments*) [interface between lamina lucida and densa = laminin-5/332/epiligrin = binds anchoring filaments (BPAG2 and α6β4 integrin) to anchoring fibrils (NC1 domain of type VII collagen)]

Zone 3—lamina densa (basement membrane proper) = type IV collagen, heparan sulfate, nidogen (BMZ)

Zone 4—sublamina densa (papillary dermis) = anchoring *fibrils*, type VII collagen

- Internal plaque (inside basal keratinocyte) = plectin, BPAG1 (230 kD) (plakin family); plectin (also a plakin) primarily binds β4 of α6β4, BPAG1 binds BPAG2 and β4; both BPAG1 and plectin bind to keratins as well to link the cytoskeleton to the hemidesmosome
- External plaque = BPAG2 (180 kD), integrins (α6β4) = anchoring filaments
- Internal plaque (plectin, BPAG1) connects with external plaque at α6β4 integrin connecting to BPAG2 at NC16A region to α6
- Laminin-332 (aka laminin-5 or epiligrin) connects between external plaque anchoring filaments (α6β4) and lamina densa (type IV collagen)
- Keratins (intermediate filaments), K5 and K14 in basal cells
- Type VII collagen comprises the anchoring fibrils

Defect in keratin 5 and 14 = EB simplex

Defect in keratin 5 = EB simplex with mottled pigmentation, Dowling-Degos, Galli-Galli

Defect in keratin 14 = dermatopathia pigmentosa reticularis (DPR) and Naegeli-Franceschetti-Jadassohn syndrome (NFJS)

Defect in laminin-5 = junctional EB

Defect in plectin = EB with muscular dystrophy

Defect in α6β4-integrin = JEB with pyloric atresia

18

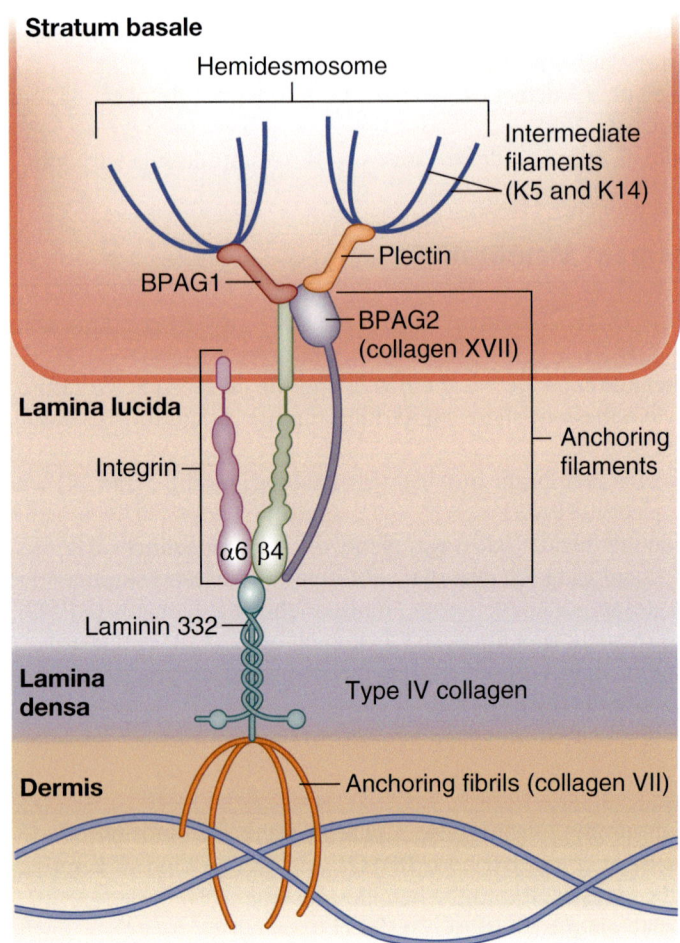

◘ **Fig. 18.2** Components and structure of the basement membrane zone (dermal-epidermal junction)

Defect in type VII collagen (anchoring fibrils) = dystrophic EB

Ab to BPAG1, 2 = bullous pemphigoid

Ab to laminin-5 ("anti-epiligrin") = cicatricial pemphigoid (Brunsting-Perry [limited to head/neck] and mucosal membrane type); can be associated with underlying malignancy

Ab to BPAG2 = bullous pemphigoid, herpes gestationis, cicatricial pemphigoid (C-terminal portion), linear IgA bullous dermatosis (97 kD segment)

Ab to α6β4-integrin (specifically β4) = ocular-specific cicatricial pemphigoid

Ab to BPAG2 (97 kD segment), NC16A of BPAG2 = linear IgA

Ab to type VII collagen = EB acquisita, bullous lupus

Note: the "plakin family" includes BPAG1 (BP230), plectin, desmoplakin, envoplakin, periplakin (may see Ab against any or all in paraneoplastic pemphigus)

Plakoglobin (a catenin) = may be part of both desmosome and adherens junctions

18.3 Cornified Envelope

- Keratinocytes mature up the epidermis and ultimately form the stratum corneum/cornified envelope (■ Fig. 18.3).
- Principal mechanical barrier of the skin = stratum corneum
- Important in regulation of water release (TEWL = trans-epidermal water loss)
- Bricks and mortar model = bricks (corneocytes or protein envelope), mortar (lipid envelope = extracellular lipid matrix from lamellar bodies)
- Cornified envelope consists of protein envelope and lipid envelope
- Granular layer contains keratohyalin granules = involucrin, loricrin (70–85% of corneum mass), profilaggrin (proteins), which become the main components of the cornified envelope
- Profilaggrin → filaggrin, proteins cross-linked bytransglutaminases
- Corneocytes formed from keratinocytes losing their lipids (that become the lipid envelope lamellar bodies), leaving the proteins (filaggrin, loricrin) behind
- Odland bodies (lamellar bodies, keratinosomes) made in spinous layer, make ceramides, contain glycolipids; these become the lipid components of the envelope
- In final stage of keratinocyte differentiation (from basal layer maturing up), keratins are aligned into arrays by filaggrin (FILament AGGRegating), and cross-linked by transglutaminases
- As filaggrin matures up stratum corneum, dehydration triggers filaggrin degradation by cathepsins
- Defect in cathepsin-C = Papillon-Lefevre and Haim-Munk syndromes
- Defect in filaggrin = ichthyosis vulgaris
- Defect in loricrin = Vohwinkel syndrome with ichthyosis (no deafness), NBCIE
- Defect in transglutaminase-1 = lamellar ichthyosis, congenital ichthyosiform erythroderma (spectrum of disease includes both)
- Defect in steroid sulfatase = X-linked ichthyosis
- Defect in ABCA12 = Harlequin fetus (can also be seen in lamellar ichthyosis)
- Defect in phytanoyl-CoA hydroxylase (PEX7) = Refsum disease
- Defect in fatty aldehyde dehydrogenase = Sjögren-Larsson

18

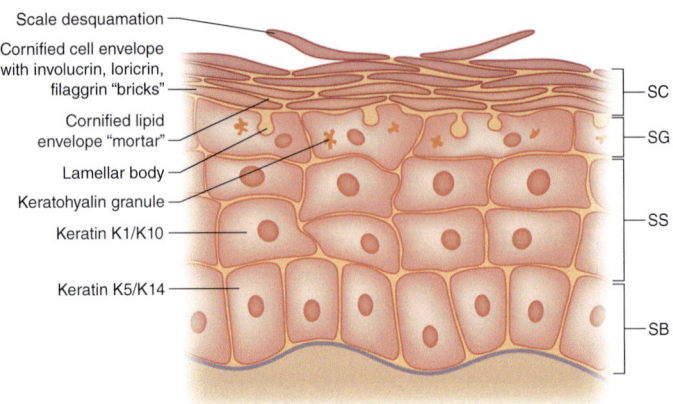

Scale desquamation

Cornified cell envelope with involucrin, loricrin, filaggrin "bricks"

SC

Cornified lipid envelope "mortar"

SG

Lamellar body

Keratohyalin granule

Keratin K1/K10

SS

Keratin K5/K14

SB

☐ **Fig. 18.3**   Keratinocyte maturation and development of the cornified envelope

— Defect in LEKTI (encoded by SPINK-5 (Serine Protease INhibitor)) = Netherton's
— Defect in corneodesmosin (component of desmosomes in the stratum corneum) = hypotrichosis simplex
— Defect in Odland bodies (lamellar bodies) = in Flegel's disease (hyperkeratosislenticularis perstans)
— Ab to transglutaminase-3 = dermatitis herpetiformis
— Keratins
  Acidic keratins (type I) (9–20), basic keratins (type II) (1–8)
  Keratin 1 and 10 = suprabasal, Keratin 5 and 14 = basal layer
  Keratin 9 (acidic) = only expressed in suprabasal palmar/plantar (partners with K1, basic)
  Defect in keratin 1 and 10 = epidermolytic ichthyosis (aka bullous congenital ichthyosiform erythroderma (BCIE) or epidermolytic hyperkeratosis (EHK))
  Defect in keratin 1 and 9 = Vorner (epidermolytic PPK) → in palmoplantar skin, 1 and 9 pair (K10 not expressed in palmoplantar)
  Defect in keratin 1 = Unna-Thost (nonepidermolytic); Mnemonic: Unna = Uno = 1
  Defect in keratin 2e = ichthyosis bullosa of Siemens
  Defect in keratin 3 and 12 = Meesmann corneal dystrophy
  Defect in keratin 4 and 13 = white sponge nevus (buccal mucosa)
  Defect in keratin 5 and 14 = EB simplex
  Defect in keratin 5 alone = Dowling-Degos, Galli-Galli
  Defect in K6a and 16 = pachyonychia congenita type 1
  Defect in K6b and 17 = pachyonychia congenita type 2 (steatocystomas)
  Defect in K14 (alone) = Naegeli-Franceschetti-Jadassohn syndrome (NFJS), dermatopathia pigmentosa reticularis (DPR)

18.4 Extracellular Matrix (ECM)

= Composed of network of collagens, elastin, glycoproteins, and proteoglycans

Collagen types
Collagen I = dermis in skin (most of ECM) and bone
Collagen II = cartilage
Collagen III = dermis in skin (especially fetal skin), vasculature, wound healing (primary component of granulation tissue)
Collagen IV = basement membrane
Collagen V = defect in classic Ehlers-Danlos syndrome
Collagen VII = anchoring fibrils
Collagen XVII = BPAG2 transmembrane protein/anchoring filaments

Collagen biosynthesis
- Collagen molecules synthesized in endoplasmic reticulum (ER); then they are assembled into triple helices composed of three polypeptide chains (α-chains) via hydroxylation (by vitamin C dependent prolyl and lysyl hydroxylases)
- Procollagen triple helix is secreted from ER across Golgi into extracellular space; it is then cleaved and assembled/cross-linked into various fibrils/superstructures (using enzymes including copper-dependent lysyl oxidase)
- Extracellular steps include cleavage and assembly into superstructures
- Enzymes involved in biosynthesis: prolyl hydroxylases and lysyl hydroxylase; these require Fe and ascorbic acid as co-factors
- Cross-linking between collagen molecules is catalyzed by lysyl oxidase, which requires copper as a co-factor

Elastin
- Elastic fibers composed of the protein elastin surrounded by mesh of microfibrils; number one component = fibrillin, which may guide elastogenesis and add structural support. Fibulin is another microfibril-associated component.
- Elastic fibers cross-linked by desmosine and isodesmosine via lysyl oxidase (the same copper-dependent enzyme that cross-links collagen)
- Elastin gene one of the largest in the human genome

Embryology
Embryonic dermis watery/cellular, ratio of collagen III: collagen I = 3:1 (opposite of adult dermis which is more collagen I). Fetal skin does not scar until this ratio changes, also related to TGF-ß isoforms

Inherited collagen/elastin disease
Defect in fibrillin-1 = Marfan syndrome
Defect in fibrillin-2 = congenital contractural arachnodactyly

18

Defect in fibulins 4 or 5 = cutis laxa
(Note: Defect in folliculin = Birt-Hogg-Dubé syndrome)
Defect in collagen I = osteogenesis imperfecta (OI)
Defect in collagen V, Tenascin X = EDS I/II (Classic)
Defect in collagen III (COL3A1), Tenascin X = EDS III (Hypermobility)
Defect in collagen III (COL3A1) (α1-chain of type III collagen) = EDS IV (Vascular)
Defect in lysyl hydroxylase = EDS Type VI (Kyphoscoliosis)
Defect in collagen I (COL1A1, 1A2) (α1 and α2 chains type I collagen) = EDS Type VII (Arthrochalasia)
Defect in ADAMTS-2 (procollagen N-proteinase) = EDS type VIIC (dermatosparaxis)
Defect in collagen type VII = dystrophic EB
Defect in ABCC6 (ATP-dependent binding cassette) = pseudoxanthoma elasticum (PXE)
Defect in ECM-1 = lipoid proteinosis
Defect in collagen IV = Alport's syndrome
Defects in copper metabolism: ATP7A (Menkes kinky hair) and ATP7B (Wilson's)

Autoimmune collagen disease
Ab to collagen IV = Goodpasture syndrome (glomerulonephritis, pneumonitis)
Ab to collagen II = relapsing polychondritis and MAGIC syndrome (mouth and genital ulcers with inflamed cartilage)
Ab to collagen XVII (BPAG2) and laminin-5 = bullous pemphigoid and cicatricial pemphigoid
Ab to collagen VII = EBA, bullous lupus
Ab to ECM-1 = lichen sclerosus

Penicillamine
= Copper chelator
- Interferes with elastin cross-linking (1. By causing low copper blood levels that cause reduced lysyl oxidase activity, 2. By directly blocking cross-linking of residues)
- Used to treat Wilson's disease
- Can cause PXE, EPS, acquired cutis laxa, pemphigus foliaceus-like drug eruption

Collagen as filler
Semi-permanent → Bovine collagen (Zyderm); no longer used in the USA
Permanent fillers → Polymethylmethacrylate beads suspended in bovine collagen (Artefill/Bellafill)

18.5 **Molecular Biology Review**

Molecular techniques
    Polymerase chain reaction (PCR) = amplifies/copies a gene or specific sequence of DNA using specific primers, DNA polymerase (e.g. Taq polymerase), and nucleotides through repeated thermal cycles
    DNA sequencing = determines exact sequence of nucleotides in a gene
    Western blot = detects protein with labeled antibodies
    Southern blot = detects DNA with radioactive DNA probe
    Northern blot = detects mRNA with radioactive DNA probe
    DNA microarray = scans an entire genome for gene expression

Other terminology
    Chromosome: composed of long arms (q) and short arms (p) = "petite", connected by centromere (site of microtubule attachment = kinetochore)
    Tumor suppressor gene = a gene that protects a cell from uncontrolled proliferation; loss-of-function mutation leads to cancer
    Proto-oncogene = a gene that if mutated (gain-of-function mutation) can become an oncogene and promote uncontrolled proliferation, leading to cancer
    Mouse models
        Transgenic mice = new gene (like a mutated proto-oncogene) can be expressed preferentially in specified cells (selected by promoter/enhancer to limit to target; e.g. melanocytes)
        Knockout mice = delete or disable a gene; good for studying tumor suppressor genes
    Gene therapy
        – Using molecular techniques for therapy, e.g. introducing gene containing tumor suppressor properties to a cancer, can be via viral vector for delivery to greater number of cells

18.5.1 **Important Tumor Suppressor Genes**

- CDKN2A (Chr 9p) = Cyclin-Dependent Kinase, regulates cell cycle progression; important tumor suppressor in melanoma; mutations associated with familial melanoma, pancreatic cancer, and astrocytomas of the brain
- NF1 (neurofibromin) directly inhibits ras
- PTEN indirectly inhibits ras via dephosphorylation of PIP3, thus preventing AKT activation; its mutation is associated with Cowden disease, Bannayan-Riley-Ruvalcaba syndrome, and possibly Proteus syndrome
- TSC1 (hamartin) and TSC2 (tuberin) are tumor suppressor genes whose products form a suppressor in the ras/AKT pathway (downstream from NF and PTEN inhibition) that inhibit mTOR (mammalian target of rapamycin); mutations in hamartin and tuberin are associated with tuberous sclerosis, and

treatment of TS with rapamycin replaces the hamartin-tuberin complex for mTOR inhibition

- PTPN11 = defect causes LEOPARD syndrome, Noonan syndrome
- PRKAR1A = defect causes Carney complex
- STK11 (LKB1) = a serine threonine kinase; defect causes Peutz-Jeghers syndrome
- p53 = can be mutated in SCC > BCC > MM
- Rb = retinoblastoma
- Note: High risk-HPVs encode oncoproteins E6 and E7, which interact with and disable p53 and Rb, respectively
- PTCH = mutated in BCCs and BCC nevus syndrome
- CYLD = CYLinDromas, mutated in Brooke-Spiegler syndrome

18.5.2 Important Oncogenes

RET—mutations in MEN2A/2B (Menin is in MEN1)

KIT—mutations in familial mastocytosis (activating), piebaldism (deactivating), and rare melanoma types (mucosal, acral, chronically sun damaged)

HRAS/KRAS—mutations in Costello syndrome, Spitz nevi may have HRAS mutation associated

BRAF, NRAS—mutations seen in melanoma

GNAQ—mutations associated with uveal melanoma, blue nevi

18.5.3 Genes in Melanoma

The molecular pathways involved with the development of melanoma can be summarized (◘ Fig. 18.4):

1. Cell proliferation (NRAS → BRAF → Mek → Erk/MAPK and PI3K/Akt pathways)
2. Tumor suppression (CDKN2A → p53 and Rb)
3. Apoptosis pathways (Bcl-2 inhibits apoptosis, BAX promotes apoptosis)
4. Melanocyte development migration (c-KIT, which can activate NRAS)

NRAS and BRAF are proto-oncogenes commonly mutated in melanoma

BRAF = most common gene mutation in melanoma, associated more with sun-protected area MM; codes for a kinase. BRAF mutations also seen in colorectal carcinoma and papillary thyroid carcinoma, but more specific for MM

BRAF inhibitors are potential MM treatments; sorafenib (soRAFenib) is a non-specific inhibitor that has not been that effective. 90% of BRAF mutations are V600E (glutamic acid for valine); vermurafenib (is a targeted specific BRAF V600E inhibitor that is still used)

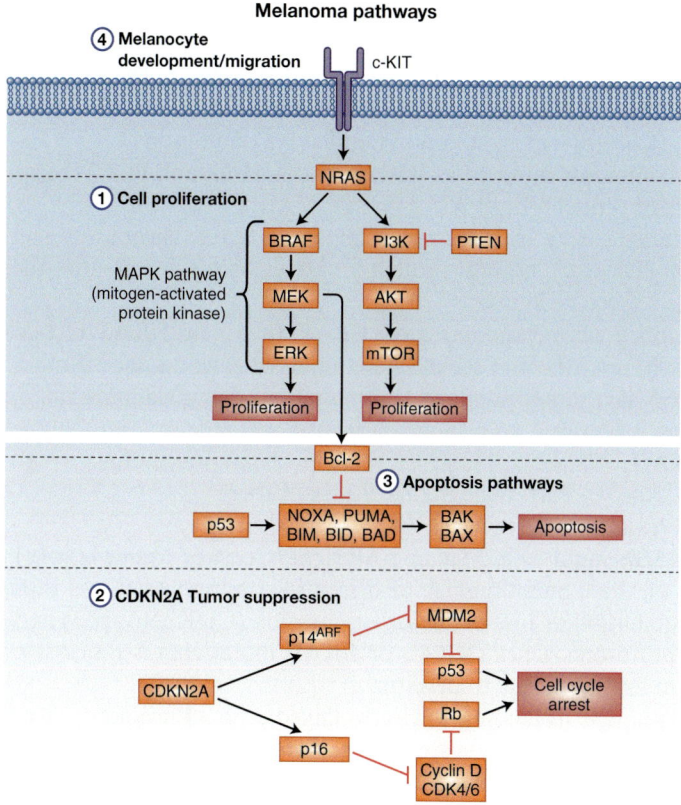

Fig. 18.4 Molecular pathways relevant to the development of melanoma

Research on treatment of melanoma has moved beyond BRAF inhibitors, but combining BRAF inhibitors with MEK inhibitors (next down the line in pathway), has improved response, overall survival, and even reduced toxicities (fewer SCCs and KAs than can be seen with vemurafenib, presumably from paradoxical MAPK activation)

The newest area of research is directed on targeting the "immunologic brakes" on T cells that limit cancer surveillance by the adaptive immune response. Blocking this interaction improves immune response against tumors (such as melanoma and many others).

Combining immunotherapy (such as CTLA-4 and PD-1 inhibitors, LAG-3 inhibitors) and targeted therapies (such as BRAF and MEK inhibitors) seems a promising idea, but toxicities have thus far limited this approach.

Using mRNA vaccine technology to prime the immune system to attack melanoma (used in combination with immunotherapy) has been recently studied and is very promising with increased response rates and minimal additional AEs

18

CDKN2A = encodes p14 and p16, which maintain activity of p53 and retinoblastoma (Rb) tumor suppressor genes, respectively, by inhibiting MDM2 (p14) and CDK4 (cyclin-dependent kinase 4) (p16), respectively. Essentially inhibiting inhibitors to keep tumor suppression going

CDKN2A (Chr 9p)—most common familial type mutation

p53 is not commonly mutated in MM, unlike in SCCs and BCCs (because of CDKN2A/p14 probably)

c-KIT = mutated only in rarer types: mucosal, acral, chronically sun damaged Imatinib (Gleevec), a multi-protein kinase inhibitor, is potential therapy since c-KIT is a tyrosine kinase

- Majority of melanomas have BRAF (60%) or NRAS (20%) mutations (would not expect to see in same tumor since have same effect)
- PTEN is a tumor suppressor often mutated in melanoma that inhibits the PI3K pathway
- GNAQ = frequent mutations seen in ocular melanoma (uveal) and blue nevi (also in Port-Wine Stains, Sturge-Weber)
- HRAS seen in Spitz nevi
- GNAS = mutated in McCune-Albright (Coast of Maine lesions)
- All of these mutations are also seen in common nevi; it is thought that a combination of loss of tumor suppression (CDK2NA, p53) and activation of proto-oncogenes (NRAS or BRAF mutations) is necessary at a minimum for melanoma to develop.
  – Although melanoma is clearly linked with ultraviolet radiation (UVR), the specific mutations seen in melanomas have not been clearly linked with UVR; they have generally lacked "UVB signature mutations" (CT → T and CC → TT, which have cyclobutane pyrimidine dimers as precursors)

18.5.4 Ultraviolet Radiation-Induced Mutagenesis

- UV radiation (specifically UVB) induces DNA damage via pyrimidine dimers
- Cyclobutane-pyrimidine dimers (CPDs) are the most common type of DNA photoproduct formed by UV irradiation, with thymine-thymine dimer (T-T) the most common of these (then T-C, C-T, C-C)
- Can be repaired by nucleotide excision repair (NER), which is defective in xeroderma pigmentosum

With regard to skin cancers:
- UVR-induced mutations aka UVB-signature mutations are seen in most NMSCs
- On the other hand, despite well-established association of melanoma with ultraviolet radiation, it is not clear how UVR causes melanoma; melanomas lack the UVB signature mutations seen in NMSCs; perhaps UVA plays a role

18.5.5 Other Important Pathways and Categories of Gene Defects

Shh-PTCH pathway
- Normally sonic hedgehog (Shh) binds to and inhibits Patched (PTCH) (the transmembrane Shh receptor), which inhibits Smoothened/SMO (a proto-oncogene). SMO promotes transcription factor Gli when Shh is present.
- Thus, Patched inactivation mutation and Smoothened activation mutations would constitutively activate Gli expression, causing BCCs ras-extracellular signal-regulated kinase (ERK) signaling pathway
- Ras (named from rat sarcoma) is an oncogene, a G protein (in a family of GTPases). Activation of ras causes to cells to grow and differentiate
- Mutations of ras proto-oncogenes are found in 20–30% of human cancers
- Ras activates 2 pathways: BRAF/Mek/ERK (MAPK) and the PI3K pathway
- NF1 is a tumor suppressor gene whose product (neurofibromin) directly inhibits ras; its mutation is associated with neurofibromatosis type I
- PTPN11 defect (a tumor suppressor) can cause LEOPARD syndrome, Noonan syndrome (these may be called RASopathies)

Wnt-β-catenin pathway
- Wnt = family of 16 secreted glycoproteins
- Wnt binds and activates Frizzled, a transmembrane G protein-linked receptor, which can then induce the accumulation of β-catenin
- When Wnt does not bind Frizzled, β-catenin is complexed with enzyme glycogen synthase kinase 3b (GSK3b) and APC (adenomatous polyposis coli) and induces rapid ubiquitin-mediated degradation of β-catenin by the cellular proteosome
- Binding of Wnt to Frizzled inhibits GSK3b, leading to β-catenin accumulation in cytosol, translocation to the nucleus where it binds transcription factors, induces Mitf and ultimately melanoblast differentiation
- β-catenin activation mutation (CTNBB1 gene) seen in pilomatricomas, and may see pilomatricoma-like changes in EICs of Gardner's (APC inactivation causes β-catenin accumulation)

18.5.6 Transmembrane Transporter Defects

Calcium pump defects (transport of Ca to ER lumen):
- Hailey-Hailey disease = ATP2C1 ("to see one Halley's comet in a lifetime")
- Darier's disease = ATP2A2 (SERCA2 pump, Sarcoplasmic Endoplasmic Reticulum Calcium ATPase 2)

18

18.5.7 Defects in Pyrin/NOD Family Related Proteins

Familial Mediterranean fever
Muckle Wells syndrome
PAPA syndrome
NOMID (neonatal-onset multisystem inflammatory disease)

18.5.8 Defects in Nuclear Envelope

Lamin A (LMNA gene) = defect causes progeria (Hutchinson-Gilford)
LEMD3 = defect causes Buschke-Ollendorff syndrome

18.5.9 Defects in DNA Repair Genes

RecQ-like helicases (DNA replication and repair)
  Note: all have premature aging, graying of hair
  - Werner syndrome; RecQL2 helicase (WRN gene)
  - Bloom syndrome; RecQL3 helicase (BLM gene)
  - Rothmund-Thomson; RecQL4 helicase (RECQL4 gene)

Nucleotide excision repair
  - Cockayne syndrome (local defect in NER)
  - Xeroderma pigmentosum (global defect in NER)
  - Trichothiodystrophy (may have some overlap with Cockayne)

Serine-threonine kinase that regulates cell cycle, senses DNA damage
  - Ataxia-telangiectasia; defect in ATM gene (a serine-threonine protein kinase that recognizes DNA damage)

Telomerase interaction
  - Dyskeratosis congenita; defect in dyskerin (gene DKC1) in most common XR form, hTERT (Telomerase Reverse Transcriptase, preserves telomeres to allow replication) and hTR mutations in AD form

Various DNA repair proteins
  - Fanconi anemia

18.6 Embryology

Specification = embryonic period (0–60 days)
Morphogenesis = early fetal period (2–5 months)
Differentiation = late fetal period (5–9 months)

Epidermis = derived from ectoderm

Dermis = derived from ectoderm and mesoderm (depends on body site)

Epidermal development

Specification = process of germ layers committing to and forming epidermis and dermis
- Gastrulation (division into 3 germ layers), bilayer formation (periderm and basal cell layer), neural tube formation (median strip of ectoderm invaginates)
- Thought to be mediated by bone morphogenetic proteins (BMPs)

Morphogenesis = committed tissues begin to form specialized structures (epidermal stratification, subdivision between dermis/subcutis, vascular formation)
- Stratification (thickening of epidermis, from expression of p63; mutation causes various ectodermal dysplasias, e.g. Hay-Wells, AEC), keratinization (in appendages first, formation of cornified layer and degeneration of periderm)

Differentiation = newly specialized tissues further develop and assume mature forms (majority of developmental errors occur here, since earlier ones are often incompatible with life)
- Granular/cornified layers complete, gland/appendage formation

Dermal development
- LMX-1B (defect causes nail-patella syndrome) and Wnt7a important for dorsal limb specification
- Embryonic dermis watery/cellular, ratio of collagen III: collagen I = 3:1 (opposite of adult dermis which is more collagen I)
- By end of 2nd trimester, elastic fibers detectable, dermis more fibrous, acellular, able to scar

18.7 Melanocyte Biology

Melanosomes = specialized lysosomes with melanin

Pheomelanosomes = spherical, globular

Eumelanosomes = elliptical, concentric rings

Eumelanin = brown/black, stimulated by binding of MSH to MC1-R

Pheomelanin = yellow/red, stimulated by binding of agouti protein to MC1-R

MC1-R = melanocortin 1 receptor
- Skin color dependent on size/distribution of melanosomes (larger in darker skin), quantity and type of melanin, rather than number of melanocytes
- Melanosomes moved along dendrites (composed of actin and microtubules) by kinesin and dynein; attached to microtubules by actin-associated myosin Va (defective in Griscelli)
- 1 melanocyte for every 10 basal keratinocytes
- 1 melanocyte for every ~30 keratinocytes (all epidermal keratinoctyes, not just basal) supplied with pigment by dendrites

18

18.8 Nail Biology

Embryology = development begins at 8–10 weeks at dorsal digital tips
The anatomy of the nail is complex (■ Fig. 18.5).
Proximal nail matrix produces dorsal nail plate; when psoriasis affects and
   makes parakeratosis, sheds cells and produces nail pits.
Distal nail matrix produces ventral nail plate
Nail plate is analogous to stratum corneum
Proximal nail fold covers proximal nail matrix, lunula = distal nail matrix

Nail-patella syndrome
 — Aka hereditary osteo-onychodysplasia (HOOD)
 — Defect in LMX-1B (transcription factor that regulates collagen synthe-
   sis, dorsal/ventral limb patterning), autosomal dominant, Chr 9
 — Clinically, see triangular lunulae (pathognomonic), hypoplastic nails,
   absent or small patellae, renal dysplasia, hyperpigmentation of papillary
   margin of iris (Lester iris)
 — Check U/A for proteinuria, pelvic XR for iliac horns

18.9 Sebum

Holocrine secretion from sebaceous glands (released with remnants of dead cells,
vs. merocrine/eccrine or decapitation/apocrine)
Largest component: triglycerides
Unique components: squalene, wax esters

18.10 Hair

Pilosebaceous unit = hair follicle + sebaceous gland ± apocrine gland
The hair anatomy can be divided into three main sections (■ Fig. 18.6):
 — Infundibulum (from surface to insertion of sebaceous duct)
 — Isthmus (from insertion of sebaceous duct to insertion of arrector pili)
   Bulge = at insertion of arrector pili thought to have the hair follicle stem
   cells, keratin 15 and 19 positive
 — Lower segment (from insertion of arrector pili to below)
   Bulb and suprabulb
 Note: apocrine gland's secretory portion is located in the deep dermis/subcu-
   taneous fat, with a straight duct that opens directly into the infundibulum
   of the hair follicle, above the entrance of the sebaceous gland

Dorsal view

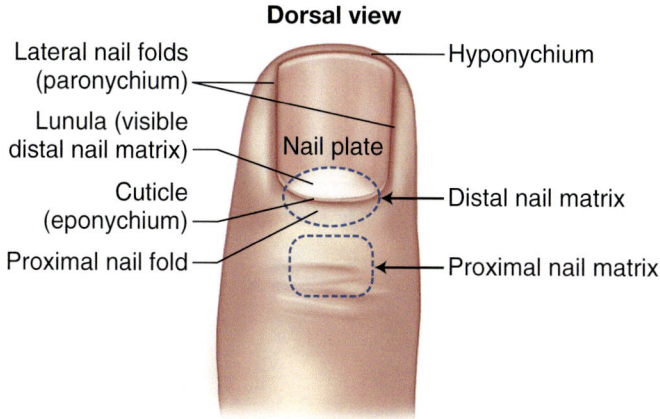

Lateral nail folds (paronychium)

Lunula (visible distal nail matrix)

Cuticle (eponychium)

Proximal nail fold

Hyponychium

Nail plate

Distal nail matrix

Proximal nail matrix

Sagittal view

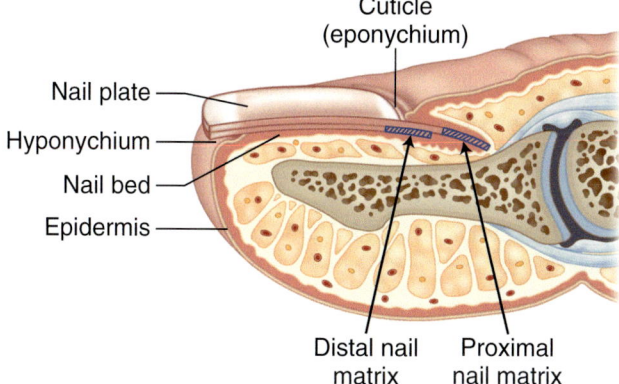

Cuticle (eponychium)

Nail plate

Hyponychium

Nail bed

Epidermis

Distal nail matrix

Proximal nail matrix

☐ **Fig. 18.5** Structure and anatomy of the nail

Anagen (85–90%), catagen (< 1%), telogen (10–15%): mnemonic for duration = 3 years, 3 weeks, 3 months; for the order, think ACT (like the high school exam)

Order of layers of hair follicle

Outer root sheath

Inner root sheath (IRS) = closely adherent to hair shaft, 3 layers

→ Henle

→ Huxley; mnemonic "Henle hugs Huxley"

→ IRS cuticle (interconnects with cells of hair shaft cuticle)

Hair shaft = 3 layers

→ Hair shaft cuticle

→ Hair cortex

→ Hair medulla

18

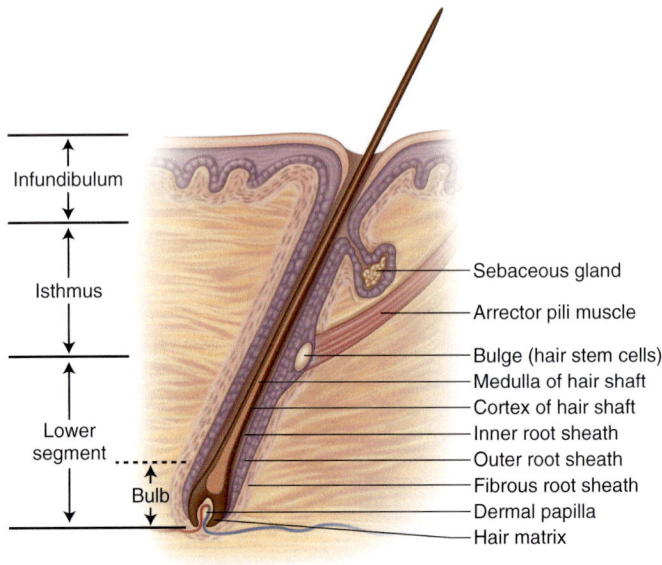

Infundibulum

Isthmus

Lower
segment

Bulb

Sebaceous gland
Arrector pili muscle
Bulge (hair stem cells)
Medulla of hair shaft
Cortex of hair shaft
Inner root sheath
Outer root sheath
Fibrous root sheath
Dermal papilla
Hair matrix

◻ **Fig. 18.6**   Structure and anatomy of the hair follicle (pilosebaceous unit)

Order of keratinization:
1. Henle's layer (1 cell thick)
2. Two cuticles (IRS cuticle and hair shaft cuticle)
3. Huxley's layer

Critical line of Auber = line through widest part of the dermal papilla in the follicle, below which is the matrix (germination center) with all the mitotically active cells

18.11   Itch Review

- Mostly C nerve fibers (slow)
- Mediators: <u>histamine</u> → but only in urticaria, arthropod bites, allergic drug
  → In most pruritus, antihistamines are ineffective
- Itch receptor nerve endings are found in the epidermis and respond to exogenous (irritants, allergens, pathogens, touch) and endogenous (various cytokines such as IL-4, 13, 31, 22 and TSLP and interferon gamma) stimuli
- Itch sensation and scratch impulse are inherently linked (brain studies show)
- Dermal mast cells: tryptase (a protease) from mast cells
  - Other proteinases are increased in atopic dermatitis, Netherton syndrome
  - Related to impaired barrier function?

- Substance P—role in itch, primes mast cells and sensory neurons
- How do opioids (morphine) induce itch?
  - Neuronal pain pathways inhibitory for itch and so when weakened by opiods allows the transmission of itch signals via spinal cord
- Heat lowers itch threshold
- Prostaglandins enhance histamine-induced itch
- Preciously felt that inflammatory itch and neuropathic itch were completely separate however as itch science involves, we see that they are interconnected and many of the inflammatory cytokines (see above) actually have receptors in the CNS

18.12 Immunology Review

18.12.1 Innate Immune Response

= Rapid, less controlled than adaptive

Neutrophils, eosinophils, NK cells, mast cells, cytokines, complement—and antimicrobial peptides

Complement

Classic pathway → Ab-Ag complex trigger

Note: IgM is the best immunoglobulin at activating complement, IgG1 and IgG3 can also activate complement; other immunoglobulins do not

Alternative pathway → polysaccharides from microbial cell walls

Lectin pathway (new) → microbial carbs with mannose-binding proteins

All three pathways activate central C3b, which helps phagocytosis (opsonization) via receptors on phagocytic cells; also complement binds to Ag-Ab complexes

C5a → attracts neutrophils

C3a, C4a, C5a = anaphylatoxins (all end in a!)
  → Induce inflammatory mediators from mast cells → vascular permeability

C5b, C6, C7, C8, C9 → form MAC (membrane attack complex)
  → Generates pores in cell membrane → osmotic lysis → death
  → Preferentially attack microbial cell

Clinical correlations

C1 esterase inhibitor deficiency
  - Inherited angioedema, never causes urticaria

C2 = most common complement deficiency, SLE-like?

C3 deficiency = can also be associated with lipodystrophy

C4 deficiency = can also be associated with PPK, SLE-like?

C5-C9 deficiency
  - Chronic *Neisseria* infections or other encapsulated bacteria

CH50 = total complement level

Acquired angioedema = see decreased C4 and C1q, associated with B-cell lymphoproliferative disorders

Hypocomplementemic urticarial vasculitis syndrome
- Defined by low serum complement levels plus presence of anti-C1q precipitin (in 100%, initiating classic pathway), decrease in C1 activity

SLE (and other collagen vascular disease)

Complement levels decreased in SLE flares because by classic pathway, complement activated by Ag-Ab complexes (as are deposited in SLE)

Toll-like receptors
- Found on dendritic cells; upon activation, may express pathogen-derived antigen to naïve T cells
- May bridge gap between innate and adaptive immunity

TLR2 → may have role in leprosy, acne; increased levels in rosacea

TLR4 → involved in nickel contact dermatitis

TLR7 → involved in imiquimod mechanism of action, ssRNA is native ligand

Anti-microbial peptides
- = Small cationic peptides important in innate immune system
- Two major family = cathelicidins (LL-37) and defensins
- Defensins include β-defensin-2, dermcidin (in eccrine sweat)
- May be upregulated in psoriasis, downregulated in atopic dermatitis (may explain why eczema and not psoriasis is superinfected easily)
- May play role in wound healing, may attract dendritic cells
- Cathelicidin is elevated in rosacea

Cytokines
- Influence proliferation, differentiation, and activation of cells
- Hard to characterize given multiple activities of each

Interleukins = made by leukocytes, affect WBCs

Interferons = interfere with viral replication

Chemokines = chemoattractants, role in leukocyte migration

Note: macrophages and neutrophils are both phagocytes

Macrophages
- Mostly for phagocytosis → recognize self versus non-self by receptors for carbohydrates usually not on vertebrate cells
- Function as antigen-presenting cells (APCs), but not as effective as dendritic cells (Langerhans cells)
- Release G-CSF and GM-CSF, which induce precursors in bone marrow → neutrophils to blood stream (also IL-8)
- Intercellular destruction by exposure to: superoxide anions, hydroxyl radicals, lysozyme, nitric oxide, hypochlorous acid
- Important in wound healing

Neutrophils
- Myeloblast is first fully committed stage in neutrophil development
- Phagocytes → kill by O_2 dependent and independent mechanisms
  O_2 dependent = "respiratory burst"—catalyzed by NADPH oxidase, which leads to superoxide anions, H_2O_2, hydroxyl radicals
  O_2 independent = myeloperoxidase, lysozyme (in azurophilic granules)

If foreign organisms covered with antibody
- → Neutrophils and Macrophages have Fc receptors (for Ab) and complement receptors which enhance adhesion to these phagocytes

Note: IL-8 = neutrophil chemoattractant primarily secreted by mononuclear phagocytes

Clinical correlations
  Chronic granulomatous disease: respiratory burst defective because of NADPH oxidase mutations; particularly susceptible to catalase positive bacteria
  Chédiak-Higashi syndrome: defective formation of lysosomes and primary granules

Eosinophils
- Role: to protect against parasite infection
- Weakly phagocytic
- Important cytokines = IL-5, and the CC chemokine, CCL11

Basophils and Mast cells = similar
  Mast cell granules: histamine, serotonin, prostaglandins, leukotrienes (enhance vascular permeability)
  Ag binds to IgE bound to mast cell → degranulation
  IgE binds to high affinity IgE receptors ($F_c \varepsilon$ receptor I)
    → Pre-formed mediators = histamine, heparin, tryptase, chymase
    → Newly formed mediators = prostaglandins, leukotrienes, PAF (platelet activating factor)
  Role in urticaria, anaphylaxis (cutaneous mast cells express C5a anaphylatoxin)

NK Cells—ADCC (antibody dependent cellular cytotoxicity)
- Recognize MHC class I molecules

18.12.2 Adaptive Immune Response

Antigen-presenting cells (APCs)
T-cells
B-cells
- Note: MHC I on every nucleated cell of body, MHC II on APCs only (can be induced on keratinocytes)

Langerhans cells (LCs)
  = Primary antigen-presenting cells; present to lymphocytes
- Derived from bone marrow, home to the epidermis, express E-cadherin

- Only identifiable by EM or histochemistry (CD45, CD1a (most useful since in epidermis, exclusive to LCs), S100, vimentin, Langerin (CD207))
- Have rod-shaped organelles—"Birbeck granules," associated with Langerin
- TGF-β seems to allow development into LCs rather than non-LC dendritic cells
- LCs actively take up antigens

CD4 → recognize antigen presented with MHC class 2 → dependent of APCs → process to present; extracellular antigens that are taken up in vesicles by endocytosis

CD8 → recognize antigen presented with MHC class 1 (like mast cells) → Usually present endogenously derived antigen, intracellular antigens (viral) that are present in the cytosol

T cells

- Develop in thymus (stem cells from bone marrow)
- TCR only recognizes short peptide fragments (B cells recognize antigen in native form)
- Development "thymic education":
  Positive selection—must recognize MHC molecules
  Negative selection—if recognizes self-antigens → apoptosis
- There are TCRs for <u>every</u> possible antigen (10^5 possible variable regions) from diverse recombination process (VDJ)
- Antigens bind to MHC class I or II molecules in V regions formed by αβ heterodimer.
- Superantigens bind directly to lateral potion of TCRβ chain and MHC class IIb chain stimulate T cells based on Vβ segment (thus, can activate 20% of immune system); this causes overproduction of cytokines and shock (like in toxic shock)
- Defects in <u>r</u>ecombinations-<u>a</u>ctivating <u>g</u>enes RAG-1, RAG-2 can cause SCID since patients can't produce antigen recognizing receptors
- Omenn syndrome = AR form of SCID with erythroderma, desquamation, alopecia, chronic diarrhea, failure to thrive, LAD, HSM
  - TCRs = associated with CD3 complex
  - TCR with peptide—MHC = first signal
  - Surface molecule interactions = second signal → without this, leads to anergy/tolerance:

– APC surface:	B7—CD28	(on T cell surface)
	LFA-1—ICAM-1	
	LFA-3—CD-2	

- Memory T cells

CD4 = T helper cells—recognize antigens, activate cell-mediated responses

CD8 = cytotoxic—crucial to antiviral and anti-tumor response

CD4 cell → will develop into either Th1 or Th2 CD4 cell; morphologically the same, differentiate by cytokine secretion pattern

B cells
   Purpose = to produce immunoglobulin
   – Primarily stimulated in T-cell dependent manner, but can secrete IgM in a T-cell independent response to certain epitopes
   – Express IgM on surface, CD40+, CD20+ (targeted by rituximab)
   – On initial exposure, antigen binds surface IgM, internalized, presented on surface with MHC II molecule to T-cell, which in turn secretes cytokines to stimulate maturation into plasma cells and production of immunoglobulins
   – Upon subsequent exposure, B-cells activated by follicular dendritic cells (in germinal centers of lymph nodes) → differentiation into plasma cells
   – In B-cells, somatic recombination of V (variable), D (diversity), and J (junctional) to make antibodies
Plasma cells
   – Produce immunoglobulin
   – May contain Russell bodies (like a pregnant plasma cell, full of immunoglobulin) or Dutcher bodies (also an intranuclear inclusion)
Immunoglobulins
   = composed of two heavy chains and two light chains
      IgM—induces agglutination, activates classical complement pathway
      IgG—majority of immunoglobulin (75%), can activate complement, maternal-fetal transfer
      IgA—mucosal, can activate alternative complement pathway
      IgE—mediates most anaphylactic/allergic reactions
      Fab = antibody-binding fragment (when digested with papain)
      Fc = constant region, determines sub-type of antibody (e.g. A, D, E, G, M)
      Hapten = coupling of host protein with allergen
Th1/Th2 paradigm
   Traditionally, T-cells were thought to fall into two main cytokine profiles, Th1 and Th2, which oppose each other. The current thought is that it is more complicated; that Th17 cells and Treg cells represent two other distinct subsets and all are intricately interconnected
   Th1 cytokines = IFN-γ, TNF-α and β, IL-2, 12
   Th2 cytokines = IL-4, 5, 6, 9, 10, 13
   Th17 cytokines = IL-17, 21, 22, 23
   Treg = recognized by CD4+, CD25+, Foxp3+
   Th1 (cell mediated immunity):
      Th1 cells produce IL-2 → more CD4, CD8 cells
      Vla IFN-γ → activate macrophages → IL-12 → more Th1
      – Activates macrophages, allowing them to kill intracellular pathogens, releases IL-12 which stimulates activation of more Th1 cells

18

Th2 (humoral immunity):

Th2 cells produce IL-4, which stimulates B cells → plasma cells → makes IgE; via IL-5, makes eosinophils, via IL-10 inhibits macrophage IFN-γ release

Th17: IL-23 stimulates Th17 cells to release IL-22 (and IL-17). IL-22 leads to keratinocyte proliferation and dermal inflammation. Levels of IL-22 correlate with disease severity.

Associations:

Th1: RA, MS, psoriasis

Th2: atopic dermatitis, SLE

Note: in past, pregnancy thought to be a mostly Th2 phenomenon, but studies have shown that an oversimplification

Immunodeficiency syndromes

1. Chronic granulomatous disease
   – Defect in NADPH oxidase, needed to make oxygen radicals for respiratory burst
2. Hyper-IgE syndrome (Job syndrome)
   – Recurrent *Candida*, *Staph* "cold abscesses," atopic dermatitis
3. Bruton's X-linked agammaglobulinemia
   – BTK (Bruton tyrosine kinase) gene defect (pre-B-cell signaling)
   – No B cells
4. DiGeorge syndrome (thymic aplasia)
   – Neonatal tetany from hypocalcemia
5. Severe combined immunodeficiency (SCID)
   – Aka "bubble boy syndrome," lack both function B and T cells
6. Leukocyte adhesion deficiency
7. Ataxia-telangiectasia
8. APECED
   – Autoimmune PolyEndocrinopathy Candidiasis and Ectodermal Dystrophy
9. Chediak-Higashi
10. Hypo-IgM syndrome
11. Thymic dysplasia with normal immunoglobulins (Nezelof syndrome)
12. Wiskott-Aldrich syndrome
    – Atopic dermatitis, thrombocytopenia, prone to infection by encapsulated bacteria
    – Defect in WASP gene

Supplementary Information

Index

A

B